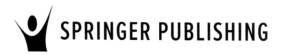

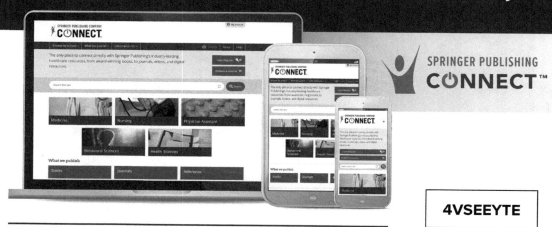
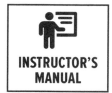
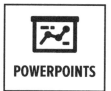
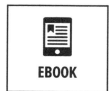
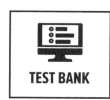

Keating's Curriculum Development and Evaluation in Nursing Education

Stephanie Stimac DeBoor, PhD, APRN, ACNS-BC, CCRN, is the Associate Dean of Graduate Programs, and Associate Professor, at the Orvis School of Nursing (OSN), University of Nevada, Reno (UNR). She oversees all of the graduate programs and specialty tracks at the OSN. She is a member of the University Courses and Curriculum Committee, and the University Research Committee. She teaches in both the undergraduate and graduate programs. In addition, Dr. DeBoor serves as a liaison to the Professional Development and Employee Engagement committee at Northern Nevada Medical Center, Sparks, Nevada. She is the recipient of several honors, including the American Association of Colleges of Nursing (AACN) 2013–2014 Fellowship Leader for Academic Nursing Program, and was honored as the Most Inspirational Teacher, UNR (2009, 2010, and 2012). She was a recent nominee for the 2021 Nurses of Achievement, Educator award and received the 2021 University of Nevada, Reno—Orvis School of Nursing Outstanding Teacher of the Year award. This award qualifies Dr. DeBoor as a nominee for the University of Nevada, Reno F. Donald Tibbitts Distinguished Teacher Award. Dr. DeBoor has published articles in *Journal of Nursing Education, Journal of Nursing Care Quality*, and *American Journal of Critical Care*. In addition to this text, Dr. DeBoor contributed a chapter, Curriculum Development in Nursing, to *Teaching in Nursing and Role of the Educator: The Complete Guide to Best Practice in Teaching, Evaluation, and Curriculum Development, Third Edition* (Springer Publishing Company).

Keating's Curriculum Development and Evaluation in Nursing Education

Fifth Edition

Stephanie Stimac DeBoor, PhD, APRN, ACNS-BC, CCRN
EDITOR

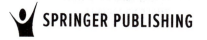

Springer Publishing Company, LLC
11 West 42nd Street, New York, NY 10036
www.springerpub.com
connect.springerpub.com/

Acquisitions Editor: Joseph Morita
Compositor: diacriTech

ISBN: 978-0-8261-8685-0
ebook ISBN: 978-0-8261-8686-7
DOI: 10.1891/9780826186867

SUPPLEMENTS:
Instructor Materials:

A robust set of instructor resources designed to supplement this text is located at **http://connect.springerpub.com/content/book/978-0-8261-8686-7.** Qualifying instructors may request access by emailing **textbook@springerpub.com.**

Instructor's Manual ISBN: 978-0-8261-8687-4
Instructor's PowerPoints ISBN: 978-0-8261-8688-1

22 23 24 25 / 5 4 3 2 1

The author and the publisher of this Work have made every effort to use sources believed to be reliable to provide information that is accurate and compatible with the standards generally accepted at the time of publication. Because medical science is continually advancing, our knowledge base continues to expand. Therefore, as new information becomes available, changes in procedures become necessary. We recommend that the reader always consult current research and specific institutional policies before performing any clinical procedure or delivering any medication. The author and publisher shall not be liable for any special, consequential, or exemplary damages resulting, in whole or in part, from the readers' use of, or reliance on, the information contained in this book. The publisher has no responsibility for the persistence or accuracy of URLs for external or third-party Internet websites referred to in this publication and does not guarantee that any content on such websites is, or will remain, accurate or appropriate.

Library of Congress Control Number: 2021918428

Contact sales@springerpub.com to receive discount rates on bulk purchases.

Publisher's Note: **New and used products purchased from third-party sellers are not guaranteed for quality, authenticity, or access to any included digital components.**

Printed in the United States of America.

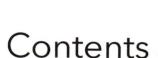

Contents

SECTION IV: PROGRAM EVALUATION AND ACCREDITATION   *247*

Stephanie Stimac DeBoor

SECTION V: RESEARCH, ISSUES, AND TRENDS IN NURSING EDUCATION   *287*

Stephanie Stimac DeBoor

Contributors

Kimberly Baxter, DNP, APRN, FNP-BC Associate Professor and Associate Dean of Undergraduate Programs, Orvis School of Nursing, University of Nevada, Reno

Stephanie Stimac DeBoor, PhD, APRN, ACNS-BC, CCRN Associate Professor and Associate Dean of Graduate Programs, Orvis School of Nursing, University of Nevada, Reno

Susan M. Ervin, PhD, RN, CNE Assistant Professor, Orvis School of Nursing, University of Nevada, Reno

Jacqueline Ferdowsali, DNP, ARNP, AGACNP-BC, ACNPC-AG Associate Professor, Track Leader and Advisor of the Adult Gerontology Acute Care Nurse Practitioner Program, Orvis School of Nursing, University of Nevada, Reno

Sarah B. Keating, EdD, MPH, RN, C-PNP, FAAN Professor and Dean Emerita, San Francisco State University, San Francisco, California, and Samuel Merritt University, Oakland, California; Endowed Professor, Orvis School of Nursing, University of Nevada, Reno (retired)

Heidi A. Mennenga, PhD, RN Associate Professor, College of Nursing, South Dakota State University, Brookings, South Dakota

Teresa Serratt, PhD, RN Associate Professor, School of Nursing, Boise State University, Boise, Idaho

Rochelle Walsh, DNP, RN, PCCN Assistant Professor, Track Leader and Advisor for the Nurse Educator program, Orvis School of Nursing, University of Nevada, Reno

Preface

It is an honor to continue the work of Dr. Sarah Keating. Her first edition of this text went to press in 2005 and almost 17 years later continues to be a mainstay for nursing educators and students. I am humbled, and excited to accept the torch that she passes to me. Sarah continues to be my friend, mentor, and advisor of all things related to nursing education and curriculum development and am very grateful for the gift she has entrusted to me.

With the onset of the COVID-19 pandemic, the face of healthcare rapidly changed. Those of us as nursing educators had to quickly pivot in adapting our courses and delivery methods to ensure ongoing education for our students. Limited contact forced us into a two-dimensional world where we learned to communicate differently. This was an unprecedented time and while the steps in the development of curriculum did not change, teaching strategies and the methods of delivery did. Evaluation methods used to assess face-to-face teaching strategies now differ when the majority of the content delivered is via online modalities. Previous advancement in technologies have allowed for increased access to education via online and distance-learning programs. Despite the impact the pandemic has had, there continues to be an increasing desire for those to advance their education toward graduate programs. What was first seen as a challenge to the day-to-day operations of education may come to serve as the norm for nursing programs. Online and distance education has become enticing as courses are offered in ways that provide flexibility in meeting the needs of the working student or those who are now homeschooling their children. It is gratifying to reflect upon nursing education and its tremendous growth that has occurred since the last edition and just within this last year.

The chapters, as with previous editions of the text, are organized in a logical manner to guide activities of development, review, and evaluation for staff development clinicians, nursing educators, and graduate nurse educator students. Content provides a discussion regarding budgetary management in relation to support for curriculum development. In the Appendix the reader finds a fictitious case study of a need's assessment and subsequent program development. It provides an opportunity for readers to review the processes involved in curriculum development. The case study brings into play international possibilities for nursing programs to build collaborative nursing curricula through the use of web-based, online platforms. There are additional data in the study for readers to develop curricula other than the one presented.

New to this edition is a chapter on curriculum development and evaluation for those in staff development. Also provided within the chapter is a case study walking the reader through the staff development or nursing professional development process of curriculum development outside of academe. Back by popular demand is a chapter on taxonomies and the relation to enhancing critical thinking. Throughout this edition are discussions of the new American Association of Colleges of Nursing's (AACN, 2021) *Essentials: Core Competencies for Professional Nursing Education* and application to curriculum development and evaluation. In addition to an overview of program evaluation, regulatory agencies, and accreditation; the text includes an example of preparation for and participation in a virtual Commission on Collegiate Nursing Education (CCNE) site visit that was implemented during the pandemic. It is necessary for nursing educators to be familiar with the various systems that either regulate, accredit, or set standards to ensure the quality of educational programs. Participating in these activities as well as routinely assessing and evaluating the program as it is implemented ensures the quality of the end product and the integrity of the curriculum. The final section of the text reviews the literature for research on nursing education as it relates to curriculum development and evaluation. Research questions are raised from the review and suggestions offered for further study. The final chapter of the text summarizes all of the chapters and identifies current and future issues and challenges for nursing educators.

For this edition, the contributors are experienced, expert nursing faculty and clinicians. They represent various nursing education levels, clinical specialties, and the geographical regions of the United States. Curriculum development and evaluation are an art and science that go beyond the methodologies of teaching. This text provides the theories, concepts, and tools necessary for curriculum development and evaluation in nursing. It serves as content essential for those in nursing professional development, nursing education students, novice educators in academe, and experienced nursing faculty to meet the challenges they face in this changing environment. The pandemic influenced the evolution of current nursing curricula and provided us with an opportunity to reexamine curriculum delivery and evaluation. As nursing educators, we continue to recognize the numerous changes and the complexity of the healthcare system; the healthcare needs of the population and more than ever the need of moving advanced practice and leadership roles into the doctoral level. Accomplished by offering programs that create nursing researchers, scholars, and faculty to keep the profession current and ready for the future. It gives me great pride to contribute to nursing knowledge and support those who pursue nursing education as their current or future path.

Stephanie Stimac DeBoor

A robust set of instructor resources designed to supplement this text is located at **http://connect.springerpub.com/content/book/978-0-8261-8686-7.** Qualifying instructors may request access by emailing **textbook@springerpub.com.**

Instructor Resources

Keating's Curriculum Development and Evaluation in Nursing Education, Fifth Edition, includes quality resources for the instructor. Faculty who have adopted the text may gain access to these resources by emailing textbook@springerpub.com.

INSTRUCTOR RESOURCES INCLUDE

- Sample Course Syllabus
- Each Chapter Includes:
  - Faculty Teaching/Learning Strategies
  - Supplemental Student Learning Activities
- PowerPoint Presentations for Lecture

SECTION I

OVERVIEW OF NURSING EDUCATION: HISTORY, CURRICULUM DEVELOPMENT AND APPROVAL PROCESSES, AND THE ROLE OF FACULTY

Stephanie Stimac DeBoor

OVERVIEW OF CURRICULUM DEVELOPMENT AND EVALUATION IN NURSING EDUCATION

The fifth edition of this text devotes itself to the underlying theories, concepts, and science of curriculum development and evaluation in nursing education as separate from the art and science of teaching and instructional processes. The textbook provides useful content for both novice and experienced faculty, those within nursing professional development, and nursing education students. The curriculum provides the goals for an educational program, guidelines for delivery, and methods for evaluating the effectiveness of the programs. Discussed are major theories and concepts that relate to instructional strategies and their contributions to the implementation of the curriculum plan.

Defining curriculum development provides a road map for beginning the process. For the purposes of the textbook, the definition is a curriculum is the formal plan of study that provides the philosophical underpinnings, goals, and guidelines for delivery of a specific educational program (Keating, 2018). The text uses this definition throughout for the *formal* curriculum while recognizing the existence of the *informal* curriculum.

The informal curriculum consists of activities that students, faculty, administrators, staff, and consumers experience outside of the formal planned curriculum. Examples of the informal curriculum include on-campus and virtual interpersonal relationships, faculty role modeling, program activity planning, such as honor pledge, pinning ceremony, and hooding; athletic/recreational activities; study groups; nursing and campus organizational activities; and personal counseling. Although the focus of the text is on the formal curriculum, nursing educators must be mindful of the role informal curriculum plays in student learning, its influence, and its ability to reinforce learning activities from the planned/formal curriculum.

While the COVID-19 global pandemic changed the way we delivered education, the principles of curriculum development remained the same. Evaluation standards were adapted for online and virtual formats. Although the pandemic has a place in educational history, to place curriculum development and evaluation in perspective, it is wise to examine the history of nursing education in the United States and the lessons it provides for current and future curriculum developers. This section examines nursing's place in the history of higher education and the role of faculty and administrators in developing and evaluating curricula. We continue to transform nursing curricula, especially with the rapid adaptation in the delivery of courses and programs through online and distance education and the application of newly developed technology to enhance instructional strategies. We continue to focus on the learner and measurement of learning outcomes. Integrating safety and quality concepts, evidence-based practice, translational science, and research into the curriculum provides exciting challenges and opportunities for nursing educators. At the national level, there is a strong call for integrating processes that are learner- and consumer-focused and, at the same time, ensuring excellence by building in outcome measures to determine the quality of the program. In addition, there is a need to cultivate our nursing scientists to stay relevant and have a voice at all tables for decision-making about healthcare. Finally, we need to pursue ongoing research on curriculum development and evaluation to provide the underpinnings for evidence-based practice in nursing education.

HISTORY OF NURSING EDUCATION IN THE UNITED STATES

Chapter 1 traces the history of American nursing education from the time of the first Nightingale schools of nursing to the present. The trends in professional education and society's needs influenced nursing programs that started from apprentice-type schools to a majority of the programs now in institutions of higher learning. As nursing faculty, we must be cognizant of the role liberal arts and sciences within institutions of higher play in nursing education by setting the foundation for developing critical thinking and clinical reasoning necessary to nursing care.

Chapter 1 reviews major historical events in society and the world that influenced nursing practice and education, as well as changes in the healthcare system. The major World Wars of the 20th century increased the demand for nurses and a nursing education system that prepared a workforce ready to meet that demand. The emergence of nursing education during the mid-20th century in community colleges continues to create debate about entry into practice. The DNP programs continue to expand throughout the United States further defining advanced practice, nursing leadership, and education, bringing educational history into focus as the profession continues to respond to the changes in healthcare and the needs of the population.

CURRICULUM DEVELOPMENT AND APPROVAL PROCESSES IN CHANGING EDUCATIONAL ENVIRONMENTS

Chapter 2 discusses the organizational structures and processes that programs undergo when changing or creating new curricula and the roles and responsibilities of faculty in realizing the changes. Chief nursing administrators and deans provide the leadership for organizing and carrying out evaluation activities. The creation of curriculum must involve consumers and users of the final product. That includes, but is not limited to, faculty and administrators, students, alumni, employers, and the people whom their graduates serve.

The chapter describes the classic hierarchy of curriculum approval processes in institutions of higher learning and the importance of nursing faculty's participation within the governance of the institution. The governance of colleges and universities usually includes curriculum committees or their equivalent composed of elected faculty members. These committees are at the program, college-wide, and/or university-wide levels and through their review and provide the academic rigor for ensuring quality in educational programs. Chapter 12 provides a view of this process outside the world of academe.

In academe, a fundamental rule is that the curriculum "belongs to the faculty." In higher education, faculty members are the experts in their specific disciplines or in the case of nursing, clinical specialties, or functional areas such as practice, administration, healthcare policy, and so forth. Nursing faculty must periodically review a program to ensure a curriculum that has its foundation in evidence-based practice is in line with the current healthcare needs of the population, the healthcare delivery system, and learners' needs. It is important to measure the program's success in preparing nurses for the current environment and for the future. While it may be unpopular to build curricula on accreditation criteria, professional standards, and national testing criteria, there is a benefit in integrating them into the curriculum. This integration helps administrators and faculty prepare for program approval or review and accreditation.

Faculty at all levels (new and experienced) have roles in curriculum development, implementation, and program evaluation. Often faculty will see only the part of the curriculum in which they are personally involved, it is necessary that all faculty have an overall view of the program as a whole. In that way, the curriculum remains true to its goals, learning objectives (student-learning outcomes), and the content necessary for reaching the goals.

REFERENCE

Keating, S. B. & DeBoor, S. S. (2018). *Curriculum development and evaluation in nursing*, (4th ed.). New York, NY: Springer Publishing Company.

CHAPTER 1

History of Nursing Education in the United States

Susan M. Ervin

CHAPTER OBJECTIVES

Upon completion of Chapter 1, the reader will be able to:

- Compare important curricular events in the 19th century with those in the 20th and 21st centuries.
- Cite the impact that two World Wars had on the development of nursing education.
- Differentiate among the different curricula that prepare entry-level nurses.
- Cite important milestones in the development of graduate education in nursing.
- Associate the decade most pivotal to the development of one type of nursing program, that is, diploma, associate, baccalaureate, master's, or doctoral degree.
- Evaluate the impact of the history of nursing education on current and future curriculum development and evaluation activities.

OVERVIEW

Formal nursing education began at the end of the 19th century when events like the Civil War emphasized the need for well-trained nurses. Florence Nightingale's model of nursing education was used to establish hospital-based nursing programs that flourished throughout the 19th century and well into the 20th. With few exceptions, however, Nightingale's model was abandoned and hospital schools trained students with an emphasis on service rather than education. Early nurse reformers such as Isabel Hampton Robb, Lavinia Dock, and Annie W. Goodrich laid the foundation for nursing education built on natural and social sciences, and by the 1920s, nursing programs were visible in university settings. World War I and World War II underscored the importance of well-educated nurses and the Army School of Nursing and the Cadet Army Corps significantly contributed to the movement of nursing education into university settings.

Associate degree programs developed in the 1950s as a result of community college interest in nursing education and Mildred Montag's dissertation outlined the preparation of the technical nurse in these settings. The situation of nursing in community colleges, along with the American Nurses Association (ANA) proposal that nursing education be located within university settings, sparked a tumultuous period in nursing education.

By the latter half of the 20th century, graduate education in nursing was established with master's and doctoral programs growing across the country. Graduate education continues to strengthen the discipline as it moves through the 21st century.

EARLY BEGINNINGS

Nursing education changed over the past 150 years in response to landmark events such as wars, economic fluctuations, and U.S. demographics. The initial milestone that catalyzed formal nursing education was the Civil War. Prior to the Civil War, most women provided nursing care to family at home. Older women who had extensive family experience and needed to earn a living might care for neighbors or contacts who were referred by word of mouth (Reverby, 1987). Although nursing practice was outside the norm for women, during the Civil War, approximately 2,000 untrained but well-intentioned patriotic women moved from the home to the battlefield to provide care to soldiers. Sadly, a lack of education, inadequate facilities, and poor hygiene contributed to more soldier deaths than bullets or battles. The need for formal education for nurses became evident. Other catalysts for formal nursing education included the transition of hospitals from places for the destitute to arenas for the application of new medical knowledge and the industrial revolution that resulted in increased slums and disease (Rush, 1992).

Earliest Attempts at Formal Training

Florence Nightingale is considered the founder of modern nursing education. She believed that education was necessary to "teach not only what is to be done but how to do it [and]…why such a thing is done" (Nightingale, 1860, p.59). The New England Hospital for Women and Children, established in 1872, was the first school in the United States to offer a formal training program. The school offered a 1-year curriculum. In addition to 12 hours of required lectures, students were taught to take vital signs and apply bandages. Interestingly, students were not allowed to know the names of medications they gave to patients, and the medication bottles were labeled with numbers. In 1875, the curriculum was extended to 16 months (Davis, 1991). Linda Richards, considered to be the first trained nurse in the United States, entered this school on the first day it opened. After her graduation, Linda Richards spent her career organizing training schools for nurses. She was superintendent of the Boston Training School for Nurses at Massachusetts General Hospital as well as at least five other schools (Kalisch & Kalisch, 2004).

First Nightingale Schools

Nightingale's educational model proposed that nursing schools remain autonomous, not under the auspices of affiliated hospitals, and were to develop stringent educational standards (Anderson, 1981; Kelly & Joel, 1996). Education, rather than service to the hospital, should be the focus. In 1873, three schools opened in the United States that provided nursing education theoretically patterned on Nightingale's model: Bellevue Training School in New York City, the Connecticut Training School in Hartford, and the Boston Training School in Boston. The Bellevue Training School opened with a 2-year curriculum. The first year consisted of lectures and clinical practice, and the second year focused on clinical practice (Kalisch & Kalisch, 2004). Although practice was primarily service to the hospital (in opposition to Nightingale's model) and learning was hit and miss, there were some interesting firsts at Bellevue. These included interdisciplinary rounds, patient record keeping, and the adoption of the first student uniform (Kelly & Joel, 1996).

The Connecticut Training School opened with four students and a superintendent of nurses. By the end of the first year, there were nearly 100 applicants, and by the end of the second year, graduates entered the field of private-duty nursing. By its sixth year of operation, the school developed a handbook titled *New Haven Manual of Nursing*. The Connecticut School is credited with the advent of the nursing cap; the wearing of large caps was instituted to contain the elaborate hairstyles of the time that were deemed inappropriate for the "sickroom" (Kalisch & Kalisch, 2004).

The initial goal of the Boston Training School, the third U.S. school, was to offer a desirable occupation for self-supporting women and to provide private nurses for the community. Initially, there was minimal focus on didactic or clinical instruction. In 1874, Linda Richards became the superintendent of the school, reorganized the school, initiated didactic instruction, and, in general, "proved that trained nurses were better than untrained ones" (Kelly & Joel, 1996, p. 27).

The Early 20th Century

By the beginning of the 20th century, more than 2,000 training schools had opened. With few exceptions, Nightingale's principles of education were abandoned, and school priorities were "service first, education second" (Kelly & Joel, 1996). The 3-year program of most nursing schools consisted of on-the-job training, courses taught by physicians, and long hours of clinical practice. Students provided nursing service for the hospital. In return, they received diplomas and pins at the completion of their training. Students entered the programs one by one as they were available, and their services were needed. From the institution's standpoint, graduates were a by-product rather than a purpose for the training school (Reverby, 1984).

Nightingale's text *Notes on Nursing: What It Is and What It Is Not* was published in 1859 and, for decades, was the sole text on nursing. If other textbooks were available to students, they were authored primarily by physicians. The first U.S. nurse–authored text, *A Text-Book for Nursing: For the Use of Training Schools, Families and Private Students*, was written by Clara Weeks (later Weeks-Shaw, 1902), an 1880 graduate of the New York Hospital and founding superintendent of the Paterson General Hospital School (Obituary, 1940). The possession of such a text led to decreased dependence of graduates on their course notes, supplied information that would otherwise have been missed because of canceled lectures or student exhaustion, reinforced the idea that nursing required more than fine character, and exerted a standardizing effect on training school expectations.

It is interesting to note that hospital training schools did not represent the sole path of nursing education in the early 20th century (Bullough, 2004). Perhaps as a harbinger of the 21st century, distance learning provided an alternative educational path. Correspondence schools emerged and were regarded by many as a satisfactory alternative to hospital schools. The best known of these schools was the Chautauqua School of Nursing in the state of New York. Founded in 1900, it offered a three-course correspondence program that included general nursing, obstetrical, and surgical nursing. It attracted students for a variety of reasons. They may have been too old (older than 35 years of age) for hospital schools, were married (hence not eligible for hospital schools), or lived in communities where no hospital school of nursing was available. Fledgling accrediting and registration bodies forced the closure of the school in the 1920s (Bullough, 2004), and it was not until the late 20th and early 21st centuries that distance learning again became an educational path for nursing.

Early Attempts of Diversity and Inclusion in Nursing Education

Mary Mahoney, the first African American nurse, entered the New England Hospital for Women and Children School of Nursing on March 23, 1878. Her acceptance at this school was unique at a time in the United States when most educational institutions were not integrated (Davis, 1991). This lack of integration, however, did not deter African American women from entering the profession of nursing. In 1891, Provident Hospital in Chicago was founded, which was the first training school for African American nurses (Kelly & Joel, 1996).

Howard University Training School for Nurses was established in 1893 to train African American nurses to care for the many Blacks who settled in Washington, D.C., after the Civil War. The school transferred to Freedman's Hospital in 1894 and by 1944 had 166 students (Washington, 2012). This rapid expansion was experienced by other African American nursing programs (Kalisch & Kalisch, 1978). Freedman's Hospital School transferred to Howard University in 1967 and graduated its last class in 1973. Howard University School of Nursing has offered a baccalaureate degree since 1974, initiated a master's degree in nursing in 1980, and recently added a Post-Master's Certificate Family Nurse Practitioner program (Howard University, College of Nursing and Allied Health Sciences, n.d.). After the *Brown v. Board of Education* decision in 1954, schools of nursing that served predominantly African American students began to decline, and by the late 1960s, nursing schools throughout the United States were fully integrated (Carnegie, 2005).

The first Native American School of Nursing was Sage Memorial Hospital School of Nursing, which was established in 1930. Located in northeastern Arizona, at Ganado, it was the first accredited 3-year nursing program on a reservation (Charbonneau-Dahlen & Crow, 2016). It was part of Sage Memorial Hospital, built by the National Missions of the Presbyterian Church, which provided care for Native Americans (Kalisch & Kalisch, 1978). By 1943, students enrolled in the school came from widely diverse backgrounds including Native American, Hispanic, Hawaiian, Cuban, and Japanese. In the 1930s and 1940s, such training and cultural exchange among minority women were not found anywhere else in the United States (Pollitt et al., 2011). The school of nursing operated through 1951; decreased funding and an increased emphasis on baccalaureate education contributed to its closure. In 1993, the first reservation-based baccalaureate nursing program was opened by Northern Arizona University at the same location as Sage Memorial School (Charbonneau-Dahlen & Crow, 2016).

One little-known legacy of the Civil War is the inclusion of men in nursing. Walt Whitman, known for his poetry, was a nurse in the Civil War. He cared for wounded soldiers in Washington, D.C., for 5 years and was an early practitioner of holistic nursing, incorporating active listening, therapeutic touch, and the instillation of hope in patients (Ahrens, 2002). There were few nursing schools in the late 19th century that accommodated men; a few schools provided an abbreviated curriculum that trained men as "attendants." The McLean Asylum School of Nursing in Massachusetts, established in 1882, was among the first to provide nursing education for men. The 2-year curriculum prepared graduates to work in the mental health facilities of the time. Treatments in those facilities included a phenomenon called "tubbing," placing the patient in a bathtub with a wooden cover locked onto the tub so only the patient's head was exposed, and it was believed this treatment required the physical power men possessed (Kenny, 2008).

The first true formal school of nursing for men was established at Bellevue Hospital in New York City in 1888 by Darius Mills. One of the best-known schools of nursing for men was the Alexian Brothers Hospital School of Nursing. It opened in 1898 and was the last of its kind to close in 1969 (LaRocco, 2011). Although the school admitted only religious brothers for most of its early history, in 1927 it began to accept lay students. In 1939, the school began an affiliation with DePaul University so students could take other science courses to apply toward a baccalaureate degree. By 1955, the school had obtained full National League for Nursing (NLN) accreditation, and by 1962, 13 full-time faculty members and eight lecturers educated a graduating class of 42 students. This was the largest class in the school's history and one of the largest classes in any men's nursing school in the country (Wall, 2009). By the mid-1960s, men were being admitted to most hospital nursing programs and the school graduated its last class in 1969.

Diverse ethnic and racial groups account for more than one third of the U.S. population (U.S. Census Bureau, n.d.) and nursing education strives to ensure the profession reflects the diversity of the nation. Strategies used for increasing diversity and inclusion in nursing education include assigning culturally similar mentors, using cohort study and project groups, and providing opportunities for students to work with diverse nurses at all levels of education (Walters & Davis, 2014). In 2019, 35.6% of baccalaureate nursing students were non-White which represents a 4% increase from 2016 (11.2% African American, 12.9% Hispanic, 0.8% American Indian, 7.8% Asian/Pacific Islander, 2.9% two or more races); in graduate programs 35.4% MSN, 33.7% PhD, and 36% DNP students were non-White (American Association of Colleges of Nursing [AACN], 2019).

REPORTS AND STANDARDS OF THE LATE 19TH AND EARLY 20TH CENTURIES

As the number of nursing schools and the number of trained nurses increased, the need for organization and standardization of education and practice was recognized. The International Congress of Charities, Correction and Philanthropy met in Chicago as part of the Columbian Exposition of 1893. Isabel Hampton, the founding principal of the Training School and Superintendent of Nurses at Johns Hopkins Hospital, played a leading role in planning the nursing sessions for the Congress. She presented a paper, *Educational Standards for Nurses*, which argued that hospitals had a responsibility to provide actual education for nursing students; the paper also urged superintendents to work together to establish educational standards (James, 2002). Hampton's paper included a proposal to extend the training period to 3 years in order to allow the shortening of the "practical training" to 8 hours per day. She also recommended admission of students with "stated times for entrance into the school, and the teaching year…divided according to the academic terms usually adopted in our public schools and colleges" (Robb, 1907, p. 24). Hampton initiated an informal meeting of nursing superintendents that laid the groundwork for the formation of the American Society of Superintendents of Training Schools (ASSTS) in the United States and Canada, which, in 1912, was renamed the National League of Nursing Education (NLNE). This was also the first association of a professional nature organized and controlled by women (Bullough & Bullough, 1978).

The year 1893 marked the publication of Hampton's *Nursing: Its Principles and Practice for Hospital and Private Use*. The first 25 pages were devoted to a description of a training school, including physical facilities, library resources, and a 2-year curricular plan for didactic content and clinical rotations (Dodd, 2001). In 1912, the ASSTS became the NLNE and their objectives were to continue to develop and work for a uniform curriculum. In 1915, Adelaide Nutting commented on the educational status of nursing and the NLNE presented a standard curriculum for schools of nursing. The curriculum was divided into seven areas, each of which contained two or more courses. There was a strong emphasis on student activity including observation, accurate recording, participation in actual dissection, experimentation, and provision of patient care (Bacon, 1987). In 1925, the Committee on the Grading of Nursing Schools was formed. The grading committee worked from 1926 to 1934 to produce "gradings" based on answers to survey forms. Each school received individualized feedback about its own characteristics in comparison to all other participating schools (Committee on the Grading of Nursing Schools, 1931).

In 1917, 1927, and 1937, the NLNE published a series of curriculum recommendations in book form. The *Standard Curriculum for Schools of Nursing* was the first, the second *A Curriculum,* and the third *A Curriculum Guide.* The first was developed by a relatively small group, but the second and third involved a long process with broad input. The published curricula were intended to reflect a generalization about what the better schools were doing or aimed to accomplish. As such, they give a picture of change over the 20-year period but cannot be regarded as providing a snapshot of a typical school. Each volume represents a substantial change from the previous, and while the same topical areas exist in all three, the level of detail and specificity increases with each decade. Indeed, the markedly increased length and wordy style of the 1937 volume appropriately carries the title *Guide.*

Each *Curriculum* book increased the number of classroom hours and decreased the recommended hours of patient care, in effect making nursing service more expensive. Each *Curriculum* increased the prerequisite educational level: 4 years of high school (temporary tolerance of 2 years in 1917), 4 years of high school in 1927, and 1 to 2 years of college or normal school in addition to high school by 1937 (NLNE, 1917, 1927, 1937).

While the NLNE advocated for changes in nursing education, there remained a need for a national association of trained nurses. Bellevue Training School founded the first alumnae association in 1889, and by 1890, there were 21 alumni associations in the United States (Kalisch & Kalisch, 2004). In 1896, with the assistance of Isabel Hampton, a national association of trained nurses became a reality. The Nurses' Associated Alumnae of the United States and Canada was established. A constitution and bylaws were prepared and, 1 year later, adopted by the organization, and Ms. Robb became the first elected president. Not one of the original attendees was an RN as there were no licensing laws in place at the time (American Nurses Association [ANA], 2021). In 1911, the Nurses' Associated Alumnae became the ANA (Kalisch & Kalisch, 2004).

MARCHING INTO SERVICE: NURSING EDUCATION IN WARTIME

Prior to World War I, nurses served in the Civil War, and the Spanish American War, which occurred between April and August of 1898. In contrast to the Civil War, only nurses who graduated from an established training school were eligible to serve in the Spanish American War. Disease again caused significant fatalities, with yellow fever claiming the lives of both soldiers and nurses (Kalisch & Kalisch, 2004). Following the Spanish American War, the need for trained nurses was reinforced and both the Army Nurse Corps and the Navy Nurse Corps were established in the early 1900s.

World War I

When the United States entered World War I, admissions to nursing schools increased by about 25% (Bacon, 1987). The two phenomena that impacted nursing education during World War I were the development of the Vassar Training Camp and the founding of the Army School of Nursing. The Vassar Training Camp for Nurses was established in 1918. Its purpose was to enroll female college graduates in a 3-month intensive course that addressed natural and social sciences and fundamental nursing skills. Following this course, students completed the final 2 years of school in one of 35 selected schools of nursing (Bacon, 1987). Of the 439 college graduates who entered the Vassar Camp, 418 completed the course, went on to nursing school, replaced nurses who had entered the armed services, and helped fill key leadership roles in nursing for the next several decades (Kalisch & Kalisch, 1978). Although short-lived, the Vassar Training Camp provided the opportunity to build nursing competencies on a college education foundation and contributed to the eventual move of nursing education into the university setting (Bacon, 1987).

In 1918, Annie W. Goodrich, president of the ANA, proposed the development of an Army School of Nursing. This was in response to extremely vocal groups who believed that, because of the war, the educational preparation of nurses should be shortened. With the backing of the NLNE and the ANA in addition to nursing leaders such as Frances Payne Bolton, the secretary of war approved the school, and Annie Goodrich became its first dean. She developed the curriculum according to the *Standard Curriculum for Schools of Nursing* published by the NLNE in 1917 (Kalisch & Kalisch, 1978).

World War II and the Cadet Nurse Corps

World War II, with its demands for all able-bodied young men for military service, mobilized available women for employment or volunteer service. From mid-1941 to mid-1943, with the help of federal aid, nursing schools increased their enrollments and postdiploma nurses completed postbasic course work to fill the places of nurses who enlisted. Some inactive nurses returned to practice (Roberts, 1954). Despite the effort necessary to bring about this increase, hospitals were floundering and more nurses were needed for the military services. Congress passed the Bolton Act, which authorized the complex of activities known as the Cadet Nurse Corps (CNC) in June 1943. It was conceived as a mechanism to avoid civilian hospital collapse, to provide nursing to the military, and to ensure an adequate education for student nurse cadets (Kalisch & Kalisch, 1978).

Hospitals sponsoring training schools recognized that CNC schools would out-recruit non-CNC schools, thereby almost certainly guaranteeing their closure or radical shrinkage. Thus, they signed on, even though hospitals had to establish a separate accounting for school costs, meet the requirements of their state boards of nurse examiners to the satisfaction of the CNC consultants, and allow students to leave for federal service during the last 6 months of their programs when they would otherwise be most valuable to their home schools. Visiting consultants looked at faculty numbers and qualifications, clinical facilities available for learning, curricula, hours of student clinical and classwork, the school's ability to accelerate course work to fit into 30 months, and the optimal number of students the school could accommodate. Schools were pressed to increase the size of their classes and number of classes admitted per year, to use local colleges for basic sciences to conserve nurse instructor time, and to develop affiliations with psychiatric hospitals, for educational reasons, and secondarily to free up dormitory space for more students to be admitted (Robinson & Perry, 2001).

Students, who were estimated to be providing 80% of care in civilian hospitals, experienced a changed practice context. In addition to providing direct care, students now decided what could safely be delegated to Red Cross volunteers and any available paid aides. With grossly short staffing, nurses had to set priorities carefully. All of these circumstances altered student learning. The intense work of the consultants, who provided interpretation and linkage between the U.S. Public Health Service (USPHS) in Washington and each school, and their strategy of simultaneously naming deficiencies and identifying improvement goals was a critical factor in the success of the programs as well as improvement in nursing education. Without the financial resources of the federal government to defray student costs, assist with certain costs to schools, and provide the consultation, auditing, and public relations/recruitment functions, the goals could not be met.

While the two World Wars had a great impact on nursing education, it is of note that nurses have served in all U.S. conflicts, including Korea, Vietnam (where eight nurses died from accidents or wounds), Desert Storm, and the ongoing Middle East crisis. Educational incentives, notably the Army Student Nurse Program and the Reserve Officer Training Corps programs, assist student nurses with educational expenses in exchange for specific years of active-duty service (Vuic, 2006).

THE EVOLUTION OF CURRENT EDUCATIONAL PATHS FOR ENTRY INTO PRACTICE

By the interwar period, the university became the dominant institution for postsecondary education (Graham, 1978). From 1920 to 1940, the percentage of women attending college in the 18- to 21-year-old age range rose from 7.6% to 12.2%. Men's attendance rose more quickly; hence, the percentage of women in the student body dropped from 43% in 1920 to 40.2% in 1940 (Eisenmann, 2000; Solomon, 1985). In the first decade of the 1900s, technical institutes such as Drexel in Philadelphia, Pratt in Brooklyn, and Mechanics in Rochester, as well as Simmons College in Boston and Northwestern University in Chicago, offered coursework to nursing students (Robb, 1907). The designers of the 1917 *Standard Curriculum for Schools of Nursing* gave some thought to the relationship of nursing education to the collegiate system. They suggested that the theoretical work in a nursing school was equivalent to 36 units, or about 1 year of college, and the clinical work another 51 units. Few voices actively campaigned for the placement of nursing education in higher learning even as late as the 1930s, despite the recommendation of the Rockefeller-funded Goldmark (1923) report *Nursing and Nursing Education in the United States* in the early 1920s. Initially, education at the university level was envisioned solely for the leaders of training schools.

Educators wanted autonomous schools of nursing with a concentration on educational goals and emancipation from hospital student apprentice, work–study curricula. These educators looked hopefully at the Yale University School of Nursing, funded by the Rockefeller Foundation starting in 1924, and headed by Annie W. Goodrich. Similarly encouraging was the program at Case Western Reserve University, endowed by Francis Payne Bolton in 1923. Vanderbilt was endowed by a combination of Rockefeller, Carnegie, and Commonwealth funds in 1930. The University of Chicago established a school of nursing in 1925 with an endowment from the distinguished but discontinued Illinois Training School (Hanson, 1991). Dillard University established a school in 1942 with substantial foundation support and governmental war-related funds. Mary Tennant, nursing adviser in the Rockefeller Foundation, pronounced the Dillard Division of Nursing education one of the most interesting in the country (Hine, 1989). Although these were milestone events, endowments did little to dissipate the caution, if not hostility, toward women on U.S. campuses. Neither did they cure-all that was ailing in nursing education. They funded significant program changes, but even these would not meet the accreditation standards of later decades (Faddis, 1973; Kalisch & Kalisch, 1978; Sheahan, 1980).

Baccalaureate Education

The diverse baccalaureate curricula of the 1930s multiplied by the 1950s, although they were still viewed as being in an experimental stage. There was little consistency among programs; they varied widely in admission and matriculation requirements, curriculum, and purpose. Some programs, for example, prepared nurses for specialty practice, while others moved toward preparing graduates for generalist practice (Harms, 1954).

Although a few programs threaded general education and basic science courses through 5 years of study, the majority structured their programs with 2 years of college courses before or after the 3 years of nursing preparation or book-ended the nursing years with the split 2 years of college work (Bridgman, 1949). Margaret Bridgman (1953), an educator from Skidmore College who consulted with many nursing schools, made favorable reference to the "upper division nursing major" in her volume directed toward both college and nursing educators. Bridgman recommended that postdiploma students be evaluated individually and provisionally with a tentative grant of credit based on prior learning, including nursing schoolwork, and successful completion of a term of academic work. The student's program would be made up of "deficiencies" in general education and prerequisite courses and then courses in the major itself. Credit-granting practices varied considerably from place to place, so a nurse could easily spend 1.5 to 3 years earning the baccalaureate.

Given the constant expansion of knowledge relevant to nursing, it was doubly difficult for programs with a history of a 5-year curriculum to shrink to 4 academic years in the 1960s and early 1970s. The expanded assessment skills expected of critical care nurses, together with the master's-level specialty emphases and certificate nurse practitioner (NP) programs, stimulated the inclusion of more sophisticated skills in baccalaureate programs in the early to mid-1970s (Lynaugh & Brush, 1996). In response to nursing service requests to narrow the gap between new graduate skills and initial employment expectations and much talk about "reality shock," baccalaureate programs structured curricula to allow a final experience in which students were immersed in clinical to focus on skills of organization and integration.

In the 1980s and early 1990s nursing experienced another shortage. Because of the severity of this shortage, accelerated or fast-track baccalaureate nursing and entry-level master's programs were developed (Keating, 2015). The purpose of these programs was to attract students with nonnursing degrees, build on learning experiences provided by these degrees, and provide a path to licensure in 11 to 18 months for the baccalaureate with an additional 12 to 24 months for the master's level (AACN, 2019a). Accelerated programs are now available in 49 states, as well as Washington, D.C.; the U.S. Virgin Islands; and Guam. In 2018, there were 282 accelerated baccalaureate programs and 64 accelerated or entry-level master's programs available with multiple new baccalaureate and entry-level master's programs planned (AACN, 2019b).

The Essentials of Baccalaureate Education for Professional Nursing Practice

AACN endorsed the original *Essentials of Baccalaureate Education for Professional Nursing Practice* in 1986; it was the first comprehensive national effort to define the essential knowledge, practice, and values that the baccalaureate nurse should have. In 1998, AACN revised the essentials. There were changes in healthcare such as increased use of technology for healthcare delivery, and changing U.S. demographics had made people 75 and older the fastest growing population. Shortened hospital stays saw the growth of managed care networks. Nurses worked in more complex and diverse environments and needed to master knowledge and skills for these environments (AACN, 1998). The 1998 *Essentials* focused on liberal education, professional values, core competencies (critical thinking, communication, assessment, technical skills), core knowledge (health promotion, risk reduction, and disease prevention, illness and disease management, information and healthcare technologies, ethics, human diversity), and role development (provider of care, designer/manager/coordinator of care, member of a profession). Changes in healthcare required nurses to. In 2008, AACN again revised *The Essentials of Baccalaureate Education for Professional Nursing Practice*. Healthcare had continued to change, and practice environments had become technologically advanced, more diverse, and global. Concern was also being expressed about healthcare outcomes. The Institute of Medicine (IOM—now known as the National Academy of Medicine—Committee on Quality of Health Care in America (2000, 2001, 2004) published a number of reports citing the role of medical errors in poor patient outcomes, calling for a safer health system, promoting evidence-based practice, and illustrating the lack of health insurance (which translated to lack of healthcare) for a growing number of people in the United States. In addition, there was a growing nursing shortage (AACN, 2008a). The 2008 *Essentials* still focused on a liberal education base and necessary knowledge and skills. But there was an increased focus on basic organizational and systems leadership for quality care and patient safety, evidence-based practice, the application of patient care technology, and interprofessional communication and collaboration.

On April 7, 2021, the AACN released the newest version of *The Essentials: Core Competencies for Professional Nursing Education*. As with previous versions, these *Essentials* provide a framework for preparing individuals as nurses (AACN, 2021). Historically, each level of nursing education was represented by separate *Essentials* documents. These included *The Essentials of Baccalaureate Education for Professional Nursing* (AACN, 2008b), *The Essentials of Master's Education in Nursing* (AACN, 2011), and *The Essentials of Doctoral Education for Advanced Nursing Practice* (AACN, 2006). In contrast, the current document addresses educational preparation for both entry-level and advanced practice. Ten domains, with delineated competencies, are applicable across four spheres of care (disease prevention/promotion of health and well-being, chronic disease care, regenerative or restorative care, hospice/palliative/supportive care) and prepare nurses to care for diverse individuals, families, and populations (AACN, 2021). While the domains and competencies are identical for baccalaureate, master's, and DNP curricula, subcompetencies move the learner from entry to advanced-level practice and knowledge.

Associate Degree Education

The NLNE held discussions during the middle and late 1940s with community colleges to discuss the possibility of associate degree nursing education (Fondiller, 2001). In 1945, the American Association of Junior Colleges (AAJC) showed an interest in nursing; at this point curriculum and recruitment were the two major challenges. In January 1946, a committee was established with representation from the Association of Collegiate Schools of Nursing (ACSN) to consider nursing education in community colleges. Between 1949 and 1950, the committee, along with NLNE and ACSN, discussed nursing education at this level. The focus was to be the "Brown" report, *Nursing for the Future*, authored by Esther Lucille Brown (1948), a social anthropologist with the Russell Sage Foundation. The immediate context for the committee, from the nursing side, was significant. In 1947, the board of NLNE adopted the policy goal that nursing education should be situated in the higher education system. Also, in 1947, the faculty at Teachers College, Columbia University (TCCU) launched a planning process that involved Eli Ginzberg, a young economist who asserted that nursing could be thought of as a whole set of functions and roles rather than a single role or type of worker. He posited that nursing needed at least two types of practitioners, one professional and one technical (Haase, 1990). Starting in the fall of 1947, Brown began her conferences with nursing leaders and visits to more than 50 schools, completing her report so that it could be disseminated in September 1948. She believed that perhaps a "graduate bedside nurse" needed more preparation than a practical nurse but less than a full-fledged professional nurse. In early 1949, NLNE sought funding for the joint work with community colleges and found the Russell Sage and W. K. Kellogg Foundations responsive with substantial support (Haase, 1990).

The committee reported that community colleges could develop one of two types of nursing programs: (a) a 2-year program that would be transfer oriented to a university program that offered a baccalaureate degree or (b) a 3-year program leading to an associate of arts or an associate of science. In 1951, Mildred Montag, whose dissertation proposed a new type of technical nursing program embedded in junior colleges, joined the committee. She was subsequently appointed to the Joint Committee in 1951 and became the project director for the anonymously funded Cooperative Research Project (CRP) in Junior and Community College Education for Nursing in early 1952 (Haase, 1990). The CRP pilot programs were 2 years long or 2 years plus a summer. Initially, they were one third general education and two thirds nursing, but they moved toward equal proportions of each by the end of the project. The curricula, although controlled by faculty in each school, tended to focus on variations in health in their first year and then deviations from normal (physical and mental illness) in the second year. These "broad fields" were accompanied by campus nursing laboratory learning and clinical learning experiences in a wide variety of settings but with a major hospital component. Students in the pilot programs were somewhat older than diploma or baccalaureate students, and some were married (a nonstarter in many diploma programs) and had children. Men were a small percentage of the students but tripled the representation in diploma programs. State board examination pass rates for graduates of the pilot group were comparable to those of other programs. Montag intended, at that time, that this program would be self-contained but stressed that graduates of this program could pursue baccalaureate education. She also recommended single licensure for nurses from all educational programs, although 25 years later, she rescinded that recommendation (Fondiller, 2001).

From the mid-1950s to the mid-1970s, when the associate degree program growth rate peaked, the number of programs doubled about every 4 years. By 1975, there were 618 associate degree programs in nursing, constituting 45% of basic nursing programs. Diploma programs constituted 31% of basic programs, although most nurses in practice still originally came from diploma programs (Haase, 1990; Rines, 1977). By 1959, W. K. Kellogg Foundation assistance to the expansion of associate degree nursing education totaled more than $3 million. The Nurse Training Act of 1964 and subsequent federal legislation funding nursing also contributed to program growth (Scott, 1972). By the 1990s, associate degree programs produced nearly 60% of newly licensed RNs. This began to shift in the 2000s. By 2011, more nurses were graduating from baccalaureate programs, and by 2012, 53% of nurses were earning baccalaureate degrees (Robert Wood Johnson Foundation, 2015).

Over the years, associate degree education lengthened in time, due in part to the expanding knowledge base needed to be "a bedside nurse." Much time was devoted to communicating with hospital nursing service representatives to identify students' competencies at graduation so that new graduate orientations and staff development plans articulated with them. Curricular offerings were fine-tuned to ensure that these baseline competencies were met. When "the bedside" noticeably moved out of the hospital in the early 1990s, questions about preparation for practice in the home care context became urgent, but the familiar condition of the hospital "nursing shortage" laid these to rest.

Programs of the 1950s in university settings had to cope with the entrenched traditions of both hospitals and universities as they struggled to make changes. By contrast, associate degree nursing programs began with a clean slate. They were initially welcomed by community colleges. The lure of having an additional supply of nurses promoted at least grudging cooperation from clinical agencies, although hospital nursing staff and administrators in many places had misgivings about the curricular arrangements and limited clinical experience of students.

The associate degree–prepared nurses of the early 1980s found expectations and mechanisms for matriculating into baccalaureate programs much more clearly defined than described by Bridgman 30 years earlier, and indeed, some baccalaureate programs were designed specifically for associate degree graduates. The ever-expanding body of nursing knowledge forced repeated decisions about which content was most essential and what clinical settings would bring about the best learning. By the 1990s, as hospital censuses plummeted and sick patients shuttled back and forth between home and ambulatory settings, programs were forced to consider increasing community-based clinical experience with its attendant challenges to find placements and provide geographically dispersed instruction.

Tumultuous Times in Nursing Education

The turbulence and cultural upheaval that characterized the mid-1960s through the 1970s was reflected in nursing education. Within nursing, a rift grew between those who believed an incremental approach would eventually get nursing education optimally situated and those who believed that the eventual goal should be clearly specified far in advance so that changes could take the goal into account. Nurses involved in day-to-day patient care and many diploma educators tended to cluster in the first group; the premise was that practice roles in nursing were rarely based on educational preparation. Graduates of all programs held the same license (Fredrickson, 1978). Those nurses, particularly educators, who were in national or regional leadership positions were in the second group. The latter group focused on the professional end of the nursing continuum, working to achieve the fullest possible academic and professional recognition for nursing so that its advocacy and action would have broad credibility and influence. They attempted to define differentiation of practice among the three levels of education (diploma, associate degree, baccalaureate) and advocated for legislation that recognized differences among graduates (Orsolini-Hain & Waters, 2009).

The ANA 1965 position paper, *Educational Preparation for Nurse Practitioners and Assistants to Nurses*, seemed like a logical step in this differentiation of practice. After all, for more than 15 years, the NLNE, reconstituted and combined with the National Organization for Public Health Nursing (NOPHN), the ACSN, and National Association of Industrial Nurses (NAIN) in 1952 to be the NLN, had been saying that education for nursing belonged in institutions of higher education. The idea that nursing was a continuum, composed of vocational, technical, and professional segments, had been talked about intermittently in those same circles during that entire period.

Unfortunately, the position paper dropped like a bomb on people who had never heard these conversations. It was said to ignore diploma schools and nurses altogether, classify associate degree–prepared nurses as technical nurses, and downgrade vocational/practical nurse preparation. Fundamental questions such as the "fit" of the three-part typology with the range of nursing work, the location and nature of the boundaries between the segments of the continuum, and the regulatory and licensure implications of such a plan could hardly be debated because of the emotionality that surrounded the specter of the loss of access to the RN title for associate and diploma nurses and what appeared to be the hijacking of the term *professional*.

Regardless of nursing program background, the term *professional* had been applied to all that was good. General usage, likewise, cast *professional* in positive terms. Students who did a project or handled a situation "professionally" knew it was well done, students who "looked professional" knew they had met certain standards (however little clean shoelaces may have had to do with actual professionalism), and students who studied to be "professional nurses" would qualify to take the state board examination, and in the years just before the position paper, thought they would give comprehensive, individualized care to patients. *Technical* just did not have the same ring to it; *technical* sounded limited and mechanical; *technical* sounded "less than." However knowledgeable, talented, and essential technical workers were in the discourse of educational macroplanners and economists, the word translated poorly to the world of nursing.

The crisis was gradually defused, partly by action on the recommendations of the next committee to study nursing, the National Commission for the Study of Nursing and Nursing Education (1970), which was commonly known as the Lysaught Commission, which reported in 1970. Among the recommendations in *Abstract for Action* were

1. statewide planning for the number and distribution of nursing education programs,
2. career mobility for individual nurses, and
3. cooperation of nursing service and education in working to improve patient care.

As the world around community colleges changed so that more and more people, particularly women, resumed formal education after a hiatus, and senior colleges had good experiences with community college graduates who sought baccalaureate degrees, the concepts of "career mobility" and "articulation" came into nursing discourse. By 1972, the NLN prepared a collection titled "The Associate Degree Program–A Step to the Baccalaureate Degree in Nursing." There were some baccalaureate educators, however, who assumed associate degree curricula were unrelated to baccalaureate curricula, and that the two curricula occupied separate universes (Haase, 1990).

In the early 2000s, partnerships between community colleges and universities set the stage for increased articulation between associate and baccalaureate programs. They developed shared curricula, admissions standards, and application processes that facilitated the movement of graduates from associate degree programs into baccalaureate education. The Oregon Consortium for Nursing Education was the first in the country to develop such an approach (Tanner et al., 2008) and acted as a model for articulation agreements between associate and baccalaureate nursing programs across the nation.

In 2010, the IOM recommended that 80% of nurses be prepared at the baccalaureate level by 2020. This would enable nurses to practice to their fullest potential, become partners with other healthcare practitioners, and enable them to advance health and lead change. This was followed by Benner et al.'s (2010) work with the Carnegie Foundation. In her work, *Educating Nurses: A Call for Radical Transformation*, she asserts that nurses work with increasingly complex patients, and with rapidly changing technology. The book calls for nurses to be educated at the baccalaureate level and practicing nurses to return to school to pursue a baccalaureate degree. As a result of the IOM (2010) report and Benner et al.'s (2010) work, there are currently more than 600 RN to BSN programs in the United States that prepare graduates for an increasingly complex healthcare system (McEwen et al., 2013).

Master's Education

Master's programs were few and relatively small in the 1950s. The 1951 report of the National Nursing Assessment Service (NNAS) Postgraduate Board of Review noted that in some instances, the same set of courses led to a master's degree for students who held a baccalaureate and to a baccalaureate for students who had no prior degree. Some of the clearly differentiated master's programs had so many prerequisites that few students qualified for admission without clearing multiple "deficiencies" by taking additional coursework. The report opined that few programs focused on nursing "in its broadest sense," as contrasted to teaching and administration (National Nursing Accrediting Service Postgraduate Board of Review, 1951).

A Work Conference on Graduate Nurse Education, sponsored by the NLN Division of Nursing Education in the fall of 1952, concluded that master's graduates needed competencies in interpersonal relations, communication skills, their selected functional area (e.g., teaching or administration), and promotion of community welfare. Master's graduates also needed knowledge about the research process so they could participate in the investigation of nursing problems, evaluate research, and translate research findings into practice (Harms, 1954). However, a 1954 study comparing six leading schools' master's curricula identified wide variability in actual practice. Program lengths were nominally 1 year for students without deficiencies; however, this ranged from 24 to 38 semester credits. Although research was an agreed-upon master's focus, only one of the six schools had one course that by title could be identified as addressing this area (Harms, 1954).

Given the relatively few students seeking admission, and the small size of programs, regional planning became important, particularly in the southern and western United States. In regional activity that was the precursor to the formation of the Southern Council on Collegiate Education for Nursing, it was agreed in 1952 that six universities—Universities of Alabama, Maryland, North Carolina, Texas, Vanderbilt, and Emory University—would come together to plan five new master's programs to serve the South. This regional project in graduate education in nursing garnered funding from both the W. K. Kellogg and Commonwealth Foundations. By 1955, all six programs were admitting students (Reitt, 1987).

In western states, the Western Conference of Nursing Education was convened in early 1956 by the Western Interstate Commission for Higher Education (WICHE). Nursing educators, nurse leaders in various other positions, and nonnurse representatives from higher education gathered to advise WICHE on the development of nursing education programs in the area. A 2-month study of nursing education in western states, conducted by Helen Nahm, laid the groundwork for the meeting. This report provided the group with the essence of hundreds of interviews conducted with educators in nursing and related fields in the eight states, as well as nurse manpower data by state for 1954. Respondents reportedly believed that graduate programs in nursing should contain more work in social science fields, advanced preparation in physical and biological sciences, strong foundations in education, and courses in research and philosophy. Graduate programs also needed strong clinical and research foci (WICHE, 1956). Subsequently, the Western Interstate Council for Higher Education in Nursing (WICHEN) sponsored joint work that developed early master's-level clinical content and terminal competencies in the early and mid-1960s (Brown, 1978; WICHE, 1967).

Enrollment in master's programs almost doubled between 1951 and 1962, growing from 1,290 to 2,472 (Harms, 1954; Kalisch & Kalisch, 1978). During the 1960s, clinical area emphases replaced functional specializations as the organizing frames for curricula. This shift in focus to nursing itself not only clarified and enriched baccalaureate curricula in later decades (Lynaugh & Brush, 1996) but also freed doctoral-level training to focus directly on nursing knowledge development.

Political pressure for access to care, interacting with the shortage and maldistribution of physicians and the recognition that nurses could competently do a subset of physician work, led to federal support for the spread of NP programs (Bullough, 1976; National Commission for the Study of Nursing and Nursing Education, 1971). Until the mid-1970s most NP preparation was offered as non-degree-related continuing education. The first national conference on family NP curricula convened in January 1976. At that point, programs ranged from 4-month certificate-level offerings to specialties set within master's programs, with divergent characteristics depending on rural or urban settings. Certificate programs accounted for 71% of NP program grants funded by the Division of Nursing of the USPHS that year. Just 9 years later, in 1985, 81% of NP program grants went to master's-level programs without any change in the authorizing law and presumably the award criteria. Multiple factors drove or accommodated this change. Practice settings had higher expectations, fears of educators about preserving the essence of nursing subsided, enough potential students saw value in a graduate degree, and faculty members who reconceptualized the curricula were persuasive. Not insignificantly, federal funds were available to assist with the costs of transition (Geolot, 1987).

Most large master's programs had multiple specialties by the mid-1980s, but these only weakly correlated with the major specialty organizations and with certification mechanisms (Styles, 1989). The clinical expertise and interest of nursing faculty, links to local resources, community needs for a particular specialty, and federal/state/local voluntary organization financial initiatives to address specific health problems all drove the pattern of specialty development (Burns et al., 1993). Nursing specialty organizations, reflecting current practice perspectives, exerted a substantial influence on specialty curricular content in their respective areas. The rapid expansion (27%) in the number of master's programs in the last half of the 1980s (Burns et al., 1993) may have spurred the creative naming of specialties for purposes of student recruitment. Efforts to rationalize the relationships of the specialties to one another and where possible, to achieve common use of resources, were the natural response to this proliferation.

By the 1990s, clinical specialist content was combined with NP approaches. Advanced practice nurses of both types were beginning to question whether the two roles were, after all, so different from one another (Elder & Bullough, 1990). Changes in healthcare financing and delivery were prompting clinical nurse specialist programs to include content to prepare graduates to deal with cost and reimbursement dimensions of care for populations (Wolf, 1990), and pressuring practitioner programs to prepare graduates to care for patients with less stable conditions. By the end of the first decade of the 21st century, this trend coalesced into an advanced practice regulatory model that has standardized graduate-level educational requirements (ANA, 2017; Trossman, 2009).

In 2001, the IOM published a report calling for increased attention to the provision of safe patient care environments. AACN, in response to that report, envisioned the clinical nurse leader (CNL) role (AACN, 2003). The CNL is a role that provides leadership at the point of care. Advanced practice preparation and clinical leadership competencies, both acquired at the master's level, prepare this nurse leader to ensure the delivery of safe, evidence-based care targeted toward quality patient outcomes. The AACN developed standards for the CNL and has a certification program for graduates of CNL programs (AACN, 2007, 2013 and 2017; Reid, 2011).

The Essentials of Master's Education in Nursing

The Essentials of Master's Education for Advanced Practice Nursing (AACN, 1996) represented agreement among educators about master's preparation for advanced practice nurses. The document also served to assist programs in the development of common curricular characteristics. In the early 21st century, as specialty advanced practice nursing education transitioned to the doctoral level, AACN (2011) developed the *Essentials of Master's Education in Nursing*. There was recognition that masters' preparation remained an important component of nursing education and masters' prepared nurses contribute significantly to current and emerging roles in healthcare. These essentials did not address preparation for a specific role; rather, they delineated outcomes expected of all master's program graduates (AACN, 2011). The current essentials, *The Essentials: Core Competencies for Professional Nursing Education* (AACN, 2021) delineate 10 domains that enfold entry- and advanced-level education. The domains include Knowledge for Nursing Practice, Person-Centered Care, Population Health, Scholarship for Nursing Practice, Quality and Safety, Interprofessional Partnerships, Systems-Based Practice, Information and Health Care Technologies, Professionalism, and Personal, Professional, and Leadership Development. Each domain has competencies applicable to entry- and advanced-level education; for example, the first competency in Knowledge for Nursing Practice is "Demonstrate an understanding of the discipline of nursing's distinct perspective and where shared perspectives exist with other disciplines" (AACN, 2021, p. 28). Subcompetencies, however, delineate entry from advanced knowledge and practice. While a baccalaureate graduate may identify concepts of nursing science, the master's (or DNP) graduate would be expected to translate concepts of nursing science into practice (AACN, 2021).

Doctoral Programs

The first doctoral programs tailored for the preparation of nursing faculty began in the 1920s and 1930s. Columbia University and New York University (NYU) offered an EdD and a PhD in their departments of education. There was, currently, little coursework specific to nursing (Carter, 2009). By the 1950s, educators began to focus on the development of doctoral work in nursing. The need for doctorally prepared faculty to teach master's students who, it was hoped, would graduate and teach in the multiplying baccalaureate programs, fueled part of the interest in this topic. But for leaders already involved in higher education, it was painfully clear that nursing needed some capacity for its own research that would focus on questions related to nursing interventions to create a coherent body of tested knowledge and improve care.

In 1954, with Martha Rogers as chair of the Department of Nursing Education at NYU, the doctoral program was redirected to become a PhD in nursing. The University of Pittsburgh established a PhD with a focus in pediatric or maternal nursing in 1954. In contrast to Martha Rogers's view that theory was the starting point that would lead to knowledge development in the "applied" field of nursing, Florence Erickson and Reva Rubin at Pittsburgh believed that extensive exposure to clinical phenomena, along with skilled faculty guidance, would develop a true nursing science (Parietti, 1979). In the West, in the early WICHE/WICHEN conversations, the temporary need for help from other disciplines for research training was posited as a mechanism to build nursing knowledge and a critical mass of investigators (WICHE, 1956). The journal *Nursing Research* became available in 1952 as a mechanism for systematic communication (Bunge, 1962).

In 1955, the Nursing Research Grants and Fellowship Program of the USPHS allocated $500,000 for research grants and $125,000 for fellowships, the first such funding for nursing. From 1955 to 1970, 156 nurses were supported by special predoctoral research fellowships for doctoral study, and from 1959 to 1968, 18 schools of nursing received federally funded faculty research development grants to stimulate research capacity. The nurse scientist graduate training programs, which provided federal incentive funding to disciplines outside of nursing to accept nurses as students and provided fellowships to the students, were designed to create a critical mass of faculty and a climate conducive to establishing doctoral programs in nursing (Grace, 1978). The program continued from 1962 to 1976 and funded more than 350 nurse trainees (Berthold et al., 1966; Murphy, 1981).

Three additional doctoral programs were established in the 1960s (Boston University, 1960, DNS, psychiatric/mental health focus; University of California, San Francisco [UCSF], 1964, DNS, multifocus; Catholic University, 1968, DNS, medical–surgical and psychiatric/mental health foci). The Boston program took a clinical immersion approach analogous to the University of Pittsburgh. UCSF's program was structured as a research degree but identified clinical involvement as the base for knowledge development, influenced both by faculty with a strong clinical identity and by the grounded theory perspectives of the several social scientists who were a part of the faculty.

A federally funded series of nine annual ANA-sponsored research conferences was initiated in 1965, and WICHEN sponsored the first of its annual Communicating Nursing Research conferences in 1968, thus creating space for face-to-face research exchange. The Medical Literature Analysis and Retrieval System made its debut in 1964, the first in a series of databases that would aid dissemination. Essential components for school of nursing research centers were identified (Gunter, 1966). A series of three federally funded conferences in Kansas City, Kansas, on nursing theory in 1969 and 1970 provided further opportunity to work through the divergent views of the relationships of theory, practice, and research to one another (Murphy, 1981).

In 1971, the Division of Nursing and the Nurse Scientist Graduate Training Committee (NSGTC) convened an invitational conference to address the type(s) of doctoral preparation. In this setting, Joseph Matarazzo, chair of the NSGTC, presented a paper arguing that nursing was ready as a discipline to launch PhD study, citing its body of knowledge and the qualifications of trainees (Matarazzo & Abdellah, 1971; Murphy, 1981). Comprehensive information about the state of nursing doctoral resources became available by the mid-1970s (Leininger, 1976), and by the late 1970s, national doctoral forums, open to schools with established programs, provided a mechanism for exchanging viewpoints about doctoral education. Three additional research journals began publication in 1978 (Gortner, 1991). "The Discipline of Nursing" (Donaldson & Crowley, 1978) was a milestone paper. It differentiated the discipline of nursing from the practice of nursing but related the two as well and proposed a productive interrelationship of research, theory, and practice. It shifted the terms of the debate away from the dichotomous basic/applied categories.

The body of knowledge in nursing was still, relative to the old disciplines, rather modest in the late 1970s, but the progress in two decades was amazing, and the infrastructure to support further development was substantial (Gortner & Nahm, 1977). Students were focusing their dissertation research on nursing clinical issues (Loomis, 1984). However, the DNS and PhD degrees, the two dominant degree titles, although differently named, were indistinguishable in their objectives and end products (Grace, 1978). Finally, themes related to the challenge of mentoring students who are dealing with what is not known and fostering "humanship" between students and faculty to encourage student growth were beginning to come to print at the end of this decade (Downs, 1978).

Fifteen additional doctoral programs opened their doors during the 1970s (Cleland, 1976; Parietti, 1979). From 1980 to 1989, the number of programs grew from 22 to 50, prompting the editorial comment "as dandelions in spring, more and more doctoral programs are appearing" (Downs, 1984, p. 59). Other observers surveying the situation recommended regional planning to sponsor joint programs but conceded that the resources were in individual universities and states and that the mechanisms for making such efforts were nonexistent. They predicted stormy waters for programs that launched without adequate internal and external supports in place (McElmurray et al., 1982). At the end of the 1980s, doctoral educators were examining the balance between theory and research methods on the one hand and "knowledge" or "substance" in the curriculum on the other (Downs, 1988).

Programs expanded from 50 to 70 from 1990 to 1999. By the early 1990s, as the research programs were more numerous and robust in the older and larger schools, with a greater emphasis on research team participation (Keller & Ward, 1993), and mentoring into the range of activities doctoral graduates became visible themes (Katefian, 1991; Meleis, 1992). Postdoctoral study became more feasible and attractive (Hinshaw & Lucas, 1993).

The perennial question from the 1960s to the 1980s, that is, whether nursing should adopt the PhD or the DNS, was answered by the hundreds of individual choices of applicants and the program choices of numerous schools: By 2000, only 12% of nursing doctoral programs conferred the DNS or variants thereof (McEwen & Bechtel, 2000). Much less clear, however, was the difference between the two. Concerns about attention to "substance," that is, organized analysis of the body of nursing knowledge, the adequacy of research programs to provide student experience, and preparation for the teaching component of graduates' expected academic roles, occupied curriculum planners in research-focused doctoral programs at the end of the century.

Questions about the desirability and feasibility of developing clinical or practice-focused doctoral programs in nursing were perennial but intermittent until 2004 when AACN adopted a proposal that would move preparation for advanced practice nursing from the master's degree framework to the doctoral level by 2015 (AACN, 2004, 2020a). Such programs are currently designed to articulate with both nursing baccalaureate and nursing master's (first professional degree and second). The four postbaccalaureate academic years include core areas for all students, as well as clinical specialty-focused study. The research-training component emphasizes the translation of research into practice, practice evaluation, and evidence-based practice improvement. Following on from that, several possible forms of end-of-program practice-focused projects and project reporting formats demonstrate the student's synthesis and expertise while laying the groundwork for future clinical scholarship (AACN, 2006). The AACN (2006) created *The Essentials of Doctoral Education for Advanced Nursing Practice* to guide schools in the development of curricula for the practice-focused doctorate. Based on changes in nursing education, learner expectations, and the U.S. healthcare system, the AACN adopted the revised *Essentials* in 2021. *The Essentials: Core Competencies for Professional Nursing Education* (AACN, 2021) delineates domains with competencies for entry- and advanced-level nursing education. Subcompetencies for each domain enable the learner to build on entry-level education for advanced knowledge and practice.

In 2020, 357 DNP programs enrolled students nationwide, and 106 new DNP programs were planned. From 2018 to 2019, the number of students enrolled in DNP programs increased from 32,678 to 36,079, and graduates increased from 7039 to 7944 (AACN, 2020a). There were 135 PhD programs in 2019, with 4,568 students enrolled and 804 graduates. While not growing as rapidly as DNP enrollment, PhD enrollment has increased 9.4% since 2009, and graduates have climbed to 41% (AACN, 2020b). What the long-term, steady-state allocation of nursing's academic resources should be for the two types of programs is yet to be determined. DNP–PhD programs were developed that enable nurses to combine skills gained in DNP education with research abilities offered through the PhD; some DNP–PhD programs also offer courses in pedagogy to assist in the transition from practitioner to faculty role.

ACCREDITATION OF NURSING EDUCATION PROGRAMS

From the standpoint of the ordinary nursing school, the possibility of actual accreditation became a reality in the 1950s. The NLNE developed standards for accreditation and made pilot visits from 1934 to 1938. By 1939, schools could list themselves to be visited in order to qualify to be on the first list published by NLNE. Despite the greatly increased work, turnover, and general disruption created by the war, 100 schools mustered both the courage and energy required to prepare for accreditation evaluation and judged creditable by 1945. Many schools that qualified for provisional accreditation, however, were due for revisiting by the end of World War II. The NOPHN had been accrediting postbasic programs in public health since 1920 but more recently had considered specialty programs at both baccalaureate and master's levels and the public health content in generalist baccalaureate programs (Harms, 1954). By 1948, these organizations, along with the Council of Nursing Education of Catholic Hospitals, ceded their accrediting role to the NNAS, which published its first combined list of accredited programs just 1 month before the survey-based interim classification of schools was published by the National Committee for the Improvement of Nursing Services in 1949 (Petry, 1949).

The NNAS, much like the cadet nurse program before it, elected a strategy designed to entice schools with at least minimal strengths to improve. It published the first list of temporarily accredited schools in 1952, giving these schools 5 years to make improvements and qualify for full accreditation. During the intervening time, it provided many special meetings, self-evaluation guides, and consultant visits to the schools. By 1957, the number of fully accredited schools increased by 72.4% (Kalisch & Kalisch, 1978). Changes in hospital school programs were catalyzed and channeled by accreditation norms (Committee of the Six National Nursing Organizations on Unification of Accrediting Services, 1949). But ultimately, the forces that drove change were primarily external, ranging from public expectations of postsecondary education mediated through hospital trustees and physicians to competition among programs for potential students, who now had access to information about accreditation. By 1950, all states participated in the state board test pool examination, another measuring rod that induced improvement or closure of weaker schools.

Despite the influential Carnegie- and Russell Sage–funded *Nursing for the Future* in 1948, which recommended a broad-based move of nursing education into general higher education, nursing's earliest centralized accreditation mechanism concentrated considerable energy on improving diploma schools, as had the Grading Committee before it (Brown, 1948; Roberts, 1954). Why this seeming mismatch between aspirations and effort? Partly, it sprang from realism: Students were in hospital schools, whether ideal or not, so they needed the best possible preparation because nursing services would reflect this quality. Furthermore, the quality of many of the baccalaureate programs left a great deal to be desired and their capacity for more students was limited, so these could not be promoted as an immediate or ideal substitute for diploma programs. Although by 1957 there were 18 associate degree programs (Kalisch & Kalisch, 1978), no one foresaw the speed of their multiplication in the next decade. Finally, nursing's collective sense of social responsibility burdened it with finding ways to continue providing essential services, both within the hospital and elsewhere, as its educational house moved from the base of the hospital to the foundation of higher education (Lynaugh, 2002).

END-OF-CHAPTER RESOURCES

DISCUSSION QUESTIONS

- The Nightingale model of nursing education was used to develop early nursing programs in the United States. What social and cultural phenomena were occurring in the United States during the 19th century that impacted the development of these and, subsequent, nursing education programs? Do similar phenomena impact nursing education today? If so, what are they, and how do they impact education?

- Associate degree programs were developed in the 1950s as a result of Mildred Montag's dissertation. Their intent was to prepare a different type of nurse than the one who was prepared at the baccalaureate level. That was not the reality, however, and debate continues (into the 21st century) about educational programs for entry-level nurses. What might nursing education, at both the associate degree and baccalaureate levels, look like today if Montag's plan for a different type of nurse had been followed?

- The AACN adopted a proposal in 2004 that would move preparation for advanced practice nursing from the master's to the doctoral level by 2025. In order to facilitate a nonstop pathway from completion of the BSN to the DNP, programs have been implemented within schools of nursing. What effect might these programs have on other doctoral programs in nursing? DNP–PhD programs are being developed to assist advanced practice nurses' transition from practice to research and academic settings. What are the risks and/or benefits of having these programs to nursing faculty and the students they teach?

LEARNING ACTIVITIES

Student-Learning Activity

Choose teams and debate the wisdom and feasibility of setting the doctoral degree as the minimum level of education for advanced practice nurses. Given the hindsight gained from the efforts to transfer prelicensure education into university settings, how would you go about assisting state boards of nursing with this transition?

Faculty Development Activity

Trace your school of nursing's history and link major curricular changes to events external to the nursing programs.

 A robust set of instructor resources designed to supplement this text is located at **http://connect.springerpub.com/content/book/978-0-8261-8686-7.** Qualifying instructors may request access by emailing **textbook@springerpub.com.**

REFERENCES

Ahrens, W. D. (2002). Walt Whitman, nurse and poet. *Nursing, 32*(5), 43–44.

American Association of Colleges of Nursing. (1986). *Essentials of college and university education for professional nursing.*

American Association of Colleges of Nursing. (1996). *The essentials of master's education for advanced practice nursing.*

American Association of Colleges of Nursing. (1998). *The essentials of baccalaureate education for professional nursing practice.*

American Association of Colleges of Nursing. (2003). *Brief history of the CNL.* http://www.aacnnursing.org/CNL-Certification/Commission-of-Nurse-Certification/History

American Association of Colleges of Nursing. (2004). *AACN position statement on the practice doctorate in nursing October 2004.* http://www.aacnnursing.org/Portals/42/News/Position-Statements/DNP.pdf

American Association of Colleges of Nursing. (2006). *The essentials of doctoral education for advanced nursing practice.* http://www.aacnnursing.org/Portals/42/Publications/DNPEssentials.pdf

American Association of Colleges of Nursing. (2007). *Clinical nurse leader education models being implemented by schools of nursing.* http://www.aacnnursing.org/Portals/42/AcademicNursing/CurriculumGuidelines/CNL-Competencies-October-2013.pdf

American Association of Colleges of Nursing. (2008a). *The essentials of baccalaureate education for professional nursing practice.* https://www.aacnnursing.org/Education-Resources/AACN-Essentials

American Association of Colleges of Nursing. (2008b). *CNL frequently asked questions.* http://www.aacnnursing.org/CNL/About/FAQs

American Association of Colleges of Nursing. (2011). *The essentials of master's education in nursing.* https://www.aacnnursing.org/Education-Resources/AACN-Essentials

American Association of Colleges of Nursing. (2013). *Competencies and curricular expectations for clinical nurse leader education and practice.* http://www.aacnnursing.org/Portals/42/AcademicNursing/CurriculumGuidelines/CNL-Competencies-October-2013.pdf

American Association of Colleges of Nursing. (2017). About the CNL. Retrieved from https://www.aacnnursing.org/CNL/About

American Association of Colleges of Nursing. (2019). *2019–2020 race and ethnicity of students enrolled in nursing programs.* https://www.aacnnursing.org/Diversity

American Association of Colleges of Nursing. (2019a). Accelerated Baccalaureate and Master's Degrees in Nursing. Retrieved from https://www.aacnnursing.org/Nursing-Education-Programs/Accelerated-Programs

American Association of Colleges of Nursing. (2020a). *DNP fact sheet*. http://www.aacnnursing.org/News-Information/Fact-Sheets/DNP-Fact-Sheet

American Association of Colleges of Nursing. (2020b). *PhD in Nursing*. https://www.aacnnursing.org/News-Information/Research-Data-Center/PhD

American Association of Colleges of Nursing. (2021). *The essentials: Core competencies for professional nursing education*. https://www.aacnnursing.org/Portals/42/AcademicNursing/pdf/Essentials-2021.pdf

American Nurses Association. (1965). *Educational preparation for nurse practitioners and assistants to nurses: A position paper*.

American Nurses Association. (2017). *APRN consensus model*. http://www.nursingworld.org/consensusmodel

American Nurses Association. (2021). The history of the American Nurses Association. Retrieved from https://www.nursingworld.org/ana/about-ana/history/

Anderson, N. E. (1981). The historic development of American nursing education. *Journal of Nursing Education*, 20, 18–36. https://doi.org/10.3928/0148-4834-19810101-05

American Nurses Association. (2021). The history of the American Nurses Association. Retrieved from https://www.nursingworld.org/ana/about-ana/history/

Bacon, E. (1987). Curriculum development in nursing education, 1890–1952. *Nursing History Review*, 2, 50–66.

Benner, P., Sutphen, M., Leonard, V., & Day, L. (2010). *Educating nurses: A call for radical transformation*. The Carnegie Foundation for the Advancement of Teaching.

Berthold, J. S., Tschudin, M. S., Peplau, H. E., Schlotfeldt, R., & Rogers, M. E. (1966). A dialogue on approaches to doctoral preparation. *Nursing Forum*, 5, 48–104. https://doi.org/10.1111/j.1744-6198.1966.tb00332.x

Bridgman, M. (1949). Consultant in collegiate nursing education. *American Journal of Nursing*, 49, 808.

Bridgman, M. (1953). *Collegiate education for nursing*. Russell Sage Foundation.

Brown, E. L. (1948). *Nursing for the future*. Russell Sage Foundation.

Brown, J. M. (1978). Master's education in nursing, 1945–1969. In J. Fitzpatrick (Ed.), *Historical studies in nursing* (pp. 104–130). Teachers College.

Bullough, B. (1976). Influences on role expansion. *American Journal of Nursing*, 76, 1476–1481. https://doi.org/10.2307/3424083

Bullough, V. (2004). How one could once become a registered nurse in the United States without going to a hospital training school. *Nursing Inquiry*, 11, 161–165. https://doi.org/10.1111/j.1440-1800.2004.00226.x

Bullough, V., & Bullough, B. (1978). *The care of the sick: The emergence of modern nursing*. Prodist.

Bunge, H. L. (1962). The first decade of nursing research. *Nursing Research*, 11, 132–137. https://doi.org/10.1097/00006199-196201130-00004

Burns, P. G., Nishikawa, H. A., Weatherby, F., Forni, P. R., Moran, M., Allen, M. E., & Booten, D. A. (1993). Master's degree nursing education: State of the art. *Journal of Professional Nursing*, 9, 267–277. https://doi.org/10.1016/8755-7223(93)90052-E

Carnegie, M. E. (2005). Educational preparation of Black nurses: A historical perspective. *The ABNF Journal*, 16, 6–7.

Carter, M. (2009). The history of doctoral education in nursing. In A. M. Barker (Ed.), *Advanced practice nursing: Essential knowledge for the profession* (pp. 31–41). Jones & Bartlett.

Charbonneau-Dahlen, B., & Crow, K. (2016). A brief overview of the history of American Indian nurses. *Journal of Cultural Diversity*, 23, 79–90.

Cleland, V. (1976). Developing a doctoral program. *Nursing Outlook*, 24, 631–635.

Committee of the Six National Nursing Organizations on Unification of Accrediting Services. (1949). *Manual of accrediting educational programs in nursing*. National Nursing Accrediting Service.

Committee on the Grading of Nursing Schools. (1931). *Results of the first grading study of nursing schools*.

Davis, A. T. (1991, April). America's first school of nursing: The New England hospital for women and children. *Journal of Nursing Education, 30,* 158–161.

Dodd, D. (2001). Nurses' residences: Using the built environment as evidence. *Nursing History Review, 9,* 185–206. https://doi.org/10.1891/1062-8061.9.1.185

Donaldson, S., & Crowley, D. (1978). The discipline of nursing. *Nursing Outlook, 26,* 113–120.

Downs, F. S. (1978). Doctoral education in nursing: Future directions. *Nursing Outlook, 26,* 56–61.

Downs, F. S. (1984). Caveat emptor. *Nursing Research, 33,* 59.

Downs, F. S. (1988). Doctoral education: Our claim to the future. *Nursing Outlook, 36,* 18–20.

Eisenmann, L. (2000). Reconsidering a classic: Assessing the history of women's higher education a dozen years after Barbara Solomon. In R. Lowe (Ed.), *History of education: Major themes* (Vol. 1, pp. 411–442). Routledge & Falmer.

Elder, R. G., & Bullough, B. (1990). Nurse practitioners and clinical nurse specialists: Are the roles merging? *Clinical Nurse Specialist, 4,* 78–84.

Faddis, M. (1973). *A school of nursing comes of age.* Howard Allen.

Fondiller, S. H. (2001). The advancement of baccalaureate and graduate nursing education: 1952–1972. *Nursing and Health Care Perspectives, 22,* 8–10.

Fredrickson, K. (1978). *The AD graduate: Excellence in practice—fantasy or reality?* National League for Nursing.

Geolot, D. H. (1987). NP education: Observations from a national perspective. *Nursing Outlook, 35,* 132–135.

Goldmark, J. (1923). *Nursing and nursing education in the United States.* Macmillan.

Gortner, S. R. (1991). Historical development of doctoral programs: Shaping our expectations. *Journal of Professional Nursing, 7,* 45–53. https://doi.org/10.1016/8755-7223(91)90074-U

Gortner, S. R., & Nahm, H. (1977). An overview of nursing research in the United States. *Nursing Research, 26,* 10–33. https://doi.org/10.1097/00006199-197701000-00005

Grace, H. (1978). The development of doctoral education in nursing: An historical perspective. *Journal of Nursing Education, 17,* 17–27.

Graham, P. A. (1978). Expansion and exclusion: A history of women in higher education. *Signs, 3,* 759–773. https://doi.org/10.1086/493536

Gunter, L. M. (1966). Some problems in nursing care and services. In B. Bullough & V. Bullough (Eds.), *Issues in nursing* (pp. 152–156). Springer.

Haase, P. T. (1990). *The origins and rise of associate degree nursing education.* Duke University.

Hanson, K. S. (1991). An analysis of the historical context of liberal education in nursing education from 1924 to 1939. *Journal of Professional Nursing, 7,* 341–350. https://doi.org/10.1016/8755-7223(91)90011-9

Harms, M. T. (1954). *Professional education in university schools of nursing* [Unpublished dissertation]. Stanford University, Stanford, CA.

Hine, D. C. (1989). *Black women in white: Racial conflict and cooperation in the nursing profession, 1890–1950.* Indiana University.

Hinshaw, A. S., & Lucas, M. D. (1993). Postdoctoral education—A new tradition for nursing research. *Journal of Professional Nursing, 9,* 309. https://doi.org/10.1016/8755-7223(93)90002-T

Howard University, College of Nursing and Allied Health Sciences. (n.d.). https://cnahs.howard.edu/departments/nursing.

Institute of Medicine. (2010). *The future of nursing: Leading change, advancing health.* https://www.ncbi.nlm.nih.gov/books/NBK209880/

Institute of Medicine Committee on Quality of Health Care in America. (2000). *To err is human: Building a safer health system.* National Academies Press.

Institute of Medicine Committee on Quality of Health Care in America. (2001). *A new health system for the 21st century.* National Academies Press.

Institute of Medicine (US) Committee on Quality of Health Care in America. (2004). *America's uninsured crisis: Consequences for health and health care.* National Academies Press.

James, J. W. (2002). Isabel Hampton and the professionalization of nursing in the 1890s. In E. D. Baer, P. O. D'Antonio, S. Rinker, & J. E. Lynaugh (Eds.), *Enduring issues in American nursing* (pp. 42–84). Springer.

Kalisch, P. A., & Kalisch, B. J. (1978). *The advance of American nursing*. Little, Brown.

Kalisch, P. A., & Kalisch, B. J. (2004). *American nursing: A history* (4th ed.). Lippincott Williams & Wilkins.

Katefian, S. (1991). Doctoral preparation for faculty roles: Expectations and realities. *Journal of Professional Nursing, 7,* 105–111. https://doi.org/10.1016/8755-7223(91)90094-2

Keating, S. B. (2015). Looking back to the future: Current issues facing nursing education from the reflections of a member of the silent generation. *Nursing Forum, 15,* 153–163. https://doi.org/10.1111/nuf.12133

Keller, M. L., & Ward, S. E. (1993). Funding and socialization in the doctoral program at the University of Wisconsin-Madison. *Journal of Professional Nursing, 9,* 262–266. https://doi.org/10.1016/8755-7223(93)90051-D

Kelly, L. Y., & Joel, L. A. (1996). *The nursing experience: Trends, challenges, and transitions* (3rd ed.). McGraw-Hill.

Kenny, P. E. (2008, June). Men in nursing: A history of caring and contribution to the profession. *Pennsylvania Nurse, 63* (Pt. 1), 3–5.

LaRocco, S. (2011, February). The last of its kind: The all-male Alexian Brothers hospital school of nursing. *American Journal of Nursing, 111,* 62–63.

Leininger, M. (1976). Doctoral programs for nurses: Trends, questions, and projected plans. *Nursing Research, 25,* 201–210. https://doi.org/10.1097/00006199-197605000-00013

Loomis, M. (1984). Emerging content in nursing: An analysis of dissertation abstracts and titles: 1976–1982. *Nursing Research, 33,* 113–199. https://doi.org/10.1097/00006199-198503000-00014

Lynaugh, J. E. (2002). Nursing's history: Looking backward and seeing forward. In E. D. Baer, P. O. D'Antonio, S. Rinker, & J. E. Lynaugh (Eds.), *Enduring issues in American nursing* (pp. 10–24). Springer.

Lynaugh, J. E., & Brush, B. L. (1996). *American nursing: From hospitals to health systems*. Blackwell.

Matarazzo, J., & Abdellah, F. (1971). Doctoral education for nurses in the United States. *Nursing Research, 20,* 404–414.

McElmurray, B. J., Kreuger, J. C., & Parsons, L. C. (1982). Resources for graduate education: A report of a survey of forty states in the Midwest, West and southern regions. *Nursing Research, 31,* 1–10. https://doi.org/10.1097/00006199-198201000-00002

McEwen, M., & Bechtel, G. A. (2000). Characteristics of nursing doctoral programs in the United States. *Journal of Professional Nursing, 16,* 282–292. https://doi.org/10.1053/jpnu.2000.9458

McEwen, M., Pullis, B. R., White, M. J., & Krawtz (2013). Eighty percent by 2020: The present and future of RN-BSN education. *Journal of Nursing Education, 52,* 549–557. https://doi.org/10.3928/01484834-20130913-01

Meleis, A. I. (1992). On the way to scholarship: From masters to doctorate. *Journal of Professional Nursing, 8,* 328–334. https://doi.org/10.1016/8755-7223(92)90095-G

Murphy, J. F. (1981). Doctoral education in, of, and for nursing: An historical analysis. *Nursing Outlook, 29,* 645–649.

National Commission for the Study of Nursing and Nursing Education. (1970). *An abstract for action*. McGraw-Hill.

National Commission for the Study of Nursing and Nursing Education. (1971). *Nurse clinician and physician's assistant: The relationship between two emerging practitioner concepts.*

National League of Nursing Education. (1917). *Standard curriculum for schools of nursing.* Waverly.

National League of Nursing Education. (1927). *A curriculum for schools of nursing.*

National League of Nursing Education. (1937). *A curriculum guide for schools of nursing.*

National Nursing Accrediting Service Postgraduate Board of Review. (1951). Some problems identified. *American Journal of Nursing, 51,* 337–338. https://doi.org/10.2307/3459422

Nightingale, F. (1860). *Notes on nursing: What it is and what it is not*. D. Appleton & Co. http://www.digital.library.upenn.edu/women/nightingale/nursing/nursing.html

Obituary. (1940). Mrs. Clara S. Weeks Shaw. *American Journal of Nursing, 40*, 356.

Orsolini-Hain, L., & Waters, V. (2009). Education evolution: A historical perspective of associate degree nursing. *Journal of Nursing Education, 48*, 266–271. https://doi.org/10.3928/01484834-20090416-05

Parietti, E. S. (1979). *Development of doctoral education for nurses: An historical survey*. University Microfilms International.

Petry, L. (1949). We hail an important first. *American Journal of Nursing, 49*, 630–633. https://www.jstor.org/stable/i304264

Pollitt, P., Streeter, C., & Walsh, C. (2011, Fall). A nurse's journey: Viola Garcia, RN: Lieutenant, nurse. *Minority Nurse*, 23–27. http://www.minoritynurse.com/article/nurses-journey#sthash.cTtXookM.dpuf

Reid, K. B. (2011). The clinical nurse leader: Point of care safety clinical. *Online Journal of Issues in Nursing, 16*(3), 1–12. https://doi.org/10.3912/OJIN.Vol16No03Man04

Reitt, B. B. (1987). *The first 25 years of the southern council on collegiate education for nursing*. Southern Council on Collegiate Education for Nursing.

Reverby, S. M. (1984). "Neither for the drawing room nor for the kitchen": Private duty nursing in Boston, 1873–1914. In J. W. Leavitt (Ed.), *Women and health in America* (pp. 454–466). University of Wisconsin.

Reverby, S. M. (1987). *Ordered to care: The dilemma of American nursing, 1850–1945*. Cambridge University.

Rines, A. (1977). Associate degree education: History, development, and rationale. *Nursing Outlook, 25*, 496–501.

Robb, I. H. (1907). *Educational standards for nurses*. Koeckert.

Roberts, M. M. (1954). *American nursing: History and interpretation*. Macmillan.

Robert Wood Johnson Foundation. (2015). *In historic shift, more nurses graduate with bachelor's degrees*. https://www.rwjf.org/en/library/articles-and-news/2015/09/more-nurses-with-bachelors-degrees.html

Robinson, T. M., & Perry, P. M. (2001). *Cadet nurse stories: The call for and response of women during World War II*. Center Press.

Rush, S. L. (1992). Nursing education in the United States, 1898–1910: A time of auspicious beginnings. *Journal of Nursing Education, 31*, 409–414. https://doi.org/10.3928/0148-4834-19921101-08

Scott, J. (1972). Federal support for nursing education, 1964–1972. *American Journal of Nursing, 72*, 1855–1860. https://doi.org/10.2307/3422325

Sheahan, D. A. (1980). *The social origins of American nursing and its movement into the university: A microscopic approach*. University Microfilms.

Solomon, B. (1985). *In the company of educated women*. Yale University.

Styles, M. M. (1989). *On specialization in nursing: Toward a new empowerment*. American Nurses Foundation.

Tanner, C. A., Gubrud-Howe, P., & Shores, L. (2008). The Oregon consortium for nursing education: A response to the nursing shortage. *Policy, Politics & Nursing Practice, 9*, 203–209. https://doi.org/10.1177/1527154408323043

Trossman, S. (2009). APRN regulatory model continues to advance. *The American Nurse, 41*(6), 12–13. http://ojin.nursingworld.org/MainMenuCategories/ANAMarketplace/ANAPeriodicals/TAN/2009-TAN/TAN-NovDec09.pdf

U.S. Census Bureau. (n.d.). *American fact finder*. https://factfinder.census.gov/faces/tableservices/jsf/pages/productview.xhtml?pid=ACS_15_5YR_CP05&prodType=table

Vuic, K. D. (2006). "Officer. Nurse. Woman." Army nurse corps recruitment for the Vietnam War. *Nursing History Review, 14*, 111–159. https://doi.org/10.1891/1062-8061.14.111

Wall, B. M. (2009, May/June). Religion and gender in a men's hospital and school of nursing, 1866–1969. *Nursing Research*, *58*, 158–165. https://doi.org/10.1097/NNR.0b013e3181a308fe

Walters, S. E., & Davis, C. (2014). Promoting diversity in nursing. *Nursing Made Incredibly Easy*, *12*(6), 10–14. https://doi.org/10.1097/01.NME.0000454753.66874.32

Washington, L. C. (2012). Preserving the history of Black nurses. *Minority Nurse*, 28–31. https://minoritynurse.com/preserving-the-history-of-black-nurses/

Weeks-Shaw, C. (1902). *A text-book of nursing: For the use of training schools, families, and private students* (3rd ed.). D. Appleton.

Western Interstate Commission for Higher Education. (1956). *Toward shared planning in western nursing education.*

Western Interstate Commission on Higher Education. (1967). *Defining clinical content: Graduate programs* (pp. 1–4).

Wolf, G. A. (1990). Clinical nurse specialists: The second generation. *Journal of Nursing Administration*, *20*, 7–8. https://doi.org/10.1097/00005110-199005000-00003

CHAPTER 2

Curriculum Development and Approval Processes in Changing Educational Environments

Stephanie Stimac DeBoor

CHAPTER OBJECTIVES

Upon completion of Chapter 2, the reader will be able to:

- Analyze facilitators for and barriers to effective curriculum development and redesign.
- Apply knowledge of potential barriers to curricular innovations in obtaining approvals for innovative curricular redesign.
- Participate in faculty development activities to increase knowledge and skills in curriculum development and evaluation.
- Analyze the role and responsibilities of faculty in curriculum development and evaluation.

OVERVIEW

Regarding curriculum, one must consider the important role faculty plays in relation to development, ongoing evaluation, and redesign. The determination of which best practices must be implemented in nursing education dictates the mastery of student's knowledge and skills necessary for them to become proficient nurses. The ever-changing and complex healthcare systems clearly identify the need for collaboration with other disciplines within the college or university. Often requirements of regulatory and accreditation agencies can present a challenging process with curriculum development and redesign. During the COVID-19 pandemic, technology expanded in both academic and healthcare settings and changed the landscape of nursing education and faculty practices. Faculty must consider the innate complexity of nursing education, navigating multilevel internal curriculum approval processes, and adherence to the requirements of regulatory and accrediting agencies that may impact the overall plan when developing or redesigning nursing curricula. This chapter provides an overview of the preparation and support necessary for curriculum development/change, innovations in curriculum development, and approvals and accreditations that inform the nursing curriculum. It discusses the essential role of faculty in nursing curriculum development and evaluation.

THE PROCESS OF CURRICULUM DEVELOPMENT

Determining the Need for Curriculum Development or Change

New faculty or community stakeholders who have a vested interest in the school of nursing and its outcomes might hold beliefs that the curriculum is outdated and no longer adequate to prepare students to meet their professional roles in the current healthcare environment. Nursing programs develop their own standard procedures of evaluation for curriculum. This can include a review of individual courses on a yearly basis or a complete program evaluation every 3 to 5 years. These along with changes to regulatory and accreditation standards may lead to the evaluation and assessment of the goals, mission, philosophy, framework, and student-learning outcomes of the curriculum, as well as course content and learning activities that identify areas of needed curricular revision or new program development.

Preparation and Support for Curricular Change

Nursing education evolved from the use of a variety of theories from other disciplines as well as middle-range theories developed specifically for their application to nursing practice. Roles in nursing continually develop to meet the needs of healthcare in order to better serve individuals, families, and the communities where they live (American Association of Colleges of Nursing [AACN], n.d.; National Academy of Medicine, 2020; Quality and Safety Education for Nurses [QSEN], 2020). Nursing faculty must be active in the scholarship of teaching by evaluating the curriculum and programs in their institutions to ensure quality education (Oermann, 2014). The need for change in nursing education requires a multifaceted approach that includes, but is not limited to, an emphasis on evidence-based practice, quality improvement, safety standards, leadership, competency frameworks, healthcare technology, and interprofessional education (Altmiller & Hopkins-Pepe, 2019; Dickow, 2021; Kirby & Good, 2020; Lopez & Cleary, 2019; Miles & Scott, 2019; Smart et al., 2020; Timm & Schnepper, 2021).

Faculty, administration, and stakeholder support is imperative for curriculum change success. According to Billings and Halstead (2020), curriculum change is inevitable as new evidence, ideas, and healthcare policies emerge. As we have experienced most recently, situations may arise as a result of a global pandemic, changes in community needs, policy, or accreditation changes, programmatic funding and resources, personnel changes, or simply that the existing curriculum is no longer effective. Faculty must realize they have a role and responsibility to create an environment that supports a dynamic process of continual quality improvement in order for effective change to take place.

In addition to recognizing and embracing the need for curriculum change, faculty members need the knowledge and skills to engage in this endeavor. Faculty should be encouraged to participate in program curriculum committee(s). The engagement of faculty in ongoing curriculum development and assessment should begin with an orientation to the university or college. Faculty must participate in regular program evaluation in order to evaluate if program objectives, outcomes, and the vision and mission are being accomplished. For each quarter, term, and semester that a course is taught, it is customary for faculty to update courses with the latest evidence-based practice and pertinent information. Updating individual courses over time, however, may impact the overall curriculum, resulting in content gaps. Thus, it is important that programs develop an overall content map to be a guide for ongoing updates and evaluation of curriculum to avoid educational gaps.

Faculty members benefit from serving on their school's curriculum committee and engaging in ongoing, open dialogue about the continuous process of curriculum evaluation. Novice faculty or faculty who have not engaged in curriculum redesign benefit from mentoring by faculty with more experience in the curriculum processes (Gentry & Vowell Johnson, 2019; Rogers et al., 2020; Webber et al., 2020). Support is necessary to implement proposed changes and include administrative assurance of needed resources: physical space, administrative assistant support, workload considerations, expert consultants, and internal administrative assurance and encouragement that the work toward curricular change is valued and needed by the organization and, most important, for successful student outcomes. Successful curriculum change requires support from all levels of the organization, faculty, and students. If not already involved, student representatives should be included as members of the curriculum committee. Students bring a unique perspective to curriculum discussions, particularly when faculty members are charged to design a rigorous program while creating an environment conducive to a variety of student-learning preferences. Students at all levels of a program are constructive facilitators for the successful implementation of a new curriculum.

An individual faculty member or a group of faculty can put forward the need for curriculum assessment, development, and reform. Work begins at the level of the school curriculum committee. This may be a formal committee within the school or for smaller schools; it may consist of the entire nursing faculty. In most institutions of higher education, curriculum development and redesign must go through an extensive, multilevel approval process. Despite the number of levels in the approval process, a proposal for curriculum approval should be completed with the expectation that it will eventually be sent to the highest review body in the parent institution. Although this process varies at each institution, Figure 2.1 depicts an example for sequencing. Consideration should be given as to whether or not this is a proposal for undergraduate- or graduate-level curricular change as they may have different processes. When submitting a proposal for curricular change, completeness, accuracy, and acceptable institutional formatting are extremely important to successfully navigate all levels of the curriculum approval.

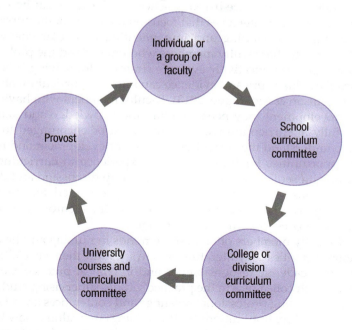

Figure 2.1 Example of curriculum approval process sequencing.

ISSUES RELATED TO CURRICULAR DEVELOPMENT OR REDESIGN

Faculty Development

It is the responsibility of the administrators and faculty in the school of nursing to build in faculty development activities to ensure the integrity of the curriculum and the quality of instruction in its implementation. These activities ultimately lead to the realization of the program goals and student-learning outcomes that ensure a quality nursing program. Curriculum development is in itself a faculty development activity (Elliott, 2015). With the current ongoing nursing faculty shortage (AACN, 2020a), schools of nursing continue to recruit new faculty from healthcare institutions and recent graduates of master's or doctoral programs. Although these new faculty may have been expert clinicians in their field, they are once again novices who will need time and mentorship to develop their new skill set as an educator. They may lack experience in academe and have no experience in curriculum evaluation or design. An orientation program for developing these clinicians is essential for their successful transition.

Orientation to the curriculum is one of the first steps for faculty development. It should not be assumed that all faculty members are familiar with the entire curriculum or underpinnings of the mission and vision, accreditation, and regulatory requirements. Other topics for faculty development related to curricular activities include the provision of knowledge on faculty governance, the processes of curriculum development and program evaluation, application of learning theories, instructional design and strategies including technology, and student assessment methods. To meet the role expectations of service and scholarship, workshops can be offered to review service opportunities within the institution and in the community for writing grants, supporting research, and preparing manuscripts for publications. Ideas that apply specifically to research related to curriculum development, program evaluation, and evidence-based practice in education can be shared in faculty meetings, workshops, and conferences that focus on the needs of the curriculum.

To be successful in developing and implementing curricular change, Billings and Halstead (2020) indicate that faculty members who understand the problems inherent in the current curriculum can effectively evaluate strategies for solving concerns within the curriculum. Scholarly literature and evidence can inform a curriculum about the scholarship of teaching (Faison & Montague, 2013). Faculty members who have less experience in curriculum development may need to attain the knowledge and skills necessary to engage successfully in curriculum work. They should be encouraged to attend curriculum meetings to understand the current processes for development and revision. Faculty development opportunities for those with less experience in curriculum development include working with senior faculty, engaging in group discussion and debate, knowing that their contributions to the process will be heard and valued, and providing ongoing administrative support. These activities are all part of the mentoring of less experienced faculty to learn the process for curriculum change.

Experienced faculty members often observe trends in nursing and healthcare through their professional activities and literature reviews within their specialties, professional organizations, and academic responsibilities and in clinical practice. Continued clinical practice, working with colleagues in the practice setting, supervising students or conducting research, and attending professional meetings and conferences are all stimuli for identifying changes and future implications for the nursing curriculum. New faculty members are usually immersed in assuming the new role of educator and, thus, may not have the time or experience to observe these implications for curriculum development and evaluation. At the same time, experienced faculty can take the opportunity to mentor new faculty and demonstrate the importance of assessing trends and changes in the healthcare system or education that influence the curriculum. As mentioned previously, the role of mentor to new faculty is a responsibility of practiced faculty and can be an expected formal assignment as part of an orientation plan or, informally, as part of the expectations for faculty.

Budgetary Constraints

Nursing has always been considered one of the costlier programs in institutions of higher education due to the lower faculty-to-student ratio. The COVID-19 pandemic has had a significant impact on all aspects of higher education, including nursing. Retirements of older faculty and the shortage of nurse educators stretch human, fiscal, and physical resources in nursing education. While the relentless echo of the growing need for more nurses at all levels of education continues, funding for many nursing programs has been significantly impacted. When developing or redesigning nursing curricula, an assessment of current and future resources is crucial. Budgetary constraints on hiring faculty and other resources, such as the availability and use of high-fidelity simulation, have a major impact on the curriculum design change and/or implementation of the curriculum. In 2019, more than 80,407 qualified applicants were turned away from U.S. nursing schools due to insufficient numbers of faculty, clinical sites, classroom space, clinical preceptors, and budget constraints (AACN, 2020b). At an unprecedented time in healthcare and current budgetary constraints, it is more important than ever that we maintain local, state, and regional partnerships with nurse employers, healthcare organizations, foundations, and other stakeholders as a sustainability strategy.

Amount of Curricular Content

Essential knowledge acquisition relevant to nursing is another issue impacting curriculum development and change in the management of the curricular content. The nursing literature provides an overwhelming amount of evidence indicating that faculty and students are besieged with enormous amounts of content (AACN, 2019; Massey et al., 2020; Tan et al., 2018). As the information explosion in health sciences education continues to flourish, an increasing amount of content is deemed essential to include in all nursing curricula (Accreditation Commission for Education in Nursing [ACEN], 2020a; AACN, 2021a, 2021b; Bove, 2020; National Council of State Boards of Nursing [NCSBN], 2016). One example of essential knowledge content in nursing curricula relates to the need to continuously improve the overall quality and safety of healthcare delivery in all areas of specialty areas. As nursing practice embraced the focus on improved quality and safety, it became clear that graduating nurses were missing critical competencies. The result was a major national initiative, the QSEN, which centered on patient safety and quality topics, with a primary goal to address the challenge of preparing future nurses with the knowledge, skills, and attitudes necessary to continuously improve the quality and safety of the healthcare systems in areas where they practice (AACN, 2021c; Levett-Jones et al., 2020; National League for Nursing [NLN], 2017). As the amount of essential knowledge and content increases, there tends to be an inherent faculty perception that they must teach everything to their students in great detail. Consequently, "content saturation" is a major problem in many nursing curricula. Giddens (2017) surmises that faculty should learn how to teach conceptually and, subsequently, minimize the emphasis on the *amount* of content students learn. Repsha et al. (2020) suggest the introduction of concept-based learning as a way to reduce the laborious content focus on concepts and instructional designs that foster intellectual development. Concept-based learning promotes the transfer of theoretical knowledge into the clinical practice site. This allows for attention to applying conceptual understanding of the complexities of human health rather than memorizing vast amounts of content.

Technology

The advance of technology and its application to healthcare and the educational arena allowed for both faculty and students to quickly pivot from face-to-face learning to online and distance education during the COVID-19 global pandemic. For well over a year now, this teaching method quickly became the standard practice in higher education. The methods of curriculum delivery and the use of technology must be addressed in any curriculum analysis, development, or redesign, including to what extent technology will be used, resources to obtain and sustain technology, and faculty development to use technology effectively to meet programmatic outcomes. For example, the use of high-fidelity simulators increased as an adjunct and replacement when students were displaced from their clinical experiences during the pandemic. High-fidelity simulation requires a significant up-front financial investment as well as ongoing costs for routine maintenance and upgrades of simulators, and for ancillary staff for simulation suites or centers. In addition, effective use of high-fidelity simulation requires a significant investment for faculty development in the use of the equipment, as well as training on how to maximize learning outcomes and incorporate simulation experiences into the curriculum. Chapter 13 provides a more in-depth view of the use of technology in face-to-face, distance, and online learning.

Faculty Issues

The shortage of nursing educators has been discussed as an issue related to curriculum development and change, yet several other faculty issues arise that could impact curriculum development or redesign. Challenges to curriculum revision often occur when working with faculty members who are resistant to change. At this moment, we are navigating recent challenges. We have all experienced work/life changes in response to the pandemic, and many are reluctant to have one more thing changed. Yet, maybe never before has there been a better time to reevaluate the current educational content and models of teaching. When considering curriculum revision, Oermann (2019) proposed four topics for consideration. First, review the literature. Decisions regarding curriculum changes need to come from the most current evidence-based practices. Second, faculty must consider what is happening within the clinical setting. Curriculum and clinical practice must be jointly considered. Third, examine current pedagogy. In some cases, a new teaching strategy may be more effective than redesigning the actual content. Finally, empower the curriculum committee and faculty who will be most affected by the change to make the decisions. Most programs have multiple approval levels that can significantly impact the time it takes to move change forward. Empowering the faculty and curriculum committee can lessen that impact.

Fear of and resistance to change are the most influential barriers to progress in curriculum development and redesign. While not an exhaustive list by any means, the following have been identified as barriers to successful curriculum development and redesign:

- Differing faculty values about nursing education
- Fear of losing control of certain aspects of the curriculum
- Differing views about priorities in the curriculum
- A lack of embracing the need for curricular change
- Uncertainty about how to begin the change process
- A lack of resources
- Incivility
- A lack of rewards
- Feeling that the curricular change process is too overwhelming given the current resources, workload, and time constraints
- Feelings of inadequacy in the area of curriculum analysis, development, and redesign (Billings & Halstead, 2020)

The work of faculty with the curriculum must consider not only a tumultuous and complex healthcare environment but also the pressures to maintain currency in both clinical expertise and teaching technologies to optimize student learning (Hande et al., 2020). Many nursing faculty members are no longer employed in healthcare facilities, and in many instances, this creates an "education–practice gap." Although clinical supervision of students helps some faculty stay connected to current clinical practices, many nursing faculty find it challenging to balance their full-time roles as educatord with the need for ongoing clinical practice. Faculty may find it difficult to access clinical practice experiences, even on a part-time or per diem basis, to maintain current practice knowledge and skills. Complex healthcare systems and practices, cost implications, and risk management considerations further complicate faculty practice arrangements. Faculty members struggle with work–life balance as they struggle to maintain academic, personal, professional, and home life, which, consequently, inhibits their willingness to take on additional responsibilities in curriculum design (AACN, 2020c).

RESEARCH IN CURRICULUM DEVELOPMENT AND EVALUATION

Issues and Trends

Some of the major internal and external issues and trends affecting nursing education today as they apply to the nursing faculty role in curriculum development and evaluation are as follows:

- Political atmosphere
- Socioeconomic concerns
- An ongoing nursing faculty shortage
- Increasing ratios of part-time to full-time faculty
- Changing ratios of tenure, tenure-track, and nontenured faculty
- A lack of faculty members at both the master's and PhD levels with formal preparation in education
- Increasing numbers of doctorally prepared graduates, especially DNP graduates, who may not have the pedagogy required for the faculty role
- Rapid changes in instructional designs prior to and during the pandemic including online platforms, distance education, high-technology simulations, and other technological advances that are changing instructional design and the implementation of the curriculum
- Healthcare system changes that influence the preparation of nurses and, therefore, the role of faculty in keeping the curriculum relevant

Ashcraft et al. (2021) address some of these issues in their paper regarding the perceptions among tenure, tenure-track, and nontenured faculty roles in nursing. Historically, nursing education focused on the development of clinical skills in the care of patients. It then moved into the academic setting with an emphasis on the sciences, social sciences, and liberal arts integrated into the science and clinical skills of the profession. As a result, nursing found itself with many challenges surrounding the nursing faculty role. More recently, institutions that are research-focused expect tenured/tenure-track faculty to generate research, as well as to fund their teaching positions with research grants. This results in increasing numbers of clinical faculty members who are part-time and who have a minimized role in faculty governance activities and scholarship of teaching. Yet these instructors (clinical faculty) are the bedrock of the prelicensure programs in delivering practical supervision, while tenure-track or tenured faculty members deliver the didactic courses and teach in graduate-level courses, resulting in lower teaching loads to provide time for research and scholarly activities. This trend in nursing education has implications for how education will be delivered and curricula designed.

Research Implications for Evidence-Based Curriculum Development and Evaluation

Nursing faculty members have boundless opportunities for educational research as it relates to curriculum development and evaluation. There is a scarcity of recent research related to nursing education due to nursing's move to provide its own doctoral education, through either research-focused (PhD/DNSc) or practice-focused (DNP), applied science doctoral degrees. Much of nursing research focuses on practice issues and healthcare policy, which is beneficial for the profession, healthcare, and the public. However, there is a paucity of research focused on nursing education, its processes, and outcomes. In Chapter 16, Serratt further delineates research from the last 10 years pertinent to curriculum design and evaluation.

ROLES AND RESPONSIBILITIES OF FACULTY

Implementation of the Curriculum

Implementation is a critical component of curriculum development and/or redesign and is the responsibility of the faculty. To ensure that the curriculum is implemented as planned, intense oversight is necessary. Rapid changes in technology and economics, along with the ever-changing evidence-based practice and the need for multiculturalism, dictate that ongoing review and redesign of nursing curricula must occur at regular intervals. One of the greatest challenges is to resist the temptation to make changes to the new curriculum too quickly before it has been thoroughly evaluated for effectiveness.

All faculty members should be thoroughly acquainted with the total curriculum, specifically its mission, philosophy, organizational framework, student-learning outcomes, and plan of study. Full-time faculty should have a working knowledge of these components for all levels of the school of nursing programs. While teaching opportunities may focus on graduate studies or undergraduate levels, it is necessary for faculty members to know how each program informs one another and builds on the other. The new AACN (2021a) *Essentials* Domains, Components, and Competencies provide a framework of the transition between undergraduate and graduate nursing education. While it is not essential that part-time faculty members know the details of the entire curriculum, they should understand the relationship of the course(s) they teach to the curriculum, its framework, program goals, and terminal student-learning outcomes.

Schools of nursing curricula generally have an organizational framework that acts as the roadmap for all levels of degree work and demonstrates the rationale for the preparation of professional nurses at each of the various levels. Critical to the integrity of the curriculum is that faculty members are able to articulate how the courses they teach fit into the organizational and programmatic framework. Thus, the temptation to independently change course content without having a conversation with the curriculum committee beforehand is less likely to occur. A course coordinator can assume the responsibility for a new faculty member's orientation to the course and its relationship to the curriculum and to the periodic assessment of the delivery of the course content to ensure it remains relevant to the curriculum. Periodic meetings of faculty members in the courses, levels, or programs to review teaching strategies, learning activities, and student-learning outcomes are vital to the implementation of the curriculum and to overall quality control. In addition, accreditation standards may require progress reports and define how often an entire program's curricula are reviewed.

Innovations in Nursing Education

A major aspect of the nursing curriculum development and redesign process is the consideration of current and future resources and needs for implementation, including the nature of the healthcare environment in which future nurses will work. It is widely noted in the literature that due to the complexities of today's healthcare system and healthcare delivery, transforming nursing education with a health systems framework is necessary to adequately prepare nurses to practice safely (AACN, 2019; IOM, 2010; National Academy of Medicine, 2020; NLN, 2017; NCSBN, 2009b, 2021; Phillips et al., 2013). Nursing education must have innovative approaches to prepare graduates at all levels of education for the nursing practice and healthcare leadership of the future. Spector and Odom (2012) defined *innovation* as "a dynamic, systematic process that envisions new approaches to nursing education" (p. 41). Innovations reported in the nursing literature include the use of dedicated educational units for clinical education (Dominio et al., 2020); pedagogical approaches such as narrative pedagogy (Christopher et al., 2020); an amalgamation of simulation, classroom, and clinical experiences (Weston et al., 2021); and gaming (McEnroe-Petitte& Farris, 2020). Other innovations in nursing education include partnering with clinical agencies or with other educational institutions to form a consortium for sharing resources for the delivery of nursing education.

Developing innovation in nursing education is an essential strategy to meet the needs of future nurses and the demands of today's healthcare environment. However, when planning an innovative curriculum, faculty should be aware of potential deterrents that may prolong the approval and implementation process. Each university has an approval process of changes in curriculum, whether at the unit, division, or university level. These processes at times can impede curricular changes by multilevel institutional committee proceedings lengthening the time to obtain approval. As a practice profession, nursing education's relationship with healthcare institutions is critical. Clinical practice settings, community partners, and educational institutions may have different perspectives about their role regarding curriculum development; thus, examining potential barriers assists in avoiding competing agendas (Virgolesi et al., 2020). In addition, there may be real or perceived regulatory barriers to novel nursing education. Although Halstead (2020), debunks that myth by identifying how accreditation standards can actually be a benefit in the development of innovative educational change. Recent changes to the AACN Essentials support innovative teaching strategies to develop student competencies. Standard III of the NLN-Commission for Nursing Education Accreditation (2016) clearly identifies that faculty innovation enables the nursing program to achieve expected outcomes. In 2008, the NCSBN established the Innovations in Education Regulation Committee. The charge to this committee was to identify real and perceived regulatory barriers to educational innovations and to develop a regulatory model for innovative educational proposals (NCSBN, 2009a). Potential regulatory barriers included specified numbers of clinical or didactic hours in the nursing curriculum, faculty–student ratios, full- and part-time ratios of faculty, disallowance of dedicated educational units due to a lack of faculty oversight or qualifications of nursing staff, and simulation limitations, all reducing the flexibility to allow for nursing innovation (NCSBN, 2009b; Spector & Odom, 2012). However, advanced knowledge of potential barriers may assist faculty in negotiating with internal or external stakeholders to overcome these obstacles and create a curriculum that is innovative, resource-friendly, and forward thinking. Before planning curricular changes, faculty must be mindful of compliance with the U.S. Department of Education, state board of nursing practice acts, and state nursing regulations. It is always advisable to consult at the conceptual stages of planning for any innovative teaching strategy proposal to curriculum redesign or the planning of a new program.

Need for Revision or New Programs

As the curriculum is implemented, faculty members continually observe and assess the effectiveness of learning activities, methodologies, student-learning outcomes, and the relationship of courses to the curriculum. When gaps or concerns are detected, it is the faculty member's responsibility to report the observations to the course leader or level coordinator. Together, faculty should further investigate and analyze the concern and then with input from students and other stakeholders bring the matter to the curriculum committee (or academic committee that has responsibility for curricular change) for its consideration. A root-cause analysis with suggestions for remediation should accompany the report to facilitate the needs identified for curricular evaluation and possible revision. Many times, faculty, students, and stakeholders identify the need for new programs based on their experiences and interactions in the healthcare system. The processes for bringing the information to the attention of the curriculum committee are the same, that is, following a needs assessment, a summary of the identified need accompanied with documentation, and a possible proposal for the development of a new track or program.

Faculty Activities Related to Curriculum Development, Evaluation, and Accreditation

Many of the roles and responsibilities of faculty in curriculum development have been reviewed. They include, on an individual level: familiarization with the components of the curriculum, developing and carrying out instructional designs and strategies that are congruent with the curriculum, observation, assessment, and reporting of needs for either curricular revision or development of new programs, participation on curriculum/academic/evaluation/accreditation committees, and developing or participating in scholarly activities that relate to curriculum development and evaluation. As academic faculty, the group should participate in orientation of new faculty members to ensure the integrity of the curriculum; review faculty governance structures to maintain faculty ownership of the curriculum; identify trends and issues in healthcare, curriculum development, and evaluation; generate research ideas; identify program development grants; actively participate in the scholarship of teaching and learning; and build on ideas for evidence-based educational practice.

Accrediting agencies such as the ACEN (2020b) and the Commission on Collegiate Nursing Education (2017) standards/criteria include the educational preparation and qualifications for nursing faculty. As part of their role, faculty members should be familiar with these expectations and ensure that they meet the qualifications and expectations for the role of faculty. Participation in accreditation activities and program evaluation activities is expected for all faculty members. Program evaluation for the academic institution usually takes place every 5 years, while accreditation takes place from every 5 to 10 years, depending on the program's history, type of program, and level of accreditation granted. Knowing the curriculum components such as the mission, vision, philosophy, organizational framework, student-learning outcomes, and the program of study are crucial responsibilities of faculty in the evaluation and accreditation processes. They should be able to articulate where the courses in which they teach fall into the curriculum framework. The faculty should be familiar with processes of continual program analysis and identifying curriculum and individual course needs for possible revision when necessary to ensure the quality and consistency of the program.

SUMMARY

Curriculum development and ongoing evaluation and redesign are core activities for nursing faculty. Faculty participation in planning for accreditation can expand their capacity to implement curriculum evaluation and design processes that have direct relevance to program outcomes. The significance of curriculum evaluation and design extends far beyond the curriculum itself. Determining how to best facilitate the curriculum process by working together as a group to identify and overcome potential barriers and being innovative to meet the challenges of educating future generations of practicing nurses in an ever-changing health system are key elements for successful curriculum development or redesign. Ongoing challenges of the collective volume of information in nursing and health sciences, the trend toward developing interdisciplinary curricula, closing the faculty–student gap in technology knowledge, and meeting the requirements of regulatory and accrediting agencies are all important issues to address as we develop nursing curricula for the future and embrace a continuous process improvement plan for curriculum design that will ensure quality education for nurses.

END-OF-CHAPTER RESOURCES

DISCUSSION QUESTIONS

- Some programs state that the curriculum is the property of the faculty. Do you agree or disagree with that statement; why or why not?

- During the pandemic, universities across the country adapted to online learning. How did that affect current curriculum approval processes?

- Why do you think faculty members have the ultimate responsibility for curriculum development and evaluation? List at least five reasons for this responsibility.

- Describe the barriers of accreditation or regulatory agencies impose on curricular development or redesign?

- Based on a current issue in nursing education, develop a research question for investigating the issue and possible solutions. Explain why you chose the issue and what implications it has for the future of nursing education.

LEARNING ACTIVITIES

Student-Learning Activities

1. Imagine yourself in the role of a new faculty member in a school of nursing. List the topics that you believe you need to know in order to be an effective teacher. Prioritize the list and explain the rationale for the order of priority.

2. Assess how the local state board of nursing reviews new or revised curricula of nursing programs. Attend a state board of nursing meeting and describe how the process of nursing program approval relates to the board's mission of protecting the public's health and welfare in your state.

 SPRINGER PUBLISHING CONNECT™ A robust set of instructor resources designed to supplement this text is located at **http://connect.springerpub.com/content/book/978-0-8261-8686-7.** Qualifying instructors may request access by emailing **textbook@springerpub.com.**

Faculty Development Activities

1. Assess your school's orientation and faculty development programs. Identify any gaps in the programs as they relate to curriculum development and evaluation. How would you develop or change the programs to meet the needs of new and experienced faculty?

2. Describe two innovations in curriculum and/or teaching strategies for implementation of your curriculum. What constraints or barriers can you identify that would delay or prohibit you from implementing these innovations?

3. Develop a list of five key facilitators and five key barriers to curriculum development and/or redesign in your school of nursing. How can you as a faculty member assist your school or other faculty members to overcome the barriers you identified?

REFERENCES

Accreditation Commission for Education in Nursing. (2020a). *ACEN history of ensuring educational quality in nursing.* http://www.acenursing.org/acen-history

Accreditation Commission for Education in Nursing. (2020b edited). *ACEN accreditation manual 2017 standards and criteria.* https://www.acenursing.org/acen-accreditation-manual/

Altmiller, G., & Hopkins-Pepe, L. (2019). Why quality and safety education for nurses (QSEN) really matters in practice. *The Journal of Continuing Education in Nursing, 50*(5), 199–200. https://doi.org/10.3928/00220124-20190416-04

American Association of Colleges of Nursing. (2019). *Fact sheet: The impact of education on nursing practice.* https://www.aacnnursing.org/Portals/42/News/Factsheets/Education-Impact-Fact-Sheet.pdf

American Association of Colleges of Nursing. (2020a). *Nursing faculty shortage.* https://www.aacnnursing.org/Portals/42/News/Factsheets/Faculty-Shortage-Factsheet.pdf

American Association of Colleges of Nursing. (2020b). *Fact sheet: Nursing shortage.* https://www.aacnnursing.org/Portals/42/News/Factsheets/Nursing-Shortage-Factsheet.pdf

American Association of Colleges of Nursing. (2020c). *Nursing faculty shortage. Factors to address the faculty shortage.* https://www.aacnnursing.org/news-information/fact-sheets/nursing-faculty-shortage

American Association of Colleges of Nursing. (2021a). *The essentials: Core competencies for professional nursing education.* https://www.aacnnursing.org/Portals/42/AcademicNursing/pdf/Essentials-2021.pdf

American Association of Colleges of Nursing. (2021b). *Understanding the re-envisioned essentials: A roadmap for the transformation of education.* https://www.aacnnursing.org/Portals/42/AcademicNursing/pdf/Roadmap-to-New-Essentials.pdf

American Association of Colleges of Nursing. (2021c). *AACN's vision for academic nursing.* https://www.aacnnursing.org/News-Information/Position-Statements-White-Papers/Vision-for-Nursing-Education

American Association of Colleges of Nursing. (n.d.). *Clinical nurse leader tool kit.* https://www.aacnnursing.org/Portals/42/AcademicNursing/Tool%20Kits/CNL-Tool-Kit/CNLToolKit.pdf

Ashcraft, A., Andersen, J. S., Rogge, M. M., Song, H., & Opton, L. (2021). Academic tenure: Perceptual variation among tenured, tenure-seeking and non-tenured faculty. *Journal of Professional Nursing, 17,* 578–587. https://doi.org/10.1016/j.profnurs.2021.03.002

Billings, D. M., & Halstead, J. A. (2020). *Teaching in nursing* (6th ed.). Elsevier Saunders.

Bove, L. A. (2020). Integration of informatics content in baccalaureate and graduate nursing education. An updated status report. *Nurse Educator, 45*(4), 206–209. https://doi.org/10.1097/NNE.0000000000000734

Christopher, R., de Tantillo, L., & Watson, J. (2020). Academic caring pedagogy, presence, and *Communitas* in nursing education during the COVID-19 pandemic. *Nursing Outlook, 68*(6), 822–829. https://doi.org/10.1016/j.outlook.2020.08.006

Commission on Collegiate Nursing Education. (2017). *Achieving excellence in accreditation: The first 10 years of CCNE.*

Dickow, M. (2021). Leadership qualities for nursing education. *Teaching and Learning in Nursing, 16*(2), 191. https://doi.org/10.1016/j.teln.2020.12.005

Dominio, K., Louie, K., Banks, J., & Mahon, E. (2020). Exploring the impact of a dedicated educational unit on new graduate nurses' transition to practice. *Journal for Nurses in Professional Development, 36*(3), 121–128. https://doi.org/10.1097/NND.0000000000000622

Elliott, R. (2015). Faculty development curriculum: What informs it? *Journal of Faculty Development, 28*(3), 35–45.

Faison, K., & Montague, F. (2013). Paradigm shift: Curriculum change. *Association of Black Nursing Faculty Journal, 24*(1), 21–22. https://search.ebscohost.com/login.aspx?direct=true&db=mfi&AN=85894972&site=eds-live

Giddens, J. (2017). *Concepts for nursing practice.* Elsevier.

Gentry, J., & Vowell Johnson, K. (2019). Importance of and satisfaction with characteristics of mentoring among nursing faculty. *Journal of Nursing Education, 58*(10), 595–598. https://doi-org.unr.idm.oclc.org/10.3928/01484834-20190923-07

Halstead, J. A. (2020). Fostering innovation in nursing education: The role of accreditation. *Teaching and Learning in Nursing, 15*(1), A4–A5. https://doi.org/10.1016/j.teln.2019.10.003

Hande, K., Jessee, M. A., Christenbery, T., Zsamboky, M., & Kennedy, B. (2020). Optimizing the student learning environment: A framework to select faculty for teaching courses. *Journal of Professional Nursing, 36*(5), 404–411. https://doi.org/10.1016/j.profnurs.2020.03.002

Institute of Medicine. (2010). *The future of nursing: Leading change, advancing health.* https://www.ncbi.nlm.nih.gov/books/NBK209880/

Kirby, K. F., & Good, B. (2020). From education to practice: Incorporating quality improvement projects into baccalaureate nursing curriculum. *AORN Journal, 111*(5), 527–535. https://doi-org.unr.idm.oclc.org/10.1002/aorn.13015

Levett-Jones, T., Andersen, P., Bogossian, F., Cooper, S., Guinea, S., Hopmans, R., McKenna, L., Pich, J., Reid-Searl, K., & Seaton, P. (2020). A cross-sectional survey of nursing students' patient safety knowledge. *Nurse Education Today, 88,* 1–6. https://doi.org/10.1016/j.nedt.2020.104372

Lopez, V., & Cleary, M. (2019). Integrating evidence-based practice into nursing curriculum. *Issues in Mental Health Nursing, 40*(4), 365–368. https://doi.org/10.1080/01612840.2019.1565880

Massey, D., Craswell, A., Ray-Barruel, G., Ullman, A., Marsh, A., Wallis, M., & Cooke, M. (2020). Undergraduate nursing students' perceptions of the current content and pedagogical approaches used in PIVC education. A qualitative, descriptive study. *Nurse Education Today, 94,* 1–6. https://doi.org/10.1016/j.nedt.2020.104577

McEnroe-Petitte, D., & Farris, C. (2020). Using gaming as an active teaching strategy in nursing education. *Teaching and Learning in Nursing, 15*(1), 61–65. https://doi.org/10.1016/j.teln.2019.09.002

Miles, J. M., & Scott, E. S. (2019). A new leadership development model for nursing education. *Journal of Professional Nursing, 35*(1), 5–11. https://doi.org/10.1016/j.profnurs.2018.09.009

National Academy of Medicine. (2020). *The future of nursing 2020–2030: Charting a path to achieve health equity.* https://nam.edu/publications/the-future-of-nursing-2020-2030/

National Council of State Boards of Nursing. (2009a). *Innovations in education regulation committee: Recommendations for boards of nursing for fostering innovations in education.* https://www.ncsbn.org/Recommendations_for_BONS.pdf

National Council of State Boards of Nursing. (2009b). *Tips for planning nursing education innovative approaches.* https://www.ncsbn.org/Tips_for_Faculty.pdf

National Council of State Boards of Nursing. (2016). *FY 2015–16 nursing education trends committee.* https://www.ncsbn.org/2016_Nursing_Ed_Trends_Comm_Report.pdf

National Council of State Boards of Nursing. (2021). *Innovations in nursing education.* https://www.ncsbn.org/669.htm

National League for Nursing. (2017). *Advocacy teaching: Nursing is social justice advocacy.* http://www.nln.org/professional-development-programs/teaching-resources/toolkits/advocacy-teaching

National League for Nursing, Commission for Nursing Education Accreditation. (2016). *Accreditation standards for nursing education programs.* http://www.nln.org/docs/default-source/accreditation-services/cnea-standards-final-february-201613f2bf5c78366c709642ff00005f0421.pdf?sfvrsn=12&_ga=2.207835675.809511687.1619978878-261853293.1584815032

Oermann, M. (2014). Defining and assessing the scholarship of teaching in nursing. *Journal of Professional Nursing*, *30*(5), 370–375. https://doi.org/10.1016/j.profnurs.2014.03.001

Oermann, M. (2019). Curriculum revisions. Making informed decisions. *Nurse Educator*, *44*(1), 1. https://doi.org/10.1097/NNE.0000000000000630

Phillips, J. M., Resnick, J., Boni, M. S., Bradely, P., Grady, J. L., Ruland, J. P., & Stuever, N. L. (2013). Voices of innovation: Building a model for curriculum transformation. *International Journal of Nursing Education Scholarship*, *10*(1), 1–7. https://doi.org/10.1515/ijnes-2012-0008

Quality and Safety Education for Nurses. (2020). *QSEN competencies.* http://qsen.org/competencies/pre-licensure-ksas

Repsha, C. L., Quinn, B. I., & Peters, A. B. (2020). Implementing a concept-based nursing curriculum: A review of the literature. *Teaching and Learning in Nursing*, *15*, 66–71. https://doi.org/10.1016/j.teln.2019.09.006

Rogers, J., Ludwig-Beymer, P., & Baker, M. (2020). Nurse faculty orientation: An integrative review. *Nurse Educator*, *45*(6), 343–346. https://doi.org/10.1097/NNE.0000000000000802

Smart, D., Ross, K., Carollo, S., & Williams-Gillbert, W. (2020). Contextualizing instructional technology in the demands of nursing education. *Computers, Informatics, Nursing*, *38*(1), 18–27. https://doi.org/10.1097/CIN.0000000000000565

Spector, N., & Odom, S. (2012). *The initiative to advance innovations in nursing education: Three years later.* https://www.ncsbn.org/InitiavetoAdvanceInnovations.pdf

Tan, K., Chong, M. C., Subramaniam, P., & Wong, L. P. (2018). The effectiveness of outcome-based education on the competencies of nursing students: A systematic review. *Nurse Educator Today*, *64*, 180–189. https://doi.org/10.1016/j.nedt.2017.12.030

Timm, J. R., & Schnepper, L. L. (2021). A mixed-methods evaluation of an interprofessional clinical education model serving students, faculty, and the community. *Journal of Interprofessional Care*, *35*(1), 92–100. https://doi.org/10.1080/13561820.2019.1710117

Virgolesi, M., Marchetti, A., Pucciarelli, G., Biagioli, V., Pulimeno, A. M. L., Piredda, M., & Grazia De Marinis, M. (2020). Stakeholders' perspective about their engagement in developing a competency-based nursing baccalaureate curriculum: A qualitative study. *Journal of Professional Nursing*, *36*(3), 141–146. https://doi.org/10.1016/j.profnurs.2019.09.003

Webber, E., Vaughn-Deneen, T., & Anthony, M. (2020). Three-generation academic mentoring teams: A new approach to mentoring faculty in nursing. *Nurse Educator*, *45*(4), 210–213. https://doi.org/10.1097/NNE.0000000000000777

Weston, J., Kimble, L., Kaplan, B., & Dyer, A. (2021). An innovative educational approach integrating simulation, classroom and clinical practice for teaching pediatric nursing. *Nurse Educator*, *46*(2), 71–72. https://doi.org/10.1097/NNE.0000000000000865

SECTION II

NEEDS ASSESSMENT AND FINANCIAL SUPPORT FOR CURRICULUM DEVELOPMENT

Stephanie Stimac DeBoor

OVERVIEW

When contemplating a new educational program or revising an existing curriculum, a needs assessment is indicated. There are two purposes for conducting an assessment. The first is to validate the currency, the academic and professional relevance, and the continued need for an existing program. The second is to establish the feasibility for a new nursing program including the demand for it, available resources, academic soundness, and financial liability.

Even though justifying revising a current program usually exists, it is wise to survey stakeholders and collect information relative to the same factors that are examined in a needs assessment for a new program. This information either reaffirms assumptions about the curriculum on the part of program planners or identifies gaps or problems that indicate a need for change. The assessment is also useful for accreditation and program review purposes and can serve as the organizing framework for a master plan of evaluation (see Section IV). Chapter 3 discusses the essential components of a needs assessment and offers a model for collecting and analyzing information that is preliminary to new program development, expansion, or revision of an existing curriculum. Chapter 4 reviews the need for financial support and the budgetary planning and management necessary for curriculum development and evaluation.

THE FRAME FACTORS MODEL

Johnson (1977) presented a conceptual model for curriculum development, instructional planning, and evaluation that is similar to the nursing process. Although it is a simple and linear model (P [planning]—I [implementation]—E [evaluation]), Johnson expanded it into a complex step-by-step logical process. The process includes examining the frame factors or context within which the program exists, setting goals, identifying curriculum content, structuring the curriculum, planning for instruction, and finally, evaluation. Johnson speaks of frame factors as the context in which the curriculum exists. Furthermore, he classifies the context into natural, cultural, organizational, and personal elements (Johnson, 1977, p. 36). Keating (2006) chose the term *frame factors*, external and internal, from Johnson's discussion and adapted it to curriculum development in nursing education. It includes the elements that Johnson identified and adds other components that specifically apply to nursing education, healthcare systems, and the profession.

Frame factors for this text are defined as the external and internal factors that influence, impinge on, and/or enhance educational programs and curricula. As a conceptual model, it collects, organizes, and analyzes information that is useful for the development and evaluation of curricula. There are two major categories of frame factors: external and internal factors. *External frame factors are those that influence curriculum development from the larger environment and outside the parent institution. Internal frame factors are those factors that influence curriculum development and are within the environment of the parent institution and the program itself.* Figure II.1 illustrates the frame factors conceptual model.

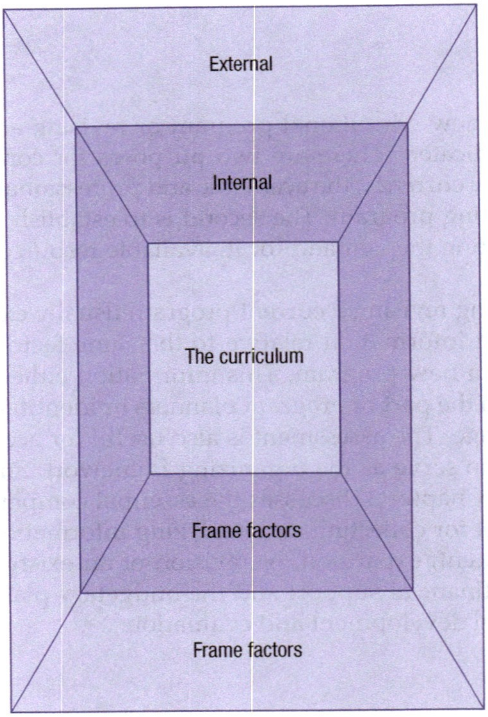

Figure II.1 Frame factors conceptual model.

Source: Adapted from Johnson, M. (1977). *Intentionality in education.* Center for Curriculum Research and Services.

To begin, one should conduct a needs assessment with faculty involvement. The principal role of the needs assessment focuses on the necessity or desire for curriculum improvement based on an assessment of its implementation and program outcomes. Faculty members cognizant of the factors that impact and influence the program have an advantage in promoting the program by an awareness of the program's financial security, its position within the healthcare system and the profession, and its role in meeting healthcare needs. In addition, data from the needs assessment are useful to individual faculty seeking grants and other funding to support research and program development activities.

It is recommended that nursing educators use the frame factors model when evaluating programs, considering revisions of existing programs, or initiating new ones. While administrators take the leadership role in conducting needs assessments, faculty should participate in the decisions for what type of and how much data to collect and for proposed changes that could affect the curriculum.

EXTERNAL AND INTERNAL FRAME FACTORS

Chapter 3 describes the factors that influence the curriculum from the environment external to the parent institution and the nursing education program. The factors include the community, population demographics, competition for clinical placements, the political climate, the healthcare system, the characteristics of the academic setting, the need for the (nursing) program, the nursing profession, regulation and accreditation requirements, and external financial support. All of these factors influence the curriculum in positive and negative ways, and although they may not be in the control of the faculty, they are important to recognize and analyze for their impact on the program. They can "make or break" a program. For example, a lack of accreditation for a nursing program can prohibit its graduates from career opportunities and continuing education.

The environmental factors within the parent institution and the nursing program that influence the curriculum are termed the "internal frame" factors. They include a description of the organizational structure of the parent academic institution; mission, philosophy, and goals; economic situation and its influence on the curriculum; resources within the institution (laboratories, classrooms, library, student services, etc.); and existing and potential faculty and student characteristics. Similar to the external frame factors, the internal factors influence the curriculum and play a major role in the development, revision, and expansion of programs. Faculty use the information gleaned from the assessment to arrive at decisions regarding the curriculum. The same data collected for a needs assessment are, in fact, related to total quality management of the curriculum and contribute to the evaluation of the program. A case study that utilizes the external and internal frame factors needs assessment model and results in the development of a new program that is provided in the Appendix.

RELATIONSHIP OF NEEDS ASSESSMENT TO CONTINUOUS QUALITY IMPROVEMENT OF THE CURRICULUM

Establishing a new program is not an exercise that occurs in a vacuum. Information from outside and within the institution can indicate a possible need for a new program or revision or expansion of its existing offerings. There are usually trigger mechanisms that initiate the need for change such as a drop in NCLEX® scores or national certification pass rates, budget cuts, community and state needs, or a nursing shortage. Rather than responding to these external stimuli in a reactive way, faculty and nursing educators should have a master plan of evaluation in place that continuously monitors the program and provides the data needed for planning for changes that are both timely and look to the future. Such activities are part of a process that provides the data for analysis and decisions leading to continuous improvement and the quality of the educational program. The factors discussed in the frame factors model in this section of the text apply to evaluation strategies as well. While Section IV discusses program and curriculum evaluation, accreditation, and strategic planning, it is useful to incorporate the notion of evaluation as a process when conducting a needs assessment, not only in terms of the present plans for program start-up and changes but also for planning for the future.

FINANCIAL SUPPORT AND BUDGET MANAGEMENT FOR CURRICULUM DEVELOPMENT AND EVALUATION

An awareness of the financial support and budgeting issues for curriculum development and evaluation is essential for nursing education administrators, managers, and faculty to ensure the success and continuation of the program. Chapter 4 provides practical guidelines for budget support, seeking funds to develop new programs through grants, endowments, and scholarships as well as managing the budget. It discusses the various roles of faculty, administrators, and staff in securing funds and planning and managing budgets for curriculum development and evaluation activities.

REFERENCES

Johnson, M. (1977). *Intentionality in education.* Center for Curriculum Research and Services.

Keating, S. B. (2006). *Curriculum development and evaluation in nursing.* Springer Publishing Company.

CHAPTER 3

Needs Assessment: The External and Internal Frame Factors

Stephanie Stimac DeBoor

CHAPTER OBJECTIVES

Upon completion of Chapter 3, the reader will be able to:

- Appreciate the value of a needs assessment for analysis of factors that influence a nursing education program and its implications for curriculum revision or development.

- Identify major external and internal frame factors for a needs assessment.

- Apply the guidelines for assessing frame factors to a simulated or actual curriculum development situation.

OVERVIEW

Curriculum development activities in the academic setting usually relate to the revision of the educational program based on feedback from various stakeholders that include, but are not limited to, staff, clients, students, faculty, administrators, alumni, and consumers of the program's participants and graduates. Whether curriculum development involves a new program or revisions of an existing curriculum, program planners and faculty must evaluate the external and internal environmental influences that affect the curriculum, their impact on the current program, and what role they play in forecasting the future.

A needs assessment for curriculum development is defined as the process for collecting and analyzing information that contributes to the decision to initiate a new program or revise an existing one (Keating, 2006, 2018). Using the frame factors conceptual model as described in the overview of Section II, collected information is organized into two major categories: external and internal frame factors (Johnson, 1977). Keating (2006) defined external and internal factors as follows: *External frame factors* are defined as those factors that influence curriculum in the environment outside of the nursing program and the parent institution. *Internal frame factors* influence curriculum from within the parent institution and the program itself. Figure 3.1 depicts the external frame factors that surround the curriculum when conducting a needs assessment, and Figure 3.2 illustrates internal frame factors.

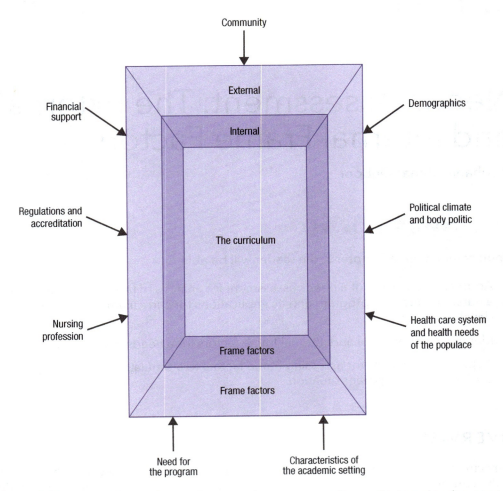

Figure 3.1 External frame factors for a needs assessment for curriculum development in nursing.

Source: Adapted from Johnson, M. (1977). *Intentionality in education* (distributed by the Center for Curriculum Research and Services, Albany, NY). Walter Snyder Printer; Keating, S. B. (2006, 2018). *Curriculum development and evaluation in nursing.* Springer Publishing Company.

EXTERNAL FRAME FACTORS

Description of the Community

The first step in developing or revising a curriculum is to provide a description of the community or context in which the program exists (or will exist). A needs assessment ensures the relevance of the program to the community and predicts its eventual financial viability. Owing to the vast differences in communities served by academic institutions and for the purposes of this discussion, *community* is defined as an entity within a larger network or system. One can view it as a microsystem within a macrosystem and how each is influential to the other. Depending on the nature of the educational program, the community can be global or as narrow as a small town within a state. Most institutions of higher education in the United States identify themselves according to classifications found in the Carnegie Foundation for Advancement of Teaching Classification. The Carnegie classification was first published in 1970 with the most recent classification

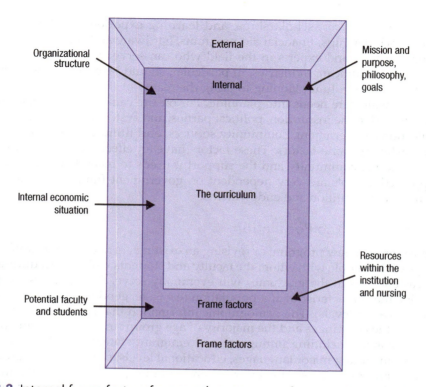

Figure 3.2 Internal frame factors for a needs assessment for curriculum development.

Source: Adapted from Johnson, M. (1977). *Intentionality in education* (distributed by the Center for Curriculum Research and Services, Albany, NY). Walter Snyder Printer; Keating, S. B. (2006, 2018). *Curriculum development and evaluation in nursing.* Springer Publishing Company.

occurring in 2018 and the next set for 2021 (Indiana University Center for Postsecondary Research, 2020). The 2018 designations are according to Basic, Undergraduate, and Graduate Instructional Program, Enrollment Profile and Undergraduate Profile, and Size and Setting. A listing with a detailed description of each type of classification and revisions through May 24, 2019, is available online at carnegieclassifications.iu.edu/downloads/CCIHE2018-FactsFigures.pdf.

Large universities or colleges with research notoriety often attract international scholars to campus or to an online program, while some state-supported and private programs attract students who live nearby and intend to spend their professional lives in their home community. The COVID-19 pandemic clearly identified the need for web-based programs and adaptation to remote learning opportunities. MOOCs (massive open online courses) are making a revival; campuses have become worldwide and attract students from many different countries and cultures who may never set foot on the physical campus. For some web-based programs that offer degree programs, there may be no physical campus, only a location at which the administration functions, with student services, library resources, classroom participation, and so forth available online. In those instances, a definition of the served community is according to its functional structure as a community, for example, a group of international nurses wishing to advance their education and practice in their home countries who enroll in an online degree program.

Both web-based and on-site campuses should survey major industries and educational systems in their communities (or networks, in the case of international and internet programs) as possible sources for students into the program and for potential partnerships such as online resources, scholarships, and learning experiences. The industry has resources for scholarships, financial aid programs, hardware and software resources for web-based learning, and experts in the field who can serve as consultants, faculty, or adjunct faculty. Healthcare industries, in particular, should be participants in the needs assessment and curriculum planning to bring the reality of the practice setting and the community's healthcare needs into planning. For on-site campuses, the major religious affiliations linked to the institution, political parties, and systems such as transportation, communications, government, community services, and utilities in the community are additional external frame factors. These factors have an effect on the curriculum as to its relevance to the community and the support it needs to meet its goal. For example, state-supported schools are very dependent on government funding, whereas private schools must rely on tuition and endowments.

Demographics of the Population

When considering a new program, or revising an existing curriculum, it is useful to have knowledge of the people with whom the faculty and students will interact during clinical experiences and whom the graduates will eventually serve. *Demographics* are the data that describe the characteristics of a population (e.g., age, gender, socioeconomic status, ethnicity, education levels). The demographic information that is vital to program planners includes the age ranges and the majority of age groups in the population, predicted population changes including immigrant and emigrant statistics, and ethnic and cultural groups, including major languages, educational levels, socioeconomic groups, and health issues and disparities. This information identifies potential students, their characteristics, and the needs of the population that the students and graduates will serve. This information will vary if being assessed for a face-to-face program or one taught completely online.

The needs of the learner guide educational programs and curricula. Conducting an analysis of the characteristics of the students for special learning needs if the student body comes from the region surrounding the institution is an important step of the process. For example, if there are nurses seeking to advance their careers, the curriculum needs to focus on adult learning theories and modalities. Younger students about to embark on their first professional degree will need curricula that focus on their developmental needs as young adults as well as the content necessary for gaining basic nursing knowledge, clinical skills, and socialization into the professional role. Meeting the learning needs of different generations of learners is a major challenge for curriculum planning. Chapter 6 addresses this issue with several ideas on learning approaches and strategies for reaching various types of learners while implementing the curriculum.

Surveying students who are coming to the institution from great distances or internationally as to why they selected the program provides useful information for program planning and recruitment. Faculty should identify potential students with needs for learning resources beyond the usual, for example, a need for tutoring for students whose primary language is not English or translators for internationally broadcast programs. It is useful to learn about the financial requirements of the program and resources available for the potential student body, such as if there is a need for major financial aid programs. Ethnicity and cultural values in the community and its beliefs about higher education have an impact on recruitment strategies and are especially important in light of the need for increasing the diversity of the nursing workforce and the educational level of nurses worldwide. Another demographic consideration is the existence of potential faculty and the identification of people who have the credentials to teach. Identifying potential faculty through partnerships with industry and the community is helpful if the program needs to recruit new faculty or seek adjunct faculty and preceptors for clinical experiences.

Political Climate and Body Politic

When assessing the community, part of the data describes the public governing structure. Governing bodies may vary between urban, suburban, and rural locations. For example, if it is urban, it is useful to know if there is a mayor, a chief executive, and a city governing board. Likewise, if it is rural or suburban, vital information includes the type of county or subdivision government, who the chief executive is, if the officials are elected or appointed, and what is the major political party. If the program educates an international clientele, the types and structures of the government involved and the place of nursing and education in governmental regulations are vital sources of information.

Equally, if not more, important is information about the "body politic." A simple definition for *body politic* is the people power behind the official government within a community (Keating, 2018). It is composed of the major political forces and the people who exert influence within the community, a group that shares a unified purpose. The assessors should identify the major players, their visibility, that is, the informal and formal powers behind the scenes. There should be consideration given to the relationships between those in political positions and those leaders of the academic institution. Additional information is how those in power influence decisions in the community and how they exert their power by using financial, personal, political, appointed, or elected positions. Specific information useful to educators is how key politicians view the college or university and during elections or other crucial times, if they recognize the power of its people (i.e., students, faculty, staff).

Relative to nursing, the politicians' and the body politics' specific interests in the profession are helpful. For example, if they have family members who are nurses or they have been recipients of nursing care, they are more apt to support nursing education programs. All educational programs need the support of the community and its power structure. Therefore, the information from the assessment of the political climate is vital to planning for the future and seeking assistance when the call comes for additional resources or for political pressure and support to maintain, revise, or increase the program.

The Healthcare System and Health Needs of the Populace

Educating nurses to care for the healthcare needs of the populace is of critical interest to the healthcare system and the consumers of care. It is obvious that information about these two factors is essential to program planning and curriculum development. To assess the international, national, or regional healthcare systems, it is necessary to identify the major healthcare providers, types of organizations, and financial bases for the delivery of healthcare. In the United States with the ongoing and further potential revisions of the Affordable Care Act (ACA), it is unwise to discuss at length the U.S. healthcare delivery system. Assessors should check governmental and healthcare systems' websites for the current and projected future of the system. An overview of the ACA is available at www.hhs.gov/healthcare/rights/index.html through the U.S. Department of Health and Human Services.

A list of major U.S. healthcare organizations and their websites is provided for the readers' convenience in searching for the latest information regarding healthcare services.

The following list provides resources that can provide information on the healthcare system or systems for the locality, region, or nation that the educational program serves:

- Major governmental healthcare systems such as Medicare, Medicaid, TRICARE (formerly, Civilian Health and Medical Program of the Uniformed Services [CHAMPUS]), Indian Health Service, Veterans Affairs (VA), and so forth
- Nonprofit or for-profit healthcare systems and agencies and eligibility for services
- Sectarian and nonsectarian health-related agencies and eligibility for services
- City, county, regional, state, and national public health services
- Services for the underserved or unserved population groups
- Major primary healthcare systems and agencies and providers
- Voluntary healthcare agencies and their services
- Other community-based health-related services staffed by nurses, for example, schools, industry, state institutions, and forensic facilities

The assembled list provides an overview of the healthcare system within which the program is located. It describes the healthcare resources that are available or not available to the population including the nursing school and institution's populations. It identifies the gaps of services in the community and the possibilities for community partnerships, including school-based services for the underserved and unserved populations. It recognizes trends in healthcare services and anticipated changes for the future that can influence curriculum development.

It is useful to know if resources within the system such as healthcare libraries are available to students and faculty during clinical experiences or as resources for students enrolled in distance education programs. A review of the list pinpoints existing clinical experience sites and the potential for new ones. Personnel in the agencies with qualifications as preceptors, mentors, and adjunct faculty are additional resources for possible collaboration opportunities. Scholarship and research opportunities for students and faculty may emerge from the review and can influence curriculum development as well as foster faculty and student development.

An overview of the major health problems in the region contributes to curriculum development as exemplars for healthcare interventions. The National Center for Health Statistics website (www.cdc.gov/nchs) provides general information on leading causes of death and morbidity. Vital statistics, health statistics, and objectives for *Healthy People 2030* are located at the following website (health.gov/healthypeople). For international facts on health in specific countries, the World Health Organization (WHO) website (www.who.int/en) is a good resource. It provides information about the various member countries' health systems and major health problems.

Characteristics of the Academic Setting

Other institutions of higher learning in the nearby community, region, or online competitors have an influence on the program and its curriculum. Identifying other institutions, their levels of higher education (technical schools, associate degree, baccalaureate, and higher degree), financial base (private or public), and affiliations (sectarian or nonsectarian) gives the assessors an idea of the existing competition and the need for programs to continue their graduates' education. Information about other institutions' intentions for the future enables developers to understand the gaps in the types of programs and the nature of the competition from other programs. For example, if the institution's curriculum offers a nurse practitioner program and two other programs in the region offer similar programs, perhaps the curriculum should be revised (e.g., as a specialty primary or acute care program), discontinued, or possibly a joint venture with the other schools sharing resources. A private institution dependent on tuition and endowments may question whether it should continue to offer a curriculum that is redundant with a state-supported school. Other data to consider are the need for nurses or saturation of specialties in the area and its surroundings that the institution serves, and even though there are multiple programs, the success rates of graduates finding employment in the region.

A suggested resource for collecting data on other academic institutions internationally and in the United States is the Council for Higher Education Accreditation (CHEA) website (www.chea.org). National databases may be found at the National Center for Education Statistics website (www.nces.ed.gov). Another source for identifying other nursing programs in the region is the list of approved programs provided by the state board of nursing. The National Council of State Boards of Nursing website (NCSBN; www.ncsbn.org/index.htm) provides a listing of the state boards and their websites, along with contact information. Finally, the U.S. Department of Education website (https://www2.ed.gov/rschstat/landing.jhtml?src=ft) provides data and statistics regarding colleges and universities.

The Need for the Program

An examination of the external environment informs the faculty about the increased or continued need for nurses. The following data points act as guides to document the need for the program:

- Characteristics of the nursing workforce and the extent of a nursing shortage, if it exists, or saturation of specialties within the area
- Predictions for future nursing workforce needs
- Adequate numbers of eligible applicants to the program, currently and in the future
- Specific areas of nursing practice experiencing a shortage
- Employers' projections for the numbers of nurses needed in the future
- Employers' views on the types of graduates needed

A brief survey of healthcare administrators can provide this information, although it is sometimes difficult to expect a good response rate owing to the current pressures on administrators or current healthcare issues, such as the pandemic. In addition, not all employers of graduates understand all roles of nursing, especially advanced practice primary and acute care differences. Another strategy is to conduct focus groups that take no more than 15 minutes in the health agencies. Instructors who use the facilities for students or clinical coordinators are excellent people for collecting the information. There are several resources to identify the national and regional need for nurses. They are the state nurses' associations that can be located through the American Nurses Association (ANA; www.nursingworld.org/membership/find-my-state/). For international information, the WHO website provides information on workforce issues worldwide as well as qualifications for nurses and nursing educators.

As described previously in the characteristics of the academic setting, knowledge of other nursing programs in the region and online is useful to avoid curriculum redundancies. The data on the need for the program demonstrate how many of its graduates are currently needed and in the future, the level of education necessary to provide the level of care required, and short- and long-term healthcare system needs. A current nursing workforce demand indicates the possibility for accelerated programs. Shortages in specialties indicate advanced practice curricula and increased opportunities for RNs to continue their education.

The Nursing Profession

In addition to the need for nurses, it is important to learn about the nursing profession in the region or nation. Professional organizations are rich resources for identifying leaders, mentors, and financial support such as scholarship aid. Curriculum developers should survey faculty and colleagues for a list of the nursing professions in the region. Such organizations include local or regional affiliates of the ANA; the National League for Nursing (NLN); Sigma Theta Tau International; educator organizations such as the American Association of Colleges of Nursing (AACN), the Association for Nursing Professional Development (ANDP), and the Organization of Associate Degree Nursing (OADN); and the plethora of specialty organizations. Questions to gather information about the profession include Who are the nurses in the area? Are there professional organizations with which the program can link? What is the level of education for the majority of the nurses in practice? Are there nurses prepared with advanced degrees who could serve as educators or preceptors? and Are scholarship and research activities in nursing and healthcare underway that present opportunities for students and faculty?

Regulations and Accreditation Requirements

Whether the program is new or under revision, an important step of the process is a review of state and national regulations regarding schools of nursing requirements and any recent or anticipated changes that affect the curriculum. Information on regulations is available through the state boards of nursing. For a listing of specific state boards of nursing, consult the NCSBN® website (www.ncsbn.org).

For programs offering online or distance education, it is important to review the information from the National Council for State Authorization Reciprocity Agreements (NC-SARA). In 2013, the U.S. Department of Education established SARA to help streamline regulations for programs offering distance education. States obtain approval for activities, such as practical experiences, online education, faculty who teach from states outside of the home institution state, marketing, and advertising, that are regulated. Currently 49 states, the District of Columbia, Puerto Rico, and the United States. The Virgin Islands are SARA members. The NC-SARA website (nc-sara.org/) provides additional information.

National accreditation is not required of schools of nursing; however, it provides the standards for nursing curricula and demonstrates program quality. Sophisticated applicants to the school will look for accreditation. Alumni find it advantageous to graduate from an accredited institution when applying for positions in the job market, for future advanced education, and positions in the military. Many scholarships and financial aid programs require that students enroll in accredited institutions. Nursing has two major accrediting agencies and a few specialty-accrediting bodies. The Accrediting Commission for Education in Nursing (ACEN) accredits clinical doctorate, master's/postmaster's certificate, baccalaureate, associate, diploma, and practical nursing programs. The website (www.acenursing.org/) provides detailed information on standards and the accrediting process. The ACEN website (www.acenursing.org/resources-for-international-programs/) lists the standards for international programs.

The Commission on Collegiate Nursing Education, an autonomous accrediting agency, accredits baccalaureate, graduate, and residency nursing programs. Its website (www.aacnnursing.org/CCNE) offers information regarding standards, procedures, and guidelines for accreditation.

As of this writing, the National League for Nursing Commission for Nursing Education Accreditation (NLN CNEA) is in the application process of seeing recognition from the U.S. Department of Education as a programmatic accreditor. Its website (cnea. nln.org/) provides updates to the application process.

In addition to accreditation, there are standards and competencies set by professional organizations that serve as guidelines or organizational frameworks for curricula. Several examples for prelicensure and graduate-level programs are those developed by the AACN (2021) in their newly revised and released *Essentials: Core Competencies for Professional Nursing Education* for baccalaureate and higher degree programs. The National Organization of Nurse Practitioner Faculties provides information regarding nurse practitioner competencies and the National Task Force on Quality Nurse Practitioner Education for primary and acute care nurse practitioner scope of practice.

Another external frame factor that influences the nursing curriculum in the United States is regional accreditation. The parent institution of a nursing program undergoes periodic review by its regional accrediting body. Members of the nursing faculty are involved in the regional accreditation process and should be mindful of the standards set by that organization as well as those set by the professional accrediting body. The CHEA identifies seven regional accrediting organizations. The CHEA website (www.chea.org/ regional-accrediting-organizations) provides information about the regional accrediting agencies. It is important to remember that some universities require that students who are seeking graduate education have received their degrees from a regionally accredited institution to qualify for acceptance. Section IV of this text offers a detailed description of accreditation processes and standards for educational programs.

Financial Support Systems

An analysis of the finances of the program provides those developing or revising curriculum with vital information on the economic health of the program. Indicators of financial health influence how the curriculum will be delivered. Faculty should recognize signs that demonstrate the program's financial viability. If new sources of income for the program are indicated, possible resources need to be identified. The proposed revisions in the curriculum must be realistic in terms of cost. If it is a new program, adequate resources including start-up funds for its implementation must be available. If it is an existing program, faculty and administration should consider whether to continue it at its present level of financial support or increase or decrease support. For example, if the program intends to double enrollment by adding task trainers and high-fidelity simulation to support a lack of clinical space, one must consider the return on investment. Does the additional tuition support the purchase of the equipment? A disruption of financial solvency occurred in many institutions following the pandemic, requiring close monitoring of spending for new programs.

Analyzing external frame factors in light of proposed new programs or curriculum revisions helps faculty and administrators determine the type of new program needed or, in the case of an existing program, the extent change is required in the curriculum. A review of the external frame factors provides a check with reality, including the community in which the program is located, the industry for which the program prepares graduates, and the economic viability of the program. Other items of study include how the program is financed and the major sources of revenues such as fees, tuition, state support, private contributions, grants, scholarships, or endowments. Knowing if there are adequate resources to support the program to be self-sufficient is a critical element in the analysis of the financial viability. Although this type of information is within the responsibility of the administration, those participating in the development of the curriculum must have a basic understanding of the financial support systems. Chapter 4 discusses the role of faculty and curriculum planners in procuring funds for supporting curriculum development and evaluation and an overview of budgetary planning and management.

INTERNAL FRAME FACTORS

Internal frame factors include a description of the organizational structure of the parent academic institution; its mission and purpose, philosophy, and goals; the internal economic situation and its influence on the curriculum; resources within the institution (e.g., laboratories, classrooms, library, academic services, instructional technology support, student services); and existing and potential faculty and student characteristics. An analysis of the information related to these factors offers the relevance of the program and allows the findings to show their importance of the quality of the program, its existence, and possible changes.

Description and Organizational Structure of the Parent Academic Institution

Investigating the environment of the parent institution housing the nursing education program provides the scenario it sets for the program. The physical campus and its buildings create the milieu in which the program exists, with the nursing program a reflection of its place within the institution or in the case of a web-based program, its network connectivity features. The nature of the institution influences the structure of the campus and, for nursing education programs, can be located in healthcare agencies, academic medical centers, liberal arts colleges, large research universities, land-grant universities, multipurpose state-supported or private universities, community colleges, or an independent internet entity. In small private institutions, the school of nursing can be one of the largest and most influential constituents, while in statewide university systems, nursing can be a small department within a health-related college that is within the greater university. The history of the institution is important to know such as its growth or change over the years and the role the nursing program had in its political fortunes or misfortunes.

Educational institutions and healthcare agencies usually have organizational structures of a hierarchal nature. Faculty should analyze the structure of the parent institution as well as that of the nursing program to describe the hierarchal and formal lines of communication that guide the faculty in developing and revising programs. For example, as described in Chapter 2, the approval of curriculum proposals and changes happen at the local level (the nursing curriculum committee and faculty) first, followed by the next level of the college curriculum committee and dean, and, finally, to an all-college or university-wide curriculum committee with its recommendations going to the faculty senate or the provost for final approval. There can be administrative approval along the way from department heads, deans, and perhaps academic vice presidents or provosts, especially regarding economic and administrative feasibility. Nevertheless, the major approval bodies are those that are composed of faculty and within faculty governance privileges.

At the same time, it is useful to include the major players within the faculty and administrative structures in order to discuss with them the plans and rationale for proposed new programs or curriculum revisions. Prior consultation with these key people can help smooth the way when the proposals are ready to enter the formal arena, and they can give advice related to changes that might enhance approval or advice on the best presentation formats that facilitate an understanding of the proposal. These contacts can be of a formal or informal nature; however, a word of caution, to avoid disastrous results: Never blindside an administrator or decision-maker. It is wise to keep them informed of new proposals or possible changes to place them in the advocate role as the approval process wends its way through the system.

Mission, Philosophy, and Goals of the Parent Institution

The mission/vision and purpose, philosophy, and goals of the parent institution determine the character of the nursing program. Most institutions of higher education focus their missions and philosophies on three actions: education, service, and scholarship/research. Nursing must examine the mission and philosophy of its parent institution to determine its place within these three basic activities. For example, a state-supported university may have as part of its mission and philosophy the education of the people of the state for professional, leadership, and service roles. Thus, the nursing program could focus its mission and philosophy on the preparation of nurses for leadership roles and the provision of healthcare services to the people of the state. If the statewide system is the predominant preparer of nurses within the state as compared to independent colleges, then the additional mission or purpose might be to provide an adequate nursing workforce for the state.

In contrast, independent or private colleges and universities may have missions and philosophies that have a sectarian flavor, such as preparing individuals with strong liberal arts foundations for public service or roles in the helping professions. Academic medical centers are yet another example of nursing's match to health disciplines housed in one institution whose mission is to prepare individuals for the health professions. In addition, community or junior college missions usually focus on technical education or on prerequisite preparation for entering into upper division–level colleges and universities.

Internal Economic Situation and Influence on the Curriculum

As stated previously, the economic health of the institution has a significant impact on the nursing program and curriculum. How much of the share of resources, income, and expenditures that the nursing program has can affect program stability and room for expansion. For example, nurse-managed clinics must be self-supporting or economic recessions can cause their demise. For state-sponsored programs, the parent institution is subject to the state economy during periods of recession and prosperity. Independent colleges, unless heavily endowed, depend on tuition, student fees, or other income-generating operations. Some parent institutions allow programs to charge a higher tuition rate for both in and out-of-state students to cover the additional costs of developing and maintaining web-based programs.

All institutions depend on endowments and financial aid programs for students including scholarships, loans, and grants. Nursing programs are eligible for many federal grants and have a history of securing other types of grants from private foundations, state-supported programs, and private contributions including those from alumni associations. These income-generating programs illustrate to the parent institution that the nursing program is viable, and at the same time, the institution's reputation and ability to garner external financial resources help the nursing program secure funding.

Institutions usually have support systems for assisting faculty to write grants and to seek outside financial support. Nursing programs should have close relationships with these support systems and have a plan in place for securing additional funds. Faculty plays a major role in writing grants with the benefits related to funding, including release time for program development and scholarship and research activities. Two sources for U.S. funding to support program development on the national level are the Health Resources and Services Administration (hrsa.gov) and the National Institute of Nursing Research (www.ninr.nih.gov). The latter focuses on clinical research; however, it is possible that faculty may wish to conduct curriculum and educational program research. ProposalCentral (proposalcentral.com/default.asp) provides a listing of other resources, grant, and scholarship opportunities.

Assessment of the economic status of the parent institution and the nursing program provides a realistic picture of the potential for program expansion and curriculum revision. When developing a curriculum, the first demand for financial support comes with the need for resources to conduct a needs assessment, such as the costs of released time for those who are conducting the assessment, reviewing the literature, and surveying key stakeholders. A cost analysis for revising a curriculum or mounting a new one requires a business case to justify the costs and to forecast its financial viability. Unless there is a nursing program financial officer, the nursing program administrator and faculty should work closely with the parent institution's business office or chief financial officer in developing the business case.

Resources Within the Institution and Nursing Program

An analysis of the existing resources within the institution and the nursing program supplies information related to possible program expansion and curriculum revisions. First, there should be adequate classrooms, learning laboratories, library staff and resources, computer facilities, clinical practice simulations, instructional technology support, and distance education resources for the current program. When planning for revisions of the curriculum or for new programs, the need for expanding these facilities and additional staffing should be identified. If expansion is not possible, then creative approaches to scheduling for maximizing the use of these facilities, for example, for evening classes, weekend learning experiences, and online delivery of courses, can be examined.

Academic support services such as the library, academic advisement, teaching–learning resources, and instructional technology contribute to the maintenance of a quality education program and are internal frame factors that should be assessed when developing new programs or revising existing ones. If there are to be new programs or expansion of current curricula, the library resources must be adequate. Library resources include not only those resources on campus but also services for off-campus programs and students. There should be internet and web-based library access for students and faculty, and this is especially true when the campus has a large commuter student population, distance education programs, or proposes new programs. Library and instructional technology support staffing must be large enough and knowledgeable about nursing education needs. Thus, faculty should have strong relationships with librarians and the instructional technology staff in order to build the resources needed to revise the curriculum or develop new programs.

Academic advisement services play an important role in program planning as new programs can require additional staffing. If the curriculum is revised, updates for academic advising are necessary so that the faculty and its support staff that provide the services have current information to impart to the students. Teaching–learning resources need to be available to keep faculty current in instructional strategies, particularly if the revisions to the curriculum have an effect on instructional design. For example, a baccalaureate program may decide to convert its RN program to a web-based delivery system. In this case, faculty often needs and should training in preparing and implementing web-based courses. The need to convert coursework into online learning during the pandemic gives us insight into identifying the strengths and weaknesses of current faculty in providing this mode of teaching and learning. We must examine if this is to become the norm and what training, along with review and revision of the curriculum, is now required.

Instructional support systems are part of planning as well since the nature of the proposed program or the revised curriculum may call for additional resources. These resources include programmed instructional units, audiovisual aids, hardware and software, computer technologies, high- and low-fidelity mannequins for simulated clinical situations, and so forth. They can generate large costs to the program and should be calculated into the business case and the costs associated with their maintenance and replacement expenses over time. Some instructional support systems include monthly or annual student fees as well. For new programs or revisions, these costs are often included in requests for additional student lab fees or external funding. If the updating or creation of new laboratory/simulation practice labs involves onetime-only costs, external funding through donations, grants, or endowments is possible.

Student support services are equally important to nursing education programs and are an integral part of the curriculum development process. Major student services include enrollment (recruitment, admissions, registrar activities, graduation records), maintaining student records, advising and counseling, disciplinary matters, remediation and study skills, work–study programs, career counseling, job placement, and financial aid. Depending on the size of the university or college, these services can be congregated into one department or subdivided into several. Their role in curriculum development is important, as expanding or changing educational programs require student services support. For example, if a new program is proposed, then the recruitment and admissions staff will need to be apprised of the program to best serve the needs of the new program in recruitment and admission activities.

Financial aid programs are crucial to the recruitment, admission, and retention of students. and if the proposal brings in new revenues through grants or other financial support structures, the financial aid staff must be cognizant of the proposal. They can provide useful information to program planners and thus, a partnership between the student services staff and the nursing program staff is beneficial.

Work–study programs and job placement information can supplement the curriculum if these programs are in concert with the educational plan and not in conflict with the program of study. An example of a conflict is a revised curriculum that calls for accelerated study and clinical experiences that disallow student employment and therefore prohibits enrollment in the work–study program. Another aspect is the potential influence of students' part-time employment on the curriculum and its role in intended and unintended outcomes on the educational experience. With the preponderance of adult learners in nursing programs, the reality of their outside employment while enrolled in studies must be taken into account.

The informal curriculum often takes place through the planned activities of the student services department. Again, partnerships between student services and nursing faculty increase the effectiveness of the formal curriculum. Students who could benefit from remediation or learning skills workshops should be referred to student services. Faculty members work with student services staff to identify the learning needs of nursing students and this is especially relevant when curriculum changes are taking place. Additionally, student services staff work with faculty concerning the special needs of students with learning disabilities and the accommodations they require without imperiling the student's individual needs or the safety of the clients for whom the students provide care.

Existing and Potential Faculty and Student Characteristics

When proposing new educational programs or revising existing curricula, thoughts need to go into the characteristics of the existing faculty and the student body who will participate in the educational program. If a new program is proposed, the faculty composition is reviewed. There should be adequate numbers of faculty members to represent diversity in gender and ethnic backgrounds and to reach the desired faculty-to-student ratio. Depending on the nature of the program, clinical supervision of students requires a low student-to-faculty ratio but can differ according to program. For example, master's and doctoral students are usually RNs and, therefore, may not need the close supervision required for entry-level students. Although, for some advanced practice roles, there is a need for close faculty supervision. However, in these latter cases, preceptorships or internships are the usual format, and a faculty member can supervise more students in collaboration with the clinical preceptors. In entry-level programs, the student to faculty ratio is usually 8 or 10 to 1; however, in the senior year, it is possible to have preceptorships or precepted clinical with approximately 12 to 15 students, depending on the nature of the clinical experiences and the availability of qualified/experienced preceptors. In some states, the state board of nursing regulates undergraduate student-to-faculty ratios, whereas accrediting bodies may make recommendations. While lectures can accommodate many students, seminars and learning laboratories demand fewer numbers of students and therefore additional faculty. Enrollment in online courses can vary, with as few as 10 to 12 at the graduate level and seminar-type courses to didactic online courses that accommodate as many as 30 or more students. In the case of the latter, the format for the course is modified to adjust to the larger number of students and the resultant teaching load for the instructor.

Yet another consideration related to faculty is the match of knowledge to the subject matter, clinical expertise, and pedagogic skills. Information on the numbers and types of faculty members needed, their required educational levels, and scholarship and research history feed into decisions about curriculum development. For international, web-based programs, potential faculty from the participating countries must be surveyed and identified, as well as the challenge for translation from English (if U.S.-based) into the predominant language spoken. As with faculty considerations, the characteristics of the student body and the types of students the faculty hopes to attract to the new program or the revised curriculum are important. If it is a new program, the potential applicant pool should be identified according to interest, numbers, availability, and competition with other nursing programs. If a new program is contemplated, its type dictates the kind of applicant pool that the program and the admissions department need to target.

The characteristics of the students in the program help tailor the curriculum according to their learning needs. For example, if it is an entry-level associate degree or baccalaureate program, the applicants may be a mix of new high school graduates, transfer students with some college preparation, and adult learners with some work experience. The curriculum is then planned to meet a diversity of learning needs from traditional pedagogic learning theories to adult learning theories. Diversity of racial, ethnic, and cultural characteristics is the other factor to consider and the educational program must plan to be culturally responsive to students as well as prepare professionals with cultural competence.

SUMMARY

While the external frame factors examine the macroenvironment surrounding the program, the internal frame factors look at factors that are closer to the program and include the parent institution as well as the nursing program itself. Factors to examine include the characteristics of the parent institution and its organizational structure. How the nursing program fits into this structure can determine the economic, political, and resource support for program changes. It sets the stage for the processes that the nursing faculty must undergo to gain approval for the proposed changes. The mission and purpose, philosophy, and goals of the parent institution influence the nature of the nursing program, and to ensure success, the nursing program must be congruent with those of the parent institution. The internal economic status and the available resources of both the parent institution and the nursing program are assessed for the financial viability as well as the necessary additional resources and support services for proposed revisions or new programs. Finally, the characteristics of the faculty and the potential student body are reviewed to determine their match to the proposed change.

This chapter introduced the steps for conducting a needs assessment in curriculum development and revision. Prior to revising or developing new curricula, an assessment of the factors that influence the educational program is necessary. Tables 3.1 and 3.2 serve

TABLE 3.1: Guidelines for Assessing External Frame Factors

Frame Factor	Questions for Data Collection	Desired Outcomes
Description of the Community	Is the community setting conducive to academic programs? Describe its major characteristics, i.e., distance education and/or on-site, totally or partially web-based, international, national, urban, suburban, or rural.	The institution's campus is a safe and supportive environment for its students, faculty, and staff.
		Industries are stable and have a history of financial support for the institution and employ its graduates.
	What are the major industries related to the institution and do they offer financial support as well as employment opportunities for graduates?	The public, private, and professional school systems provide graduates for the institution and are of high quality. School counselors have strong relationships with the institution's admissions department.
	What are the major educational systems, and what is the quality of the programs? How do they feed into the parent institution?	Community colleges and higher degree institutions collaborate and have articulation agreements for ease of transfer.
	What community services provide an infrastructure for the institution, i.e., transportation and communications services?	Students have access at a reasonable cost to public transportation to and from home (for commuter students) and to stores and other community services.
		The community has multiple media communication networks of high quality for marketing, public relations, and educational purposes. Internet, postal service, and other delivery systems are reliable.
	What services provide an infrastructure for the institution, i.e., recreation, housing, utilities, and human and health services?	There are varied and multiple recreational sites for students' leisure activities.
		If there are no student health services, the community has quality health and human services for which students are eligible.
	What type of government is in place in the community, and what are its politics? Is the government supportive of the institution in its midst, and does it recognize its contributions to the community?	The governmental structure is supportive of the parent institution in its community.
		Key members of the parent institution serve on advisory boards for the local government.

(continued)

TABLE 3.1: Guidelines for Assessing External Frame Factors (*continued*)

Frame Factor	Questions for Data Collection	Desired Outcomes
Demographics of the Population	What are the characteristics of the general population?	The population reflects multicultural and ethnic characteristics with a wide range of age groups.
	What indications are there that the population supports higher education?	A majority of the population and the powers structures completed high school or higher levels of education, and/or there is growing interest in and need for these levels of education.
	Within the population, what is the potential for acquiring students, faculty, and staff for the program?	There is an adequate applicant pool for the program(s). There are potential qualified faculty and staff available.
Political Climate and Body Politic	Identify the type of government and its structure. Who are the political power brokers in the community?	Key politicians and community leaders support the institution and have working relationships with the people within the educational institution.
	What are the relationships of the parent institution to the political power brokers?	
The Healthcare System and Health Needs of the Populace	Identify the major types of healthcare systems and the predominant healthcare delivery patterns.	Currently and for the future, there are ample clinical spaces for nursing student placements in the various healthcare systems and settings.
	Describe the major healthcare problems and needs of the populace in the educational program's region.	Major healthcare problems and needs match the foci of the curriculum.
	Describe the role of nursing in the healthcare system.	Nursing, as part of the healthcare workforce, has a strong representation within the healthcare system.
Characteristics of the Academic Setting	Identify other institutions of higher learning in the region or on the internet. Within those institutions, what types of nursing programs are offered, if any?	Other institutions of higher learning in the region or on the internet have programs that are not in direct competition with the curriculum and can serve as feeder schools to the program. There are no known future plans that could conflict with the program.
	Are there potential or existing competitors?	

The Need for the Program	Describe the nursing workforce in the region as well as the state and nation.
	Describe the numbers and types of nurses needed in the region, state, and nation(s) for the future.
	There is a demonstrated need for nurses in the region, state, and nation(s) currently and in the future.
	The numbers and types of nurses meet the goals and type(s) of preparation available in the educational program for the future.
The Nursing Profession	List the major professional nursing organizations in the region or nation.
	Describe the characteristics of nurses in the region.
	There are at least two major nursing organizations in the region or nation to be served that support the program and provide collegial relationships for students and faculty.
	The types of nurses in the region match the potential applicant pool for continued education and/or faculty and mentor positions.
Financial Support	Analyze the present financial health of the parent institution and the nursing program.
	Develop a list of existing and potential economic resources.
	The institution and the nursing program are in solid financial condition and there are either guaranteed state or national support or substantial endowment funds from the local and greater communities for the future.
	There are adequate economic resources for the present and the future of the program.
Regulations and Accreditation Requirements	Identify the state board of registered nursing or national regulations for educational programs.
	List accreditation agencies that impact the parent institution and the nursing education program.
	The nursing education program meets the state board or national regulations and has or is eligible for approval.
	The parent institution is accredited by its regional or national agency, and the nursing program meets the standards of a national professional accrediting body.

TABLE 3.2: Guidelines for Assessing Internal Frame Factors

Frame Factor	Questions for Data Collection	Desired Outcomes
Description and Organizational Structure of the Parent Academic Institution	In what type of educational institution is the nursing program located?	The nursing program matches the type of educational institution in its purpose, mission, and vision.
	What is the milieu of the parent institution in regard to the nursing program?	There is a supportive organizational system for program planning and curriculum revision.
	What is the organizational structure of the parent institution? What place in the institution does the nursing program hold? What influence does it have?	The nursing program is recognized in the institution for its place in education, scholarship, and service to the community.
	In what order must a program go through the approval process? Who are the major players in the various levels of approval processes?	A fair, participative, and comprehensive review process begins at the program level and moves through a logical sequence of the governing body for final approval that results in an economically sound and high-quality educational program.
	What are the layers of approval processes for program approval and curriculum revisions?	
Mission and Purpose, Philosophy, and Goals of the Parent Institution	What are the mission, philosophy, and goals of the parent institution?	The mission and purpose, philosophy, and goals of the parent institution are congruent with and supportive of the nursing program.
	Are they congruent and supportive of the nursing program?	
Internal Economic Situation and Its Influence on the Curriculum	What is the operating budget of the nursing program? Is it adequate for the support of the existing program?	The nursing program has adequate resources for supporting its educational program from the parent institution.
	Are there resources for program or curriculum development activities?	The nursing program has the resources for program or curriculum development activities.
	Does the program have a financial officer or administrative assistant who can develop a business plan for the proposed program or curriculum revision? If not, are there resources available from the parent institution?	The nursing program has a business plan, the resources, and administrative support for mounting a new program or revising the existing curriculum.

Resources Within the Institution and Nursing Program	If the program is on-campus or a combination of on- and off-site, how many classrooms, clinical practice, simulation, and computer laboratories does the nursing program have, and are they under its control? Can they accommodate additional students or newer technologies in the proposed program or curriculum revisions? Are there plans for these facilities in the proposal, and are the costs calculated in the business plan?	The current physical facilities, such as classrooms, offices, clinical practice and simulation laboratories, and computer facilities, are adequate and can accommodate curriculum revisions or new programs, OR there are plans for expansion in place that are part of the business plan and have the support of the financial bodies of the institution.
	For both off- and on-site, are the web and technology systems and staff in place for the institution and nursing program? Are they adequate and up-to-date? Are there plans for increasing and updating the systems and staff according to the revised or new program needs?	There are technology systems and faculty and staff support systems that facilitate program planning and curriculum revisions.
	What are the available resources for program planning and curriculum revision? Is there released time available for those involved? Is there staff support available? What teaching–learning continuing education programs are available to faculty?	There are adequate instructional and technology support systems and staff available for the current program and for proposed future programs.
	How many texts and journal holdings. as well as electronic databases, does the library have, and will they meet the needs of students and faculty in the future?	The current and proposed library and electronic holdings are adequate to meet the needs of the nursing program and proposed curricular revisions.
	Is there adequate librarian and technical support?	There are reasonable hours/days and staff support for students and faculty to access the library and other electronic communications.
	What are the available hours/days and staff support for students and faculty to access the library and other electronic communications?	

(continued)

TABLE 3.2: Guidelines for Assessing Internal Frame Factors (*continued*)

Frame Factor	Questions for Data Collection	Desired Outcomes
Potential Faculty and Student Characteristics	Describe the characteristics of the current student body and the history of the applicant pool to the nursing program. Has the program been able to meet its enrollment targets in the past 5 years? If not, what strategies have taken place to meet the target? What are the characteristics of the student body for the proposed program or revised curriculum? Is there an adequate applicant pool to fulfill enrollment targets? Has the nursing program a partnership and plans with the admissions department for recruiting and retaining students? Describe the characteristics of the current faculty. Are the numbers of faculty sufficient? Do they meet program requirements, educational level, clinical expertise, scholarship/research, and teaching experience qualifications? Do they represent diversity? Are there plans to recruit additional faculty if indicated?	The parent institution and the nursing program have the resources to recruit, educate, and graduate the type of student body that the new program or curriculum revision requires. There is a sufficient number of qualified faculty members who represent diversity and meet faculty-to-student ratio standards as well as academic, accreditation, and professional requirements.
Analysis of the Data and Decision-Making	Summarize the conclusions by generating a list of positive, negative, and neutral findings that can influence the curriculum and program planning.	Develop a final decision statement as to the feasibility for developing a new program or revising the curriculum based on the needs assessment and its findings of the external and internal frame factors.

as guidelines for identifying the frame factors, collecting the data for an assessment, and analyzing the findings to determine if there is a need for a new program or if changes are necessary for an existing program. The Appendix offers a case study illustrating a needs assessment and, based on the needs assessment, a proposed curriculum revision.

END-OF-CHAPTER RESOURCES

DISCUSSION QUESTIONS

1. Conducting a needs assessment is time-consuming; discuss the pros and cons of using all faculty members, a representative task force, paid consultants, or a combination of all three to conduct the assessment.

2. Curriculum development and curriculum evaluation are two different processes. How might a needs assessment apply to the appraisal of both processes?

LEARNING ACTIVITIES

Student-Learning Project

As a student group, examine the community around you for its potential for a nursing program. Use Tables 3.1 and 3.2 to collect data on the factors that you need to consider. After you collect the data, summarize your findings and compare them to the "Desired Outcomes" listed in the tables. Based on the findings, justify why or why not a new or revised nursing program is needed.

Faculty Project

Using Tables 3.1 and 3.2, assess your nursing curriculum. Collect data for each frame factor as it applies to the curriculum. Summarize your findings and compare them to the "Desired Outcomes" listed in the table. In light of your summary, is a curriculum revision or a new program indicated? Explain your reasons for the decision.

 SPRINGER PUBLISHING CONNECT™ | A robust set of instructor resources designed to supplement this text is located at **http://connect.springerpub.com/content/book/978-0-8261-8686-7.** Qualifying instructors may request access by emailing **textbook@springerpub.com.**

REFERENCES

American Association of Colleges of Nursing. (2021). *The essentials: Core competencies for professional nursing education.* https://www.aacnnursing.org/Portals/42/AcademicNursing/pdf/Essentials-2021.pdf

Indiana University Center for Postsecondary Research. (2020). *The Carnegie classification of institutions of higher education* (2018th ed.). Author. https://carnegieclassifications.iu.edu/downloads/CCIHE2018-FactsFigures.pdf

Johnson, M. (1977). *Intentionality in education.* Center for Curriculum Research and Services [Distributor]; Walter Snyder [Printer].

Keating, S. B. (2018). Needs assessment and financial support for curriculum development. In S. B. Keating and S. S. DeBoor (Eds.), *Curriculum development and evaluation in nursing* (4th ed.). New York, NY: Springer Publishing Company.

Keating, S. B. (2006). *Curriculum development and evaluation in nursing.* Springer Pubishing Company.

CHAPTER 4

Financial Support and Budget Management for Curriculum Development or Revision

Stephanie Stimac DeBoor

CHAPTER OBJECTIVES

Upon completion of Chapter 4, the reader will be able to:

- Analyze the influence that financial costs and budgetary management have on curriculum development or revision.
- Itemize the costs associated with curriculum development or revision.
- Identify resources for the financial support of curriculum development and revision activities.
- Analyze the roles of faculty, administrators, and staff in budgetary planning, management, and the procurement of funds for curriculum development and revision.

OVERVIEW

Activities associated with curriculum development for new programs or revision of existing ones require financial support for the time spent by personnel on the project and its associated costs. The costs may be major or minor depending on the extent of the changes or new program development. For example, if it is a revision, it may not call for additional faculty but, perhaps, renovation of the physical facilities, equipment (simulation, task trainers, products), and other instructional support needs. New programs usually require start-up costs associated with their initiation such as the time spent on developing the program prior to student admission, approvals from accreditation agencies and regulating bodies, and increased recruitment activities for students and new faculty. One must consider institutional and degree productivity when developing a new program. This chapter discusses the types of costs that occur, their impact on the proposed program or revision, budget planning and management, and possible resources for funding. The roles of administrators, faculty, and staff are described.

FINANCIAL COSTS AND BUDGETARY PLANNING

Financial Costs

The process for evaluating an existing program for possible revision and conducting a needs assessment for possible changes or creating a new program involves administrative, faculty, and staff time. Depending on the extent of the change or development of a new program, the time spent may be part of the usual role of these personnel. For example, faculty curriculum committee members review recommendations for change in the curriculum as part of committee activities, which, in turn, are part of the service role expectations for faculty. Another example is when planning and managing the budget, the department chair over graduate or undergraduate programs may find that one of the tracks in the overall program is losing money owing to low student enrollments while another track is turning away applicants. Analyzing the problem and bringing it to the attention of the faculty are the next steps in addressing the problem and are considered a usual administrative responsibility.

While activities associated with program changes normally take place in faculty curriculum committees and the time spent on these activities is considered a part of the faculty service role, faculty time spent over and above the usual service activities may be necessary. The costs associated with the additional time occur in the form of release time or a stipend for individual faculty members, or a consultant may be hired to coordinate the project. Staff support for the activities such as taking and recording minutes for meetings, coordination of participants' schedules for meeting times, collecting data for assessment, and so forth are included in the costs.

When calculating the costs associated with curriculum development, both direct and indirect costs must be considered. Direct costs are those that can be attributed to new costs and include: additional personnel; physical facilities such as offices, labs, classrooms, and furnishings; staff and instructional support equipment; web-based informatics and technology systems; computers and their hardware and software; office supplies; and so on. Indirect costs are those associated with the use of existing staff, physical facilities such as offices and meeting rooms, utilities, furnishings, and supplies that the institution provides from its resources. These indirect costs are usually estimated on a percentage of the total direct costs and can range from approximately 3% to 40% of the total costs. Personnel costs represent the largest expenditure for supporting curriculum change or development. However, there are a few other direct costs, such as fees associated with data collection when conducting a needs assessment, office supplies, new computer hardware and software, and travel for data collection or consultation purposes.

Costs of Nursing Programs in Academe

An important consideration when managing resources for use within a new specialty track or a new program is institutional productivity. One can examine institutional productivity through the lens of a return-on-investment basis. What are the expenditures for each student enrolled compared to tuition received? Often nursing programs must defend themselves from other disciplines that assume that nursing education is an expensive proposition. Certainly, the nursing faculty-to-student ratio required for clinical supervision in healthcare agencies is costly. However, large theory classes in which lecture prevails as the modality for entry-level programs, the use of online education, and clinical simulation help counterbalance the expense. In addition, clinical instructors are often part-time or serve as adjunct faculty who cost less than tenured or tenure-track faculty who are full-time. Retention rates and degree completion rates provide performance measures to support the creation of a new program. The literature on the costs of program development is sparse; several articles were identified that discuss how to estimate the costs and benefits for a new program. The reader may find them useful when involved in curriculum development and planning.

Tuition alone may not support the need for a new program or even revisions to an existing program. There is strong competition in capturing funding opportunities within the university system. If contemplating the addition of a new track to an existing MSN or DNP program, one must question the return on investment. Universities are looking at different business models over state funding to ensure a program will remain viable if initiated. As an example, Broome et al. (2018) examined the business development initiative undertaken by Duke University. This funding model created revenue for the program outside of the typical tuition, endowment, and grant support. By participating in outside revenue-producing activities that align with the school of nursing's and or parent institution's mission can contribute to needed funding. Components of the business model are outlined along with examples of initiatives that support funding for programs and research.

A successful partnership between practice and academe is described by Rousch et al. (2021). The partnership consisted of an internship for senior baccalaureate in nursing students in the last semester of their senior year. Benefits listed for the hospital included an increase in baccalaureate-prepared graduates in the hospital and lower costs for orientation programs, while the university experienced successful NCLEX® pass rates and highly satisfied graduates.

The knowledge and skill in creating a strong business case can be used to justify to decision-makers the need to invest resources for a new program or programmatic revisions. A business case, simply put, is the who, what, why, and how outline for justification of the project. Storer Brown et al. (2020) provide a business case template used in their description of a care coordination and transition management program. They point out that the first step is completed in the "prework." This is completing a thorough investigation of the undertaking, including the challenges and opportunities that may exist in current programs. Performing a literature review related to current trends can lend credence and support for the proposal. One must identify and have conversations early on with stakeholders who can become frontline supporters of the project. Once "prework" is completed the following steps are undertaken to develop a business case. First, write a clear and succinct description of who the program is for and its producible; for example, what is the aim of the program (e.g., creation of an adult-gerontology primary care nurse practitioner program), and what is the role in the delivery of healthcare services (increase the number of providers to rural communities)? Include a list of necessary action items, such as recruitment of students, hiring of faculty, and so forth, needed for implementation of the program. Second, identify measurables for program success (number of admissions, retention, graduates, employment). Finally, provide a spreadsheet that affords a visual of the costs for mounting the program, maintaining it, and the estimated return on the investment, including how it will be sustained over the long term. Examples of return on investment include increased student enrollments and, therefore, increased income from tuition, fees, scholarships, and possible long-term grants and endowments for the program.

Budgetary Planning and Management

The chief nursing officer (CNO; dean, director, or chair) of the educational program is responsible for managing the budget. Administrative support staff assists in the management of the budget allocation, although, in some smaller nursing programs, these responsibilities may be included in the expectations of the CNO. Planning for the future, both annually and long term, is part of the CNO role. Schools of nursing and their parent institutions have strategic goals and plans for the future, usually within a 5-year framework. In addition, most schools have a master plan of evaluation. These plans, with their goals and objectives, provide guidelines for projected curriculum revisions, new program proposals, and program and accreditation activities. Thus, a section in the budget for curriculum development and evaluation should be part of the planning process. When planning annual budgets in association with the development of short- and long-term goals, administrators should involve faculty, staff, and community stakeholders to assist in the identification of current and potential needs for curriculum revision and the development of new programs and their related costs.

Specific items in budgets that relate to curriculum planning include faculty released time to identify possible revisions or new programs, released time for conducting a needs assessment, consultant fees if indicated for major revisions or new program development, expenses related to attendance at relevant conferences/workshops, and additional staff support, office supplies, and communications and technology support. According to the program's long-range goals or strategic plan, these costs may be for 1 year or several depending on the extent of the changes. As the planning process develops, indications for change or new programs require further planning for the future based on the costs for developing new programs and, perhaps, discontinuing programs that no longer meet the goals of the program. Table 4.1 lists the elements to consider in planning annual budgets as they apply to curriculum revision or development of new programs.

TABLE 4.1: Budget Elements for Curriculum Assessment and Planning

Item	Associated Costs	Potential Benefits	Risks	Total Cost
Faculty Released Time	% of released time necessary (salary)	Faculty development in curriculum planning and assessment Faculty ownership of the curriculum	Time away from teaching activities Development of barriers and resistance to curriculum change	$
Conference Workshop Attendance	Fees, travel expenses	Faculty development for curriculum planning	Time away from teaching activities	$
Consultant	Consultation fees, travel, lodging, other identified expenses	Expert assistance for identifying needs, redundancies, and nonproductive programs	Insufficient or inadequate product compared to outlay	$
Staff	% of released time necessary (salary) *or* new temporary position	Experienced program management perspectives *or* 100% of time devoted to the activity	Time away from usual activities Temporary positions are difficult to fill	$ (Salary and benefits)
Office Supplies	Computer accessories, paper, desk supplies, etc.	Support for the process	None	$
Needs Assessment	Access to databases, travel to agencies, mailing costs, telephone charges, etc.	Documents needs for program Develops potential partnerships with community stakeholders and agencies	Time-consuming Can be slanted Missing data	$
Reports	Time of personnel Office supplies	Record for documentation and planning purposes	Time-consuming	$

(continued)

TABLE 4.1: Budget Elements for Curriculum Assessment and Planning (*continued*)

Item	Associated Costs	Potential Benefits	Risks	Total Cost
Total				$

If the school of nursing decides to offer a new program based on the findings from a needs assessment, planning for a budget to start and maintain the program is a crucial step. Costs for developing the curriculum, including recruitment of students, and additional faculty, staff, physical facilities, and supplies, must be part of the cost side of the budget, along with the revenue side of the budget to indicate sources of financial support. See Table 4.2 for a listing of the items to include in a budget when planning for a new program. The role

TABLE 4.2: Elements for Budget Planning for New Programs

Item	Year 1	Year 2	Year 3	Year 4	Year 5[a]
COSTS					
Salaries and Benefits of Existing Faculty, Administrators, and Staff for Curriculum Development					
Salary and Benefits for Coordinator of Program					
Salary and Benefits for Program Faculty					

(*continued*)

TABLE 4.2: Elements for Budget Planning for New Programs *(continued)*

Item	Year 1	Year 2	Year 3	Year 4	Year 5[a]
Consultant Fees and Costs					
Salary and Benefits for Support Staff					
Recruitment of Personnel					
Recruitment of Students					
Capital Improvements/Additions					
Supplies, Services, Technology, and Information Services and Staff					

(continued)

TABLE 4.2: Elements for Budget Planning for New Programs (*continued*)

Item	Year 1	Year 2	Year 3	Year 4	Year 5[a]
Library Additions and Staff					
INCOME					
Student Enrollments/Tuition (include admissions, anticipated attrition rate, and graduations; part-time, full-time if applicable)					
Student Fees					
Income From Grants, Endowments, Donations, Scholarships, Other					
TOTALS					

[a]*Five-year budget planning is recommended with an annual review for adjustments.*

of the CNO in this undertaking—overseeing finances, faculty, and facilities—is resource manager. They have the final say in whether to move forward with the proposal to the university's senior approval committee. In some cases, it may be the provost alone making the final decision.

Under normal circumstances, the information provided here regarding budgetary planning and management depicts a typical plan for program development. Unfortunately, the COVID-19 global pandemic presents significant challenges to the upcoming years and future budgetary plans. Friga (2020) offers strategies for managing budgets within higher education. While this plan is for top management regarding budgetary concerns, it can easily be translated to schools within the university system. This three-step plan includes conducting scenario planning, developing assumptions, and launching actions. In conducting scenario planning, one should include the mission of the institution and propose "best-," "moderate-," and "worse-" case scenarios. This can include questioning of overall freshman enrollment for the fall semester and what percentage of matriculating students will return to campus. This does not seem to be a concern for school of nursing programs across the country as the American Association of Colleges of Nursing (2020) still shows programs at capacity and turning away students. In developing assumptions, one must still rely on the current data to forecast future budgetary plans. Friga encourages that universities, as a whole, examine programs of low enrollment that are not profitable and make cuts as necessary. Is there revenue to sustain this program? If not, then the program must be suspended or eliminated completely. Finally, use the information gathered in the previous two steps and consider actions. While on a university scale this may include cuts across all faculty and program lines, at a school or program level, this may include additional cuts in the operating budget. For example, faculty may be limited in their ability to travel for faculty development opportunities and may be asked to participate in online or close-to-home activities. Overall, these steps provide an opportunity to revisit multiple areas of the current budget and explore planning for the future.

SOURCES FOR FINANCIAL SUPPORT

There are three major sources of funding for curriculum development and planning other than the home institution's support in its regular budget. Depending on the nature of the home institution, the majority of funds for the budget come from the general funds (if state-supported), tuition and fees, endowments, grants, and donations. When considering funds for curriculum development, the three major resources for funds are grants (private and public), partnerships with the community, and philanthropy (donations and endowments). Each of these sources is discussed with ideas from the literature for procurement of funds.

Grants

A major resource for program development and student and faculty support at the federal level comes from the Health Resources and Services Administration (HRSA), Division of Nursing (2021). Included in the program of grants are traineeships for advanced practice students, faculty loans, support for nurse-managed healthcare services, and program development. The program development funds, for the most part, focus on starting up new programs and a large part of the funds support curriculum development. It is not permanent funding and is intended as an incentive to increase the advanced practice nursing workforce and support other types of advanced nursing education programs, for example, education and public health. The costs for preparing a grant proposal must be factored into the planning process including faculty and staff time and additional related costs for preparation of the grant. If faculty have never written a grant before, it is important that they first identify university resources that can assist in this process. Kulage et al. (2015) list the costs associated with the preparation of a grant submitted to the National Institute of Nursing Research (NINR). The NINR (2017, 2021) supports research activities related to clinical practice and the advancement of nursing science, but not for program development.

In addition to federal grants, there are major private foundations and organizations interested in supporting nursing education programs. They include the Bill and Melinda Gates Foundation (www.gatesfoundation.org), the Robert Wood Johnson Foundation (www.rwjf.org), the W. K. Kellogg Foundation (www.wkkf.org), the Josiah Macy Jr. Foundation (www.macyfoundation.org), the Gordon and Betty Moore Foundation (www.moore.org), and many others. A listing of other resources may be found at the proposalCENTRAL (proposalcentral.altum.com). Many universities and colleges offer courses in grant writing, and those new to the process are encouraged to access those opportunities.

Partnerships

There is a long history of partnerships between nursing education programs and healthcare agencies. The purpose of these partnerships is not only to provide clinical experiences for students but also to support schools of nursing in preparing professionals for the workforce. These partnerships take many forms, including work–study, internship, or residency experiences for students who may earn a modest salary and at the same time earn academic credits; contributions of nursing clinicians to the school as instructors; the use of facilities for laboratory and simulation experiences; continuing education and research opportunities for both faculty and staff; and scholarship or loan programs for students in exchange for contracts to work for the agency upon graduation. The numbers and amount of financial support available from agencies seem to ebb and flow according to nursing workforce demands and the financial climate at the time.

An example of partnerships between healthcare systems and educational institutions is the Veterans Affairs (VA) Nursing Academy (VANA) that was established in 2007. The VANA project supplied $60 million to establish partnerships with the VA and schools of nursing. It funds faculty positions using expert clinicians from the VA system (or the community if there is a lack), provides clinical practice experiences for students, and recruits new graduates into the VA system. There are four established regions including the western, midwestern, southern, and northeastern regions of the United States. Benefits for the schools and the VA include current updates on clinical practice and an increase in the faculty workforce as well as the nursing workforce. This model serves as an example for other healthcare systems wishing to increase the nursing workforce and, at the same time, participate in updating nursing curricula and addressing the nursing faculty shortage (Bowman et al., 2011). In 2012, following the success of the VANA, the Veterans Affairs Nursing Academic Partnership (VANAP) program was launched. This program includes a number of partnerships with nursing schools throughout the United States that are selected through a competitive application process (U.S. Department of Veteran's Affairs, n.d.).

Roach and Hooke (2019) describe the VANAP program in which schools of nursing and VA hospitals collaborated providing clinical learning experiences that provide mutual benefits. Students experience a well-rounded clinical experience by participating in quality improvement projects, faculty are afforded development opportunities, and the hospital benefits from the opportunity to recruit and implement student-supported care initiatives. VA employees act as adjunct faculty providing cost savings associated with the clinical supervision of students by faculty.

Partnerships between other schools of nursing and the institution's own programs in nursing can result in common campus activities such as orientation sessions, sharing of core courses that are common to program curricula, for example, statistical methods; blended clinical experiences that provide different, yet collaborative, levels of care; and end-of-program projects that reflect varying levels of practice or role functions. These collaborative activities can lead to a savings in resources such as faculty and staff costs and facilities as is the case in a state university offering graduate courses across disciplines. Graduate courses that might be of broad interest to students in other programs are being offered university-wide. This not only proves to generate revenue and save on cost but also improves collegial relationships between multiple disciplines of students (University of Nevada, Reno Graduate School, personal communication, April 2021).

Philanthropy

The CNO (dean, director, or chair) of the educational program, along with the support of members from the development and foundation offices, is frequently responsible for the recruitment of philanthropic donors. In addition, faculty and student are often the face of the nursing program throughout the community and play a role in identifying and recruiting potential donors. Philanthropic funds come from donations to nursing programs. A large majority of these donations are earmarked for scholarships for students. However, there are times when programs receive donations for program development. A successful fundraising campaign consists of knowing the potential donors and having a personal connection. Contacts made with unknown people seldom succeed. The motivation of the donor for contributing to the program should be known, whether in response to a personal connection with the school, a desire to contribute to a good cause anonymously or not, and an opportunity to establish a memorial or tribute to someone close to the donor. When proposing a contribution to a project, it is important to point out the direct and indirect benefits for the donor from the gift and what impact it will have on the program and healthcare system currently and in the future.

Alumni organizations have in the past been a good resource of funding for nursing programs and schools. It is important to continue to nurture these relationships long after graduation and support alumni organizations through special functions, such as reunions at the time of graduation, other university and school of nursing events, and guest lectures. Fostering alumni participation can begin early in the professional socialization process through the nursing student association with faculty mentoring and support. Although Langley (2020) outlines that due to debt from student loans, increasing tuition costs, and an overall change in attitudes regarding philanthropic donations, there is a noted decline in alumni contribution dollars. We must look beyond the "status quo" and recognize that our donors have changed and so must our fundraising efforts.

ROLE OF ADMINISTRATORS, STAFF, AND FACULTY IN FINANCIAL SUPPORT FOR CURRICULUM DEVELOPMENT ACTIVITIES

Administrators and Staff

A curriculum revision or the development of a new program indicates the need for additional administrator and faculty time that is usually over and above the normal job expectations. Therefore, release time and related costs are expected and must be planned for in the budget. Administrators, with faculty input, should include a line item for program planning in the budget to cover these anticipated costs. While indirect funds from a grant can supplement salaries for required released time spent on program planning, they usually are not available until after the grant is approved and funded, sometimes long after initial activities take place. Depending on the institution's policies regarding indirect funds, administrators may have the discretion to use funds for program development generated from other grants. Otherwise, funds for program planning should be part of the regular budgeting process.

The administrator and the administrative staff have responsibility for the management of the school budget and records of expenditures for curriculum revision or new program development. The records are especially useful for illustrating how the expenditures tie to the purpose of the funding and the grant/project goals. They provide documentation for accounting purposes. Each year, the annual budget review process provides time for administrators, staff, and faculty to identify continuing and future funding needs for program development.

Faculty

Curriculum development and evaluation are ongoing processes built into the educational program activities. Nursing educators in the process of delivering the curriculum through instructional activities such as classroom lectures, seminars, conferences, laboratory practice, simulation activities, online teaching, and clinical supervision gather information on how well the curriculum is delivered. This ongoing assessment of teaching effectiveness and student-learning outcomes is part of the role of teaching and is a job expectation. Therefore, as part of the usual responsibilities, is supported through faculty salaries. Another aspect of faculty work is participation in work groups, such as course, level, and curriculum committee meetings. These activities are considered part of the service role for faculty and, from a budgetary point of view, are a part of the salary paid to faculty and the expected responsibilities of the role. If major curriculum revisions or a new program are indicated, conducting a needs assessment and developing the curriculum can require faculty time over and above the usual expectations. In that case, the administrator and faculty in the program need to identify sources of funds to support the release time for these activities and to plan for them in the budget.

SUMMARY

This chapter discusses the importance of financial support for curriculum revision and program development. It reviews the costs, benefits, and budget planning and management activities associated with curriculum development and revision. Resources for funding these activities are offered and the roles of administrators, staff, and faculty in seeking funding, planning, and managing the budget are described.

END-OF-CHAPTER RESOURCES

DISCUSSION QUESTIONS

1. Explain how the school of nursing and university resources and finances influence development, revision, and maintenance of the program's curriculum?

2. What individual or group do you believe has the responsibility for procuring funds for program development and curricular revision? Provide a rationale.

LEARNING ACTIVITIES

Student-Learning Activities

Attend an undergraduate or graduate curriculum committee meeting. Select and interview a member or chair of the curriculum committee for their perspectives on financial support for program development and curriculum revision. The following are nterview questions you might consider asking:

1. How much time do you spend on curriculum activities outside the attendance of the curriculum committee meeting?

2. Are you compensated in any way for this time, or is it an expectation of your role? Do you believe faculty should have release time for curriculum development activities? Why or why not? How would you pay for overtime?

3. When was the last curriculum revision? Do you expect a revision in the near future? Are there plans for review and revision of the curriculum in the school strategic plan?

4. Do you participate in planning for future curriculum committee activities and development, and are budgetary issues involved in the planning?

5. Are you aware of any resources to support curriculum change or new program development? If yes, what are these sources?

Faculty Development Activities

1. Survey your community/region for existing partnerships between nursing education programs and clinical agencies. Other than providing clinical experiences for students, are there any other financial support programs related to curriculum revision or new program development in the partnership?

2. Identify needs for and possible partnerships to support nursing education in your region. Indicate your strategies for developing the partnership and its maintenance over time.

A robust set of instructor resources designed to supplement this text is located at **http://connect.springerpub.com/content/book/978-0-8261-8686-7.** Qualifying instructors may request access by emailing **textbook@springerpub.com.**

REFERENCES

American Association of Colleges of Nursing. (2020). *Building capacity through university hospital and university school of nursing partnerships*. https://www.aacnnursing.org/News-Information/Position-Statements-White-Papers/Building-Capacity

Bowman, C. C., Johnson, L., Cox, M., Rick, C., Dougherty, M., Alt-White, A. C., Wyte, T., Needleman, J. & Dobalian, A. (2011). The Department of Veterans Affairs Nursing Academy: Forging strategic alliances with schools of nursing to address nursing's workforce needs. *Nursing Outlook, 59*, 299–307. https://doi.org/10.1016/j.outlook.2011.04.006

Broome, M., Bowersox, D., & Relf, M. (2018). A new funding model for nursing education through business development initiatives. *Journal of Professional Nursing, 34*(2), 97–102. https://doi.org/10.1016/j.profnurs.2017.10.003

Friga, P. N. (2020). Under Covid-19, university budgets like we've never seen before. Unprecedented times require unprecedented strategies and actions. *The Chronicle of Higher Education*. https://www.chronicle.com/article/under-covid-19-university-budgets-like-weve-never-seen-before/

Health Resources and Services Administration. (2021). *Apply for a grant*. https://bhw.hrsa.gov/funding/apply-grant

Kulage, K., Schnall, R., Hickey, K. Travers, J., Zezulinski, K., Torres, F., Burgess, J., & Larson E. L. (2015). Time and costs of preparing and submitting an NIH grant application at a school of nursing. *Nursing Outlook, 63*(6), 639–649. https://doi.org/10.1016/j.outlook.2015.09.003

Langley, J. M. (2020). *The future of fundraising. Adapting to changing philanthropic realities*. Academic Impressions.

National Institute of Nursing Research. (2021). *Research and funding*. https://www.ninr.nih.gov/#

National Institute of Nursing Research. (2017). *Mission & strategic plan (2022–2026) – Under development*. https://www.ninr.nih.gov/aboutninr/ninr-mission-and-strategic-plan

Roach, A., & Hooke, S. (2019). An academic-practice partnership. Fostering collaboration and improving care across settings. *Nurse Educator, 44*(2), 98–101. https://doi.org/10.1097/NNE.0000000000000557

Rousch, K., Opsahl, A., & Ferren, M. (2021). Developing an internship program to support nursing student transition to clinical setting. *Journal of Professional Nursing, 37*(4), 696–701. https://doi.org/10.1016/j.profnurs.2021.04.001

Storer Brown, D., Start, R., & Matlock, A. M. (2020). Creating a business case template for care coordination and transition management. *Nursing Economic$, 38*(6), 308–315. NLM UID: 8404213

U.S. Department of Veteran's Affairs. (n.d.). *Office of Nursing Services*. https://www.va.gov/NURSING/workforce/workforce.asp#vanap

SECTION III

CURRICULUM DEVELOPMENT PROCESSES

Stephanie Stimac DeBoor

OVERVIEW OF CURRICULUM DEVELOPMENT PROCESSES

Prior to discussing curriculum development, it is useful to review the definition of curriculum. For the purpose of this text, *a curriculum is the formal plan of study that provides the philosophical underpinnings, goals, and guidelines for the delivery of a specific educational program.* Chapter 5 introduces the classic components of the curriculum and the process for its development followed by Chapters 6 and 7, which describe the implementation of the curriculum through the application of learning theories, educational taxonomies, critical thinking concepts, and learner-focused, instructional strategies. Chapters 8 and 9 describe undergraduate and graduate programs with the various pathways into the profession that are linked to them including Chapter 10 on the doctorate of advanced practice and research-focused doctoral degrees. Chapter 11 depicts a proposed unified curriculum summarizing the various educational pathways in nursing. Chapter 12, new to this text, provides an overview of curriculum design and evaluation in the specialty of staff/nursing professional development (NPD). The final chapter discusses the application of technology to the implementation of the curriculum through learning strategies, distance education, and online programs.

Experienced educators understand that with changes in evidence-based practice (EBP), along with feedback from students, faculty, and consumers there is a need to update the curricular plan. Section IV describes in detail the value of evaluation activities as they apply to approval, review, and accreditation of nursing programs. Still, it is wise in this section on curriculum development processes to recognize the need for continually monitoring the program, at least annually, to ensure that it is meeting the original mission, framework, goals, and objectives of the curriculum. Feedback from regulatory and accrediting bodies indicates to faculty the need for revising the curriculum, discontinuing certain programs within it, or initiating new tracks. If this exercise is conducted every year, maintaining the integrity of the curriculum becomes easy, and there are fewer steps when seeking approval for major or minor changes. Annual review and minor revisions contribute to a curriculum that is current and prepares nursing professionals for current and future employment markets.

PURPOSE OF CURRICULUM DEVELOPMENT

The overall purpose of curriculum development in nursing education is to meet the learners' needs by ensuring that it meets educational and professional standards and that it is responsive to the current and future demands of the healthcare system. To accomplish this long-term goal, the curriculum serves as the template for faculty to express its vision, mission, philosophy, framework, goals, and objectives of the nursing program. Although curriculum development falls within the role of the faculty, consumers of the program need to be involved in the process. Consumers include the students, their families, the healthcare system that utilizes its graduates, nursing educators and staff in the practice setting, and last, but not least, the patients who receive nursing care from students and graduates.

COMPONENTS OF THE CURRICULUM

The classic components of a school of nursing curriculum include (a) the mission and vision (for the future) of the program; (b) the philosophy of the faculty that usually contains beliefs about teaching and learning processes; critical thinking, scholarship, research, and EBP; and other selected concepts, theories, essentials, and standards that define the specific nursing education program; (c) the purpose or overall goal of the program; (d) a framework by which to organize the curriculum plan; (e) the end-of-program objectives or student-learning outcomes; and (f) an overall implementation plan (program of study). The components should be congruent with the parent institution's mission and philosophy. Chapter 5 discusses the components in detail and the pros and cons of frameworks to organize the curriculum plan. Chapter 6 reviews learning theories in relation to implementing the curriculum. Chapter 7 discusses educational taxonomies, critical thinking concepts, and their application to implementing the curriculum. These major theories, concepts, and models serve to guide educators as they develop mission and philosophy statements for the program and build the curriculum plan. They are considered again in detail as faculty applies them to the implementation of the curriculum through the processes of learner-focused instructional design and student evaluation. Chapter 6 discusses course development approaches to provide state-of-the-art active learning strategies to realize the mission and goals of the curriculum.

LEVELS OF NURSING EDUCATION

Chapters 8, 9, and 10 apply the components of the curriculum to the various levels of nursing education including the associate degree, the baccalaureate, master's, DNP, and research-based doctorates (e.g., the PhD and DNS). Each chapter provides a summary of the role that each level of education plays in the mission, philosophy, organizational framework, goals, and end-of-program objectives for its parent institution. Included are the various pathways to completion and entry into practice, as well as advanced practice. Also provided is a discussion of issues that apply to each such as entry into practice, opportunities for further education, advanced practice, contributions to nursing education and the profession, EBP, and research. To summarize the various pathways into nursing at the entry and advanced practice levels, Chapter 11 proposes a unified curriculum for nonstop entry into practice, ending with a doctorate. Parallel to it is the same curriculum that allows nurses to step out when they wish to enter practice and later continue their education into advanced roles. The latter facilitates this movement by removing some of the barriers to continuing education that presently exist.

Staff Development: The Specialty of Nursing Professional Development

New to this text is Chapter 12, which examines the role of educators in staff/NPD. Readers are provided the modern history of staff development, roles, and responsibilities of those within NPD; learning theories; and curriculum development and evaluation outside of academe.

DISTANCE EDUCATION AND TECHNOLOGY

Chapter 13 examines technology's influence on nursing education. It traces the history of distance education from the early home study programs to today's high technology–based programs delivered from home campuses to distant satellite campuses, as well as virtual campuses. The pandemic is responsible for the highest growth of online education ever seen in the history of educational programs. A discussion regarding the online format offering not only individual courses but also degree programs and their impact on campus-based programs. The chapter goes on to examine realistic clinical simulation programs that allow students to acquire basic, advanced, and critical thinking nursing skills in a safe environment prior to actual clinical practice. Other high-tech devices and systems, such as electronic record systems, smartphones, electronic tablets, and advanced communication systems, add to the rapid changes in the delivery of education and the need for students and faculty to keep abreast of the newer innovations.

CHAPTER 5

The Classic Components of the Curriculum: Developing a Curriculum Plan

Stephanie Stimac DeBoor

CHAPTER OBJECTIVES

Upon completion of Chapter 5, the reader will be able to:

- Recognize the various types of educational institutions and levels of nursing education.
- Distinguish the formal curriculum from the informal curriculum.
- Analyze the components of the curriculum according to their role in producing a curriculum plan.
- Assess an existing curriculum or educational program by using Table 5.1.

OVERVIEW

This chapter provides an overview of types of educational institutions in higher education and how the various levels of nursing education fit into them. It continues with a discussion about the classic components of the curriculum from the mission to its implementation plan. Table 5.1 provides guidelines for assessing the key components of a curriculum or educational program.

TYPES OF INSTITUTIONS

Most institutions of higher education identify themselves according to classifications found in the Carnegie Classification of Institutions of Higher Education (2018). Carnegie classifies institutions into the following categories: doctoral, master's, baccalaureate, baccalaureate/associate's, associate's, special focus institutions, and tribal colleges. Within some of these categories are subcategories such as R1, R2, and R3 for doctoral programs, according to the level of research, and M1 and M2 to differentiate between larger and medium programs at the master's level. Types of higher educational institutions are classified as "private" or "public" and "undergraduate" or "graduate." For the purposes of this text, the discussion about types of higher educational institutions includes private (nonprofit and for-profit) and public institutions (federal, state, or regionally supported), as well as community colleges, small liberal arts colleges, large multipurpose or comprehensive colleges and universities, research-focused universities, and academic health science/medical centers.

"Sectarian" and "nonsectarian" institutions are yet another classification, with sectarian institutions reflecting a religious affiliation, for example, Notre Dame University, Southwest Baptist University, Brigham Young, and so on. While curriculum development activities are quite the same across types of institutions, the differences arise when examining the overall purpose and mission of the institution and the financial and human resources that are available for revising or initiating new programs.

LEVELS OF NURSING EDUCATION

The types of nursing education programs addressed in this text range from the associate degree to the doctorate level, and many nursing curricula include step-in and step-out educational programs that provide career ladder opportunities for nurses. Associate degree programs are usually housed in community colleges. These colleges are regional, public-supported institutions; however, there are some privately funded 2-year colleges that include nursing programs. Baccalaureate, master's, and doctorate nursing programs are found in both state-supported and privately funded institutions. There are a few "single-purpose" nursing-only schools. Many of these schools are or were former diploma, hospital-based programs with the latter converting to associate degrees or baccalaureates in nursing. Most hospital-based diploma programs are affiliated with higher degree programs, for example, community colleges and baccalaureate or higher degree programs. According to the National League for Nursing (NLN, 2019) Faculty Census Survey 2018–2019, hospital-based/special focus programs account for 2% of all nursing programs in the United States, with most located in the East, Midwest, and South.

For all types of programs, administrators and faculty should plan in advance for the financial support of curriculum development and evaluation activities and investigate possible external resources such as grants for curriculum changes and program development activities. Federally sponsored programs that are available for nursing program development and traineeships may be found at the Health Resources and Services Administration's (HRSA) website (www.bhw.hrsa.gov/fundingopportunities).

THE FORMAL AND INFORMAL CURRICULA

The *formal curriculum* is the planned program of studies for an academic degree or discipline. It includes the components of the curriculum that are discussed in this chapter and the curriculum plan is visible to the public through its homepage, publication in catalogs, and recruitment materials. The *informal curriculum* is sometimes termed the hidden curriculum, or co-curriculum, and is composed of extracurricular activities. These planned and unplanned influences on students' learning should be kept in mind as faculty assesses and develops the curriculum. Examples include honor pledges and special convocations with invited speakers, student organization activities that parallel coursework, alumni association activities that provide mentorship and preparation for entry to practice, and outside-of-class meetings with students and faculty to enrich learning experiences. The co-curriculum incorporates planned activities, such as collaboration and interprofessional education (IPE) with other academic units, student affairs meetings (information meetings, orientation, counseling sessions, etc.), field trips, work–study programs, service learning, and planned volunteer services in the community. Examples of extracurricular activities are athletics, social gatherings, and student organization events.

Some additional examples of the informal curriculum's influence in nursing are honor society meetings, study groups, student nursing association meetings, student-invited attendance at faculty meetings, and participation in academic committees. Many schools of nursing schedule informal student–faculty (S-F) meetings, holiday parties, and special events planning, such as pinning and hooding ceremonies and so on. These activities provide opportunities for student and faculty interchanges to enrich and supplement the formal classroom setting, as well as facilitate leadership opportunities for the students.

Effects of S-F Interactions on the Curriculum

Several studies have demonstrated the positive effects that S-F interactions have on the learning environment and, ultimately, on the success of the curriculum's purpose. Booth (2020) found that students and faculty working together to established core value statements reduced incivility and contributed to strong, positive relationships between faculty and students that help create a positive learning environment. Gazzardo et al. (2021) conducted a qualitative study that examined student perspectives related to their interactions with faculty. Recruitment was focused on students who were experiencing academic, personal, or financial hardships. The authors identified four themes that contribute to S-F relationships. The first, *Creating Pedagogical Space*, speaks to faculty flexibility with assignments and responsive communication. When both were perceived students felt supported and were successful. The second theme, *Being Inclusive and Aware*, relates to providing a welcoming space for diverse students. When this is not perceived, students often struggle within the program of study. The third theme, *Being Engaged and Engaging Students*, is about finding balance in rigor that challenges the student to reach potential versus breaking their spirit. The final theme, *Doing More Than Teaching*, refers to engagement, mentorship, and genuine caring demonstrated to the student, making them feel like they mattered. Faculty who demonstrate these actions and behaviors gleaned from this study's findings contribute to an environment that is conducive to supporting student learning, especially when students are experiencing academic, personal, and financial issues.

THE CAMPUS ENVIRONMENT

Traditionally in higher education, the physical environment (campus) is important to the image of the home institution and plays a major role in building a sense of belonging for students and alumni alike. Additional factors, such as spirituality and religious affiliations, also contribute to students' perceptions of the campus environment. Fosnatch and Broderick (2020), cite the increasing discrimination incidents on U.S. campuses are tainting students' perceptions of the overall campus environment. It's more important than ever for faculty to understand how students experience learning in an environment that they deem hostile. What draws students to the campus environment? Tyre (2020) states it is more than a "tagline or logo." Students feel like they belong because of the experiences they have. If the campus environment does not provide enjoyable experiences, then the student and their learning are impacted. The literature supports that those who have positive experiences during on-campus education have better learning outcomes. Schimek (2016) studied students' perceptions of a liberal arts college environment in relation to its mission. The study supports the notion of campus as home and its influence on the educational environment for students, especially in traditional institutions. Unfortunately, the pandemic created a situation in which students were forced to leave the physical environment of learning and move into a virtual learning environment (VLE).

The VLE presents challenges to teachers to develop an academic, online environment that includes faculty office hours, student and faculty meeting rooms, and learning strategies that foster a sense of community. While the physical environment plays a small role in programs that are delivered at a distance or completely online, some colleges and universities require periodic on-campus academic program meetings or immersions and offer special teaching and learning events for distance education students during their on-site campus experience. This aids in keeping the student feeling connected to the home campus. Another strategy is to provide program information materials that include pictures of the campus and campus life. This helps students identify with the physical location and landscape to form images unique to the home campus.

One lesson learned during the pandemic was the social distress felt by those that abruptly moved from a face-to-face environment to an online format. Langegård et al. (2021) examined nursing students' experiences with this type of transition. Findings indicated that at every level, students struggled with the change in social interaction and identified that they preferred a traditional on-campus environment to one online. The authors challenge faculty when teaching online to create learning activities that encourage social interaction and to ensure a well-designed structured course to offset any social distress. Examples of strategies to provide social interaction are to offer a "social hour" and open a chat room that allows students to check in with each other outside of a group project or a required virtual class meeting. Faculty can participate, or have a separate "group office time," during which students can gather just to chat with the faculty. Both options provide opportunities for social connection.

COMPONENTS OF THE CURRICULUM

The following discussion examines each of the major components of the curriculum from the mission and/or vision statements to the philosophy statement that embraces faculty beliefs and values about liberal education and the sciences; professional values, professionalism, and nursing practice; interprofessional communication and collaboration; social justice, advocacy, diversity, and cultural competence; the healthcare system; the prevention of disease and promotion of health; patient safety and quality healthcare; scholarship, research, translational science, and evidence-based practices (EBP); information systems and technology; critical thinking; and teaching and learning concepts and theories. A description follows on how the organizational framework and/or concept analysis/map, overall goal or purpose of the curriculum, end-of-program objectives/student-learning objectives (SLOs), and level objectives guide the implementation plan that flows from the mission and philosophy statements.

THE MISSION OR VISION STATEMENT

Traditionally, higher education institutions in the United States have three major elements included in their mission, that is, teaching/learning, service, and scholarship/research. The mission statement for each institution depends on the nature of the institution, and the three major elements are often divided into separate permutations. In more recent times, some organizations either replace or supplement the mission statement with a vision statement. For the purposes of this discussion, the *mission statement* is the institution's beliefs and purpose about its role and responsibilities for the preparation of its graduates (outcomes). A *vision statement* is outlook-oriented and reflects the institution's plans and dreams about its direction for the future. It is usually short, visionary, and inspirational.

Chief administrators (presidents) of institutions of higher learning assume much of the responsibility for ensuring that the mission and vision are current and reflect the purpose of the college or university. They provide the leadership and resources for administrators, staff, faculty, and students to implement the mission and vision, maintain its relevancy in the community, and meet future educational needs. The purpose/mission of the institution is examined and a vision statement is developed that looks into the future for the next decade or two. These activities foster creativity and a movement toward the future that provides the framework for planning. Developing or revising the mission and vision statements is usually a part of a strategic planning process that involves all of the constituents within the institution.

As with the presidents of universities and colleges, deans and directors of nursing education programs have a leadership role in developing program missions and visions that are not only congruent with the parent institutions but look to the future as well. Additionally, the mission needs to be examined frequently for its relevance to the rapidly changing healthcare system and the needs of society. Unless the nursing program is a stand-alone academic entity, the mission of the major academic division (e.g., college or school in which it resides) is examined in addition to that of the parent institution. Both the missions of the parent institution and its academic subdivision should be congruent with each other and provide guidelines for the mission statement of the nursing program.

Smaller institutions may focus on liberal arts as a basis for all disciplines and professional programs to meet societal needs, while large research-oriented universities or academic health sciences centers might espouse new knowledge breakthroughs by its faculty's and graduate students' research. In the case of the former, nursing's mission statement would reflect the graduation of well-prepared nurses to meet current and future healthcare demands; the latter would have an emphasis on nursing research and leadership in the profession.

PHILOSOPHY

For the purposes of this text, a definition of *philosophy* is <u>an analysis of the explanations for certain views or concepts as expressed into fundamental beliefs</u>. The philosophy for a curriculum should flow from the mission and vision. It gives faculty members the opportunity to discuss their <u>beliefs, values, and attitudes</u> about nursing and an education that imparts a body of knowledge and skills for the next generation of care providers. Each individual member holds their own personal philosophy of education and nursing; thus, the development of a philosophical statement can become an arduous task on which to agree. Nevertheless, the resulting statement reflects the faculty's (as a whole) rationale for the school of nursing's purpose and serves as a scaffold for the remainder of the curriculum components, their implementation, evaluation, and outcomes.

Once again, the development of the school of nursing's philosophy reflects those of the parent institution and the subdivision of the parent in which nursing is housed if not a stand-alone school within the university. The ideal nursing philosophy incorporates all the components of the parent institution and subdivision's philosophies, although at times, there are mismatches to some of the specific components. A discussion and record of the rationale as to why that incongruence exists and how the nursing program meets other components provide valuable information for members of the school and external reviewers' understanding of the fit of the nursing program within its parent institution and/or subdivision. An example of incongruence of a nursing program's philosophy with its parent institution's philosophy is when the program is within a traditional liberal arts college that has no other professional programs. In this case, the nursing program's philosophy speaks to the importance of a strong liberal arts foundation for its graduates and the role of the nursing program to produce graduates who provide healthcare for the community.

The majority of nursing education programs' philosophies include the basic theories, concepts, beliefs, and values of faculty. It should offer guiding principles for the remainder of the curriculum and should be evident in the organizational framework(s), goals, objectives, and the implementation plan through its courses.

ESSENTIALS FROM THE LIBERAL ARTS AND THE SCIENCES

The liberal arts and the sciences serve as the knowledge base for the discipline of nursing. There is value in integrating other disciplines both within and outside of healthcare (Carter Kooken & Kerr, 2018). The liberal arts and sciences provide students with critical thinking, inquiry, philosophy, writing, communications, mathematics, science, and research skills that serve as the foundation to the professional role.

Along with the traditional requisite sciences of anatomy, chemistry, microbiology, nutrition, and physiology for nursing, genomics is now included in most programs as a separate course or integrated throughout the curriculum. The American Nurses Association in 2009 published the *Essentials of Genetic and Genomic Nursing: Competencies, Curricula Guidelines, and Outcome Indicators* and the need for including this content into a nursing curriculum. The recent pandemic has clearly indicated that nursing's knowledge of genetics and genomics plays an important role in caring for the complexity of patients in healthcare (Seibert, 2020). In addition, the Omics Nursing Science and Education Network (2021) recommends and provides a knowledge matrix for the integration of omics into doctoral-level nursing curriculum, especially research doctorates. Omics include the sciences of genomics, transcriptomics, proteomics, epigenomics, exposomics, microbiomics, and metabolomics. Integrating this knowledge provides nursing scientists a way to keep pace with emerging scientific findings.

PROFESSIONAL VALUES, PROFESSIONALISM, AND NURSING PRACTICE

Nursing has the largest number of professionals in the U.S. healthcare system, and while it has many pathways for entry into professional practice, it meets the criteria of a profession, that is, a professional discipline requiring a specific body of knowledge with members who study and practice the discipline. Professional values describe the standards and beliefs accepted by the membership. Value statements provide the rationale and purpose of the mission and vision in relation to the population served. It includes specific ethics and theories, and it produces relevant research. Epstein and Turner (2015) provide an overview of the nursing code of ethics, including the history of its development, its contribution to the profession, and its value to nurses in practice in all settings.

Wentworth et al. (2020) conducted a qualitative study examining nursing students' responses when witnessing a breach in practice standards by RNs in the clinical setting. Most felt ill prepared to confront the action observed but clearly recognized violations as identified in the American Nurses Association (2015) *Code of Ethics*. These authors express concerns that current education does not prepare students to assert themselves during moral conflicts. Also of concern is whether exposure to breaches in the standards of practice transfers to new nurses entering the profession. Discovering conflicts in values and beliefs requires a discussion of the issues. As educators, we are tasked with modeling professional standards and values for our students. Thus, a curriculum must support students in developing an ethical conscience, professional values, and tools to deal with moral distress.

INTERPROFESSIONAL COMMUNICATION AND COLLABORATION

Nursing and other healthcare disciplines recognize the need for IPE, and with the complexity of the current U.S. healthcare system, it is an important concept to include in discussions and planning for the educational program. The American Association of Colleges of Nursing (AACN, 2021a) and the NLN (2021) support the National Academy of Medicine's (formerly the Institute of Medicine [IOM], 2021) recommendations that call for interprofessional collaboration to meet the healthcare needs of the population. AACN's (2021a) new essentials list *Domain 6 - Interprofessional Partnerships*, as "intentional collaboration across professions and with care team members, patients, families, communities, and other stakeholders to optimize care, enhance the healthcare experience, and strengthen outcomes" (p. 11). The NLN lists specific recommendations for administrators and faculty for interprofessional collaboration in education and practice.

Often in developing IPE for nursing, the immediate thought is to combine efforts of nursing and medical students, but several examples from the literature exemplify the collaboration among other disciplines and serve as models for developing curricular experiences that are interdisciplinary in nature. It is common to think about collaboration with other healthcare disciplines outside of medicine (e.g., social work, public health, pharmacy, dentistry), but there are also opportunities outside of healthcare that can serve as strong IPE experiences, for example, assigning a group of community health nursing students with students from business, engineering, and computer sciences to conduct a community needs assessment for a fictitious rural healthcare satellite clinic. Each of these disciplines brings a unique perspective on needs for finances, building, communications, services, and staffing. This type of collaboration supports developing skills in communication, teamwork, and problem-solving, along with building relationships among outside disciplines that contribute to the promotion of quality care outcomes.

SOCIAL JUSTICE, ADVOCACY, DIVERSITY, AND CULTURAL COMPETENCE

Many of the standards for accreditation of nursing programs and requests for proposals for educational funding refer to the notion of inequality, health disparities, and a lack of access to healthcare for some populations. Certain populations and oppressed groups suffer the consequences of discrimination and unfair treatment in the healthcare system. Implicit bias, or unintentional discrimination, contributes to health disparities and poor patient outcomes. Nursing as a prime caring profession must be cognizant of these injustices and have the power and strategies to advocate for their clients and themselves to provide quality healthcare for all. Social justice is an important concept often found in the missions and philosophies of educational programs; however, it is sometimes difficult to find evidence of its integration into the curriculum plan and its implementation.

Arthur et al. (2021) ask the question as to whether during educational discourse, the term *social justice* has "become somewhat vacuous and devoid of substantive meaning" (p. 101). These authors purport that terms associated with social justice usually present a negative connotation. Based on their findings, they challenge educators to put forward a "positive conception" of social justice. They identify that this is not an easily accomplished task, but we must differentiate between justice and injustice. In education, we often teach by presenting the injustices, thus perpetuating the negativity.

Stamps (2021) suggests integrating implicit bias–informed content into ongoing nursing education. Students who are cognizant of their implicit biases have an opportunity to make changes, or at least be better prepared for situations that spark feelings of discomfort, based on their awareness. Not knowing of or understanding implicit bias leads to disparities in care.

Integrating social justice theories and concepts into the curriculum implies not only an understanding of the concepts but also an awareness of the social injustices in society and the types of actions that nurses should take to bring about change. Woodward et al. (2016) reviewed the literature to find factors that influence the participation of nurses in political participation and social action. Three themes emerged: political education in the nursing curriculum, personal interest in political knowledge, and the value of collective action through membership in professional organizations. To ensure that social justice concepts and actions are included in the nursing curriculum, theories of social justice, political action strategies, and professional responsibilities should appear not only in the philosophy but specifically integrated into courses as well.

Diversity, cultural consciousness, and the role of nursing are major concepts within the social justice system. *Diversity* is defined in its broadest sense not only in terms of race, ethnicity, culture, language, gender, and other differences from the dominant culture but also, in terms of the diversity of opportunities in nursing. Thus, when faculty develops the philosophy, it must consider these factors and how the curriculum will meet society's diverse healthcare needs from entry-level graduates who function in all settings to those in advanced nursing roles in primary and tertiary care settings. Nursing care requires cultural consciousness (recognition, respect, tolerance) of differences among groups, while *cultural competence* denotes the knowledge and skills required for delivering care in cross-cultural situations.

The AACN (2020) issued a new white paper to support diversity, inclusion, and equity in admissions to nursing programs. Recommendations include the recruitment of students who reflect the populations they serve. They also include the following key areas for consideration:

- Adapting mission, vision, and value statements to champion diversity and inclusion
- Initiating systems redesign to support a shift in admission strategy
- Budgeting and fiscal considerations
- Staff and faculty development needs
- Best practices connected to student retention
- Using technology to enhance efficiency
- Utilizing nursing's centralized application service (NursingCAS) to support holistic admissions (AACN, 2021b)

THE HEALTHCARE SYSTEM

Knowledge of how the healthcare system is organized, financed, and regulated is essential for nurses to understand how it functions and nursing's role. Nurses must be prepared to provide leadership in the management of healthcare services and to address policy issues. The current organizational system of healthcare in the United States is in a state of flux owing to the pandemic and ongoing changes of the Affordable Care Act of 2010 (ACA; U.S. Department of Health and Human Services [HHS], 2020; HHS, Office of Civil Rights, 2021).

The COVID-19 pandemic taxed the U.S. healthcare system more than ever seen in modern history. The system often lacked the capacity, human resources, and equipment to provide quality patient care. Rationing of beds and lifesaving equipment while trying to provide equitable access to care were debated and ultimately implemented with each surge to preserve resources.

As a result of the 2020 election and the pandemic, the ACA once again faced challenges and revisions. As of February 2021, the HHS reports that 31 million people are enrolled in the ACA and Medicaid Expansion programs. Nurses must keep abreast of the changes in the healthcare system in order to advocate for people receiving services and to ensure safe and high-quality care. Curriculum planners, looking to the preparation of knowledgeable nursing professionals, should examine the history of the system for its implications on current and future healthcare services and provide the tools for political action in the healthcare arena.

DISEASE PREVENTION AND HEALTH PROMOTION

A primary resource when planning for a curriculum that includes population health, clinical prevention, and health promotion is the Healthy People Overview website (health.gov/healthypeople) that reviews the 10-year cycle agendas of the *Healthy People* from 2020 through 2030. *Healthy People 2030* launched August 18, 2020, and includes 355 core or measurable objectives (Office of Disease Prevention and Health Promotion, 2021). The high-priority health issues and actions indicated for 2030 are to promote population health, provide access to quality healthcare and services for all, and focus on individual and social determinants of health. In addition, *Healthy People 2030* offers how current objectives help the United States against future threats similar to COVID-19. Implications for nursing education come from the document and include the need for knowledge of epidemiology, population health, determinants of health, and disparities to achieve health equity for all groups.

The National Institute of Nursing Research's (NINRs, n.d.) strategic plan for 2022 to 2026 to address healthcare challenges through nursing research and provide a vision for the field of nursing science is currently under development. After a review of the literature, Ariosto et al. (2018) report a downward trend toward educating nursing students in population health. The authors suggest that acute and critical care are the focus of current preparation. They further assert a needed competency in population health for our future nurses to identify, analyze, and implement strategies for improving overall community well-being. During the recent pandemic, public/community health nurses assumed leadership roles and oversaw "safe and nondiscriminatory" care in our communities. These nurses are well versed in and prepared for responding to community crises, which supports the necessity for curriculum development or revision of this content in nursing education.

PATIENT SAFETY AND QUALITY HEALTHCARE

Patient safety and quality healthcare concepts are embedded in nursing knowledge and patient-centered clinical practice. Based on the recommendations of the IOM (2003) regarding patient safety, these concepts receive emphasis in the curricula of health professionals and the delivery of healthcare. In 2005, the AACN and the Robert Wood Johnson Foundation founded the Quality and Safety Education for Nurses (QSEN) Initiative with its goal to prepare nurses to improve patient safety and provide quality care in the healthcare system. The project continues to this day. The goal of the nationwide project is integrating the QSEN six core competencies into the curriculum to enhance patient safety and quality of care. For current information on the project, the QSEN website (qsen.org/competencies/pre-licensure-ksas/) provides information on competencies, learning modules, current conferences, and so forth.

Increased acuity levels and patients with complex physiologic and psychosocial challenges add to the challenges for providing safe and quality care. In addition, all these factors call for interdisciplinary collaboration to ensure a safe and compassionate healthcare environment. The Agency for Healthcare Research and Quality lists prevention quality indicators, inpatient quality indicators, patient safety indicators, and pediatric quality indicators on its website (www.qualityindicators.ahrq.gov).

INFORMATION SYSTEMS AND PATIENT CARE TECHNOLOGY

The integration and use of information systems and patient care technology are included in the AACN new *Essentials* (*Domain 8: Information and Healthcare Technologies*) document for baccalaureate, master's, and doctoral professional nursing education (AACN, 2021a). The domain descriptor states, "Information and communication technologies and informatics processes are used to provide care, gather data, form information to drive decision making, and support professionals as they expand knowledge and wisdom for practice. Informatics processes and technologies are used to manage and improve the delivery of safe, high quality, and efficient healthcare services in accordance with best practice and professional and regulatory standards" (AACN, 2021a, p. 11).

Information systems and patient care technology are crucial components to include in nursing curriculum in order to keep abreast of expanding developments in the field and their impact on the delivery of healthcare, research, scholarly activities, and teaching and learning modalities. It is important for faculty to be knowledgeable about and competent in these concepts and skills in order to integrate them into the curriculum and assist students in the application of informatics and technology.

Not only do technology and informatics apply to today's nursing practice and to students to gain nursing competencies in the care of clients, but they also serve as platforms for the delivery of nursing education programs such as web-based, hybrid, and web-enhanced courses. In the clinical setting, professionals and students use smartphones, patient information systems, computerized medical records, telemedicine/nursing, and high-tech devices for patient monitoring and care. Chapter 13 discusses in more detail informatics and technology as they apply to nursing education.

SCHOLARSHIP, RESEARCH, TRANSLATIONAL SCIENCE, AND EVIDENCE-BASED PRACTICES

Scholarship and Research

Scholarship and research provide the foundation for EBP. Both concepts appear in nursing curricula and are components for consideration by faculty when developing or revising the philosophy of the educational program. The new AACN *Essentials* (AACN, 2021a), include a domain-specific to the *Scholarship for Nursing Practice (Domain 4)*, which speaks to the "generation, synthesis, translation, application, and dissemination of nursing knowledge to improve health and transform health care" (p. 10).

Scholarship and research concepts begin at the associate degree level and continue in complexity to the PhD level, where new knowledge is tested and added to the body of scientific knowledge for the discipline. At the doctoral level, the AACN suggests in order for nurses to affect healthcare they must have educational preparation in leadership, teamwork, and scholarship. This skill set is essential in transforming healthcare.

Faculties identify the scholarship/research competencies expected of their graduates according to the level of the educational program and the practice areas or role functions expected of graduates to achieve. Associate degree programs may expect their graduates to understand the use of EBP, research-based nursing interventions and to challenge practices that lack data to support their use or result in quality patient outcomes. Each level of nursing thereafter should build on that basic understanding and culminate in critical evaluation and application of knowledge, up to and including participation in and dissemination of one's own scholarship.

Baccalaureate programs usually require a basic statistics course to support a nursing research course in the curriculum with expectations that graduates understand the research process so they can be discerning consumers of the research literature and use it to provide EBP. Writing assignments across the curriculum develop students' scholarly skills to review and analyze the literature in order to communicate professionally and apply evidence from the literature to practice. The use of a journal club is one way to help nursing students accomplish this task. Murrock (2020) found that implementing a journal club with undergraduate nursing students built confidence about their ability to review literature and its importance in directing nursing practice. Equally as important is faculty development for adapting teaching strategies that support students learning of the evolving demands on nursing practice in the healthcare system.

Most graduate nursing programs require graduate-level statistics and research in nursing as core courses. Depending on the nature of the institution and the degree purpose (administration, specialty advanced practice, nurse educator, informatics, etc.), the program usually has capstone options that include theses, scholarly projects, professional papers, or advanced practice projects. Some advanced practice programs include comprehensive examinations in addition to the written paper or sometimes as the only capstone requirement. Requiring a thesis at the master's level is decreasing; however, it can serve as a pathway to doctoral studies.

Both research-intensive (PhD) and applied practice (DNP) programs require supporting research and statistical analyses courses. Research-based doctoral dissertations synthesize knowledge of nursing science on a selected topic and generate new knowledge through quantitative, qualitative, or mixed-methods processes. The DNP is an applied professional/practice degree as described in the *AACN Position Statement on the Practice Doctorate in Nursing* (AACN, 2004). Depending on the institutional requirements, students may choose from a variety of options for their DNP project (e.g., translation of research, protocol development, program evaluation and intervention, community project, health promotion, etc.). DNP programs may require culminating projects that translate existing knowledge and research on a selected topic for the development of new, evidence-based strategies for advanced practice and/or their application to leadership roles that initiate change.

Translational Science

Translational science, also known as implementation science, is still a relatively new discipline in healthcare. This science applies to the analyses of research and current practice in order to apply these analyses to practice. Titler (2018) provides an introduction to translational science as a way of closing the gap between the evidence and practical use for improving patient and population health. This introduction provides defining and clarifying terms, theories, models, and implementation strategies to use in translational science. Multiple opportunities exist for students and graduates to advance the science and practice of nursing. The Titler article is useful, especially for program planners who are developing curricula for DNP programs.

Evidence-Based Practice

EBP, a systematic approach to improving patient outcomes, is the transformation of knowledge into clinically applicable care processes. Research and translational science are the base for EBP. Therefore, it is important for all levels of nursing education from undergraduate to graduate students to understand these concepts and discern between valid and reliable evidence-based nursing interventions and interventions that have no supportive data or rationale for their use. Mackey and Bassendowski (2017) trace the history of evidence-based nursing practice from the time of Florence Nightingale to the present. They review several definitions of EBP, and many versions are contained throughout the literature. The essential concepts of the practice include that it is research-based and nursing discipline–specific, reflects the entirety of nursing practice and research, applies to all levels of nursing education, is a problem-solving approach to clinical decision-making, utilizes the nurse's expertise, includes the patient's perspective, and operates within the context of caring. Its purpose is to ensure patient safety and quality of care, optimize patient outcomes, and improve clinical practice.

As with the research process, accordingly, the type of nursing education program directs the level of education for EBP. For example, Associate degree students have theory and clinical experiences that demonstrate the use of EBP. Baccalaureate students further this knowledge by raising questions related to practice and seeking answers through literature review. Master's students apply EBP in advanced roles, raise questions, and investigate current research to inform their practice. Students in applied practice (DNP) or professional doctoral programs (PhD, DNS) synthesize this knowledge and generate new interventions for EBP. Theory-based doctoral students study the domain of EBP and develop new knowledge related to its use and value.

CLINICAL JUDGMENT AND ITS APPLICATION TO NURSING

There is a mounting concern that new graduate nurses entering the workforce lack clinical judgment to practice safely. Developing clinical judgment comes from the combined mental processes of critical thinking and decision-making and is essential to the preparation of nurses. Clinical judgment is part of *The Essentials: Core Competencies for Professional Nursing Education* (AACN, 2021a) and thus should be integrated into the overall nursing curriculum.

Hensel and Billings (2020) recommend the use of a framework and multiple active learning strategies to assist students in developing clinical judgment. The National Council of State Boards of Nursing (2019) created the Clinical Judgment Measurement Model as a "framework for measuring clinical judgment and decision making within the setting of standardized, high-stakes examination" (www.ncsbn.org/14798.htm). The utilization of this framework combined with concept mapping, clinical scenarios, simulation, and on-site clinical shifts help student nurses develop clinical judgment and safe practice.

BELIEFS ABOUT TEACHING AND LEARNING PROCESSES

Beliefs about teaching and learning form the premise for the delivery of the nursing curriculum. Classroom lectures, clinical laboratory sessions, and clinical experiences in the real-life setting provided the traditional method for teaching. The emphasis was on teaching and the curriculum reflected that modality. In the last 5 to 10 years, with the focus on program outcomes and the advent of technology, the emphasis changed to learner-centered education. The role of the teacher, instead of a transmitter of knowledge, became a role of expert, mentor, and coach. The pandemic further transformed teaching and learning. Teaching strategies changed and attempted fostering of active student participation via new interactive platforms. Adaptation of typical learning activities required students to take on a more active role in their education instead of acting as passive receivers of knowledge. These changes require faculty to reexamine theories and principles of teaching and learning to guide, evaluate, and adapt to the learner characteristics and needs. Chapter 6 of this text reviews learning theories applicable to nursing education.

ORGANIZATIONAL FRAMEWORKS AND CONCEPT ANALYSIS AND MAPPING

Organizational Frameworks

Although accreditation is voluntary, most schools of nursing in the United States are accredited by a national organization, either the Accreditation Commission for Education in Nursing (ACEN, 2017/2020), the Commission on Collegiate Nursing Education (CCNE) or newly approved (May 25, 2021) the National League for Nursing Commission for Nursing Education Accreditation (NLN-CNEA). At one time, both the ACEN and the CCNE accrediting bodies required or implied that organizational frameworks were necessary to design the educational program's objectives, content, and instructional design. It was common for schools of nursing to use theoretical or conceptual models from nursing or other related disciplines as organizational frameworks. These frameworks served a useful purpose to place certain theories, concepts, content, and clinical learning experiences into the curriculum. While they are no longer explicitly required in the standards for accreditation, an implied curricular framework for both the ACEN (2020) and the CCNE (2018). The ACEN refers to professional standards and competencies while CCNE refers to the AACN *Essentials*. Many of the concepts listed under the discussion of the philosophy in this text are included in the accreditation standards for the curriculum, for example, social justice, population health, cultural diversity, patient safety, and quality healthcare.

Concept and/or Content Analysis/Mapping

The process of concept analysis or mapping is useful for ensuring that essential knowledge and skills are integrated into the curriculum. Concept mapping is a detailed analysis of a concept and its relationships within the curriculum that is depicted in a map with arrows signifying relationships. It should include the expected competencies for student achievement as well as the places in the curriculum where the concept is introduced, built on, and mastered. Concept mapping serves as a teaching and learning strategy to promote the development of critical thinking and problem-solving at all levels of nursing education.

Fowler et al. (2018) provide an example of a clinical curriculum mapping for their MSN and DNP program. The faculty identified that this process provided an "organized and consistent" way to ensure the teaching of essential content throughout the program. The process helped faculty understand the curriculum and plan for its implementation. The process of curriculum mapping helps identify where critical elements and concepts occur and at what level, eliminating redundancy or possible omission of essential content. Figure 5.1 presents a sample concept map for IPE collaboration in a baccalaureate program.

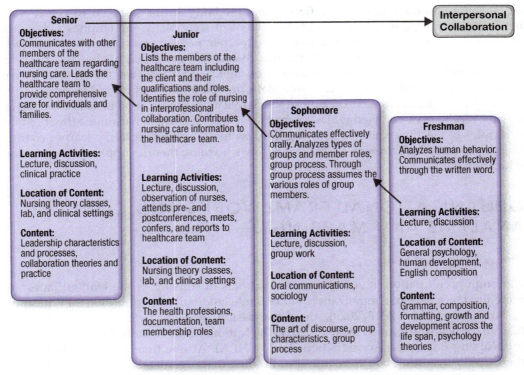

Figure 5.1 Concept map for IPE collaboration at the BSN level.

Source: Keating, S. B. (2018). The classic components of the curriculum: Developing a curriculum plan. In S. B. Keating & S. S. DeBoor (Eds.), Curriculum development and evaluation in nursing education (4th ed., pp. 81–106). Springer Publishing Company.

IMPLEMENTATION OF THE CURRICULUM

Overall Purpose and Goal of the Program

After the philosophy, mission, vision, and organizing framework/concept analysis are developed, the next logical step in curriculum development is to state the overall purpose or goal of the program. Developers must consider accountability issues that relate to graduates' competencies in meeting the healthcare systems' demands and the healthcare needs of the people they serve. Faculty must grapple with these issues as it develops statements on the purpose of the nursing program and the overall long-term goal for graduates. Whether the statement becomes global and idealistic or specific and stated in measurable terms depends on the faculty's philosophy, values, and beliefs and subsequent statements and objectives that specify the graduates' learning outcomes. Examples of concepts include statements on caring, health promotion, and other types of nursing interventions; client systems; professional behaviors and competencies; and the healthcare system. Characteristics of the graduate that are unique to the specific school of nursing can be included (e.g., "a caring, compassionate healthcare provider").

The type of nursing education program influences the overall program purpose or goal statement. Levels of clinical competence and knowledge acquisition will differ among licensed practical/vocational nursing, diploma, associate degree, baccalaureate, master's, and doctoral programs. Programs with multiple layers of preparation, including undergraduate and graduate education usually have a global statement of purpose with each program, adapting that statement to meet its specific level of education. Although the statements of purpose and overall goal can be succinct, they act as the guides for the end-of-program objectives/SLOs.

STUDENT-LEARNING OR END-OF-PROGRAM AND LEVEL OBJECTIVES

As reiterated throughout this chapter, nursing programs must demonstrate that they meet the overall program mission, purpose, and goal. SLOs, or end-of-program objectives, reflect the conceptual framework and define the specific expectations or competencies of graduates upon completion of the nursing program. In order to reach these objectives, intermediate-level or semester objectives are developed in sequential order. Such as in a 2-year associate degree program, there are end-of-first-year and end-of-second-year expectations, all of which lead to the end-of-program objectives. In a baccalaureate program, there may be freshman-, sophomore-, junior-, and senior-level objectives. Some programs prefer to divide the objectives into semesters and could be titled in that fashion, that is, first semester, second semester, third semester, and so on. Graduate programs may indicate junior or senior levels, semester levels, first year and second year, doctoral candidate, and so forth.

Chapter 7 of the text provides an overview of the educational taxonomies such as the classics developed by Bloom (1956). These taxonomies categorize domains of learning and provide guidelines for writing objectives related to the domains. The major domains are cognitive, affective, psychomotor, and behavioral. Furthermore, these domains are divided into levels of development and difficulty. For example, in nursing, the psychomotor skill of measuring blood pressure moves from recognition of the blood pressure measurement tools to mastery of the skill. At the same time, the student is utilizing the cognitive domain by first recalling the physiology of blood pressure and identifying the norms for blood pressure. The student continues to comprehend, apply, analyze, synthesize, and evaluate knowledge that results in nursing diagnoses and actions such as referral of clients for management of abnormal findings, teaching clients how to manage hyper- and hypotension or, in the case of the advanced practitioner, prescribing interventions to control hypertension.

The classic taxonomies assist in the development of end-of-program, level (intermediate), and course objectives. To develop or assess end-of-program objectives, the first task is to look at the program mission, purpose, and overall goal. Faculty members discuss what they expect of their graduates at the end of the program to meet the overall goal. A list of these expectations is developed into end-of-program objectives, which are analyzed for their specificity to meet the overall goal and the selected organizing or conceptual framework of the curriculum. To illustrate, if the program chooses the new AACN *Essentials* (AACN, 2021a) to guide the curriculum, the specific end-of-program outcome or SLO based on *Domain 3: Population Health* would state "Apply knowledge of population health factors to the care of diverse populations for the improvement of health outcomes." From that SLO, concept analysis would link it through the various levels of the curriculum with a junior-level objective stating "Analyze population health factors affecting the care of diverse populations" and, at the sophomore level, "Identify population health factors that affect the care of diverse populations." Content related to these concepts would be listed under the objectives and learning activities described in order to achieve each level objective. All levels of objectives provide the guidelines for planning, implementing, and evaluating the curriculum.

Level or semester objectives follow the same pattern as the SLOs. Faculty reviews each level for the progression of objectives toward the end-of-program objectives. Some programs start from basic knowledge and skills at the first level or semester to the complex knowledge and skills expected at the senior level of the program. Other programs expect the mastery of specific knowledge and skills earlier in the program that are reinforced throughout the program and practiced after graduation. Still other programs use a combination of both. Decisions on the patterns of progression depend on the philosophy and organizational framework or concept analysis, including the developmental stage of the learner. Documenting these decisions with a rationale for their placement in the curriculum provides aid in future evaluations of the curriculum, total quality management of the program, and accreditation reports.

PROGRAM OF STUDY

The overall goal, SLOs, level objectives, and organizing framework serve as a master plan for placing content into the curriculum and developing a program of study. Faculty are responsible for developing the curriculum plan and revising it periodically as needed. Developers examine the program prerequisites for their logical location in the curriculum. Prerequisites for prelicensure nursing programs include the liberal arts; social, physical, and biologic sciences; communications; mathematics; and other general educational requirements.

Graduate nursing programs require a baccalaureate in nursing or an associate degree in nursing and a baccalaureate in another discipline, unless a master's entry program. The same principles apply to nursing or other disciplines' doctorate programs. Each doctorate program prescribes the courses or degree work necessary to meet the equivalent of its lower degree requirements.

Once the prerequisites are completed, the nursing curriculum plan has a progressive order for sequencing nursing courses. For example, a Nursing 101–Fundamentals of Nursing course is a prerequisite for Nursing 102–Nursing Care of the Older Adult. and Nursing 501–Nursing Research is the prerequisite for Nursing 502–Master's Scholarly Project. Corequisites are courses that can be taught simultaneously and are complementary, for example, N301–Health Promotion of Children and Adolescents and N303–Nursing Care of Children and Adolescents. Again, the placement of courses depends on the curricular framework with the course objectives and content leading toward the achievement of level objectives and, eventually, the program outcomes.

The numbers of units or credits are assigned to each course keeping in mind the total allotted to the major. For associate-degree nursing programs, nursing credits average five 3-credit courses, or 15 credits, per semester with total degree requirements averaging 60 to 72 credits. It should be noted that some programs operate on quarter credits or units that are usually 10 weeks in length as contrasted to the usual spring and fall semester length of 15 to 16 weeks with a 13- to 14-week summer semester. In that case, one-quarter credit or unit is equivalent to two thirds of a semester credit or unit.

Baccalaureate programs average a total of 120 to 130 credits for the degree. The master's in nursing program ranges from 30 to 60 or more total credits depending on the nature of the program, with advanced practice roles requiring a higher number of credits. Owing to the wide range of nursing credits and the many credits required for advanced practice at the master's level, the profession is moving toward advanced practice degrees at the doctoral level. The majority of master's and doctorate degree credits are in the nursing major with only a few, if any, from other disciplines or electives.

Content experts serve as guides for nursing course placements and once the courses have been placed in a logical sequence, the course descriptions are written, usually by the content expert or the person who will serve as the "faculty of record" (in charge of the course). For instance, the content expert for the course Nursing Care of Children and Adolescents would probably be a faculty member who is a clinical expert, certified as a CNS or nurse practitioner in pediatrics. Course descriptions are brief paragraphs with several comprehensive statements that provide an overview of the content of the course. They do not contain student-centered objectives.

Course objectives follow the course description and are learner-centered, based on the content of the course, their place in the curriculum plan, relationship to the level and end-of-program objectives, and relevance to the organizational framework. Finally, an outline of the course content is listed and should be tied to the objectives of the course. A course schedule is usually included and tied to the content outline. See Exhibit 5.1 for a classic outline of components for a course syllabus.

All these components are subject to faculty approval as well as the parent institution. Once established, faculty members who are assigned to courses have the freedom to rearrange or update the content and to teach the courses in their preferred method. However, changes to the course title, credits, objectives, or descriptions must undergo the same approval processes as the original courses. Although this may appear stifling to academic freedom, it ensures the integrity of the curriculum.

Usually, new or revised course descriptions, objectives, and content outlines are presented to the program's curriculum committee for recommendations and approval, submitted to the total faculty for approval, and continue through the appropriate channels of the parent institution for final formal approval. Because of the many layers of approval, faculty members must be mindful of the initial proposals so that they will not need frequent revision, as any changes to course titles, credits, descriptions, number of credits, and objectives are subject to the same review processes.

EXHIBIT 5.1: The Major Components of a Syllabus

Parent Institution Logo

School of Nursing

Type of Program

Course # and Title

Course Description:

Credits:

Pre- or Corequisites:

(continued)

EXHIBIT 5.1: The Major Components of a Syllabus (*continued*)

Class Type: (lecture, seminar, laboratory, practicum)

Faculty Information:

Office Hours:

Required and Recommended Texts:

Course Objectives:

University/College Core Objective or Requirement Statement (e.g., Technology, Diversity, Ethics)

Teaching and Learning Strategies: (include teacher and student expectations)

Attendance and Participation Requirements:

Evaluation Methods:

Assignments:

Course Content and Weekly Schedule:

University/College Statements that may include;

Academic Dishonesty Statement:

Disability Statement:

Surreptitious Recording of Course Content

ADA Compliance Statement:

Title IX Statement:

TABLE 5.1: Guidelines for Assessing the Key Components of a Curriculum or Educational Program

Components	Questions for Data Collection	Desired Outcomes
Mission	What are the major elements of the parent institution and subdivision (if applicable) missions? Are these major elements in the nursing mission? If not, give a rationale as to why. How does the nursing mission speak to its teaching, service, and research/scholarship roles?	The nursing mission is congruent with that of its parent institution and, if applicable, the academic subdivision in which it is located. The mission reflects nursing's teaching, service, and research/scholarship role.
Philosophy	Is the nursing philosophy congruent with that of the parent institution philosophy and subdivision (if applicable)? If not, give the rationale as to why it is not. What statements in the philosophy relate to the faculty's beliefs and values about teaching and learning, critical thinking, liberal arts and the sciences, the healthcare system, prevention	The philosophy statement is congruent with that of the parent institution and academic subdivision (if applicable). The philosophy reflects the faculty's beliefs and values on teaching and learning, critical thinking, etc.

(continued)

TABLE 5.1: Guidelines for Assessing the Key Components of a Curriculum or Educational Program (*continued*)

Components	Questions for Data Collection	Desired Outcomes
	of disease and promotion of health, interprofessional collaboration, diversity and cultural competence, social justice, scholarship, research and evidence-based practice, information systems and technology, quality healthcare, and patient safety?	
Organizing Frameworks/ Concept Analysis/ Mapping	What is the organizing framework or content map for the curriculum and how does it reflect the mission and philosophy statements? To what extent does the framework or content map appear throughout the implementation of the curriculum? Are the concepts/content readily identified in all the tracks of the programs?	The curriculum has an organizing framework or content map that reflects its mission and philosophy. The concepts of the organizing framework or content map are readily identified in all tracks of the nursing education program.
Overall Purpose and Goal of the Program	Does the overall goal or purpose statement reflect the mission, philosophy, and organizing framework or concept map? Is the statement broad enough to encompass all tracks of the nursing program? Does the statement lead to the measurement of program outcomes?	The overall goal or purpose statement reflects that of the mission, philosophy, and organizing framework. The overall goal or purpose includes all tracks of the nursing program. The overall goal or purpose is stated in such a way that it is a guide for measuring outcomes of the program (program review).
Student-Learning Outcomes or End-of-Program and Level Objectives	Are the mission, overall goal or purpose, and organizational framework reflected in the objectives? Are the objectives arranged in logical and sequential order? Is each objective learner-centered, and does it include the content, expected level of behavior of the learner, feasibility, and time frame?	The objectives reflect the mission, overall purpose or goal, and organizing framework. The objectives are sequential and logical. The objective statements are learner-centered and include the content, expected learner behavior and at what level, feasibility, and time frame.
Implementation Plan	Does the curriculum plan reflect the organizing framework or concept map, overall goal, end-of-program, and level objectives? Is there documentation of approval of the curriculum plan in the permanent records?	The implementation plan for the curriculum reflects the organizing framework, overall goal or purpose, end-of-program and level objectives. The curriculum plan and its prerequisites and courses have the approval of the appropriate governing bodies.

(continued)

TABLE 5.1: Guidelines for Assessing the Key Components of a Curriculum or Educational Program (*continued*)

Components	Questions for Data Collection	Desired Outcomes
	Does each track in the program have a curriculum plan that includes course descriptions, credits, pre- and corequisites, objectives, and content outlines?	The implementation plan for each track includes all courses and credits, pre- or corequisites, descriptions, objectives, and content outlines.
Summary	Has each component of the curriculum been addressed? Is each component congruent with those of the parent institution? If not congruent, has the rationale for incongruence been addressed? Are the components of the curriculum listed and do they flow in a logical and sequential order? Does the implementation plan flow from the overall goal, student-learning objectives (SLOs), end-of-program objectives, and level objectives? Is the implementation plan congruent with the organizing framework or concept map? Is the curriculum relevant to current and future nursing practice demands and needs for nurses?	Based on an analysis of the curriculum, each component is addressed. The curriculum components are congruent with the parent institution and with each other. The components flow in a logical and sequential order. The implementation plan flows from the overall goal, SLOs, and level objectives. The implementation plan is congruent with the organizing framework or concept map. The curriculum reflects relevance to current nursing practice demands and the need for nurses and projected future changes in the healthcare system.

Source: Keating, S. B. (2018). The classic components of the curriculum: Developing a curriculum plan. In S. B. Keating & S. S. DeBoor (Eds.), Curriculum development and evaluation in nursing education (4th ed., pp. 81–106). Springer Publishing Company.

SUMMARY

This chapter reviewed the components of the curriculum and the processes faculty members undergo in developing or revising curricula. Assessing and revising (if necessary) each component of the curriculum in logical sequence helps maintain its integrity and ensure its quality. Faculty members are experts in their discipline and are, therefore, responsible for ensuring that essential knowledge, as well as the latest breakthroughs in its science, is in the curriculum. Curriculum development and revision processes must be based on information from evaluation activities; the latest changes in the profession, healthcare, and society; and forecasts for the future. Table 5.1 provides guidelines for assessing the key components of a curriculum or educational program.

END-OF-CHAPTER RESOURCES

DISCUSSION QUESTIONS

1. Which component or components of the curriculum do you believe have the most impact on the implementation of the curriculum?

2. In which ways do you believe curriculum mapping or organizational frameworks serve to ensure the quality of the educational program? Give an example of an organizational framework that illustrates your belief.

3. Why do you agree or disagree with the principle of faculty control of the curriculum?

LEARNING ACTIVITIES

Student-Learning Activities

1. Using Table 5.1, assess the educational program in which you are enrolled for the components of the curriculum. Are they easily identified? What resources do you need to locate them?

2. Attend one or more curriculum committee meetings and identify which of the components of the curriculum are addressed. Observe faculty members' interactions, their commitment to curriculum development and evaluation, and the role they play in developing or revising the curriculum. Note evidence of the routes of approval for any changes to the curriculum.

Faculty Development Activities

1. Using Table 5.1, assess the educational program in which you teach for the components of the curriculum. Are they easily identified? What resources do you need to locate them?

2. When you attend the next curriculum committee meeting, identify which of the components of the curriculum are addressed. Observe faculty members' interactions, their commitment to curriculum development and evaluation, and the role they play in developing or revising the curriculum. Note evidence of the routes of approval for any changes to the curriculum.

 A robust set of instructor resources designed to supplement this text is located at **http://connect.springerpub.com/content/book/978-0-8261-8686-7.** Qualifying instructors may request access by emailing **textbook@springerpub.com.**

REFERENCES

Accreditation Commission for Education in Nursing. (2017, edited July 2020). *ACEN accreditation manual. 2017 standards and criteria.* https://www.acenursing.org/acen-accreditation-manual/

American Association of Colleges of Nursing. (2004). *AACN position statement on the practice doctorate in nursing.* https://www.aacnnursing.org/Portals/42/News/Position-Statements/DNP.pdf

American Association of Colleges of Nursing. (2020). *Promising practices in holistic admissions review: Implementation in Academic nursing*. https://www.aacnnursing.org/Portals/42/News/White-Papers/AACN-White-Paper-Promising-Practices-in-Holistic-Admissions-Review-December-2020.pdf

American Association of Colleges of Nursing. (2021a). *The essentials: Core competencies for professional nursing education*. https://www.aacnnursing.org/Portals/42/AcademicNursing/pdf/Essentials-2021.pdf

American Association of Colleges of Nursing. (2021b). *AACN issues new white paper to support diversity and inclusion efforts*. https://www.aacnnursing.org/News-Information/Press-Releases/View/ArticleId/24743/white-paper-diversity-inclusion

American Nurses Association. (2009). *Essentials of genetic and genomic nursing: Competencies, curricula guidelines, and outcome indicators* (2nd ed.). https://www.genome.gov/pages/careers/healthprofessionaleducation/geneticscompetency.pdf

American Nurses Association. (2015). *Code of ethics for nurses with interpretive statements*.

Ariosto, D. A., Harper, E. M., Wilson, M. L., Hull, S. C., Nahm, E.-S., & Sylvia, M. L. (2018). Population health: A nursing action plan. *Journal of the American Medical Informatics Association, 1*(1), 7–10. https://doi.org/10.1093/jamiaopen/ooy003

Arthur, J., Kristtjansson, K., & Vogler, C. (2021). Seeking the common good in education through a positive conception of social justice. *British Journal of Educational Studies, 69*(1), 101–117. https://doi.org/10.1080/00071005.2020.1724259

Bloom, B. S. (Ed.). (1956). Taxonomy of educational objectives: Handbook I, cognitive domain. D. McKay.

Booth, T. (2020, March). Creating a culture of civility in academic nursing [Poster]. Sigma Theta Tau International and National League of Nursing, Nursing Education Research Conference 2020: Transforming Nursing Education Through Evidence Generation and Translation, Washington, DC, USA. https://sigma.nursingrepository.org/bitstream/handle/10755/20185/Booth_Poster.pdf?sequence=1&isAllowed=y

Carnegie Classification of Institutions of Higher Education. (2018). *Basic classification description*. http://carnegieclassifications.iu.edu/classification_descriptions/basic.php

Carter Kooken, W., & Kerr, N. (2018). Blending the liberal arts and nursing: Creating a portrait for the 21st century. *Journal of Professional Nursing, 34*(1), 60–64. https://doi.org/10.1016/j.profnurs.2017.07.002

Commission on Collegiate Nursing Education. (2018). *Standards for accreditation of baccalaureate and graduate nursing programs*. https://www.aacnnursing.org/Portals/42/CCNE/PDF/Standards-Final-2018.pdf

Epstein, B., & Turner, M. (2015). The nursing code of ethics: Its value, its history. *Online Journal of Issues in Nursing, 20*(2), Manuscript 4. https://doi.org/10.3912/OJIN.Vol20No02Man04

Fosnatch, K., & Broderick, C. (2020). An overlooked factor? How religion and spirituality influence student's perception of the campus environment. *Journal of College and Character, 21*(3), 186–203. https://doi.org/10.1080/2194587X.2020.1781660

Fowler, T., Conner, R., & Smith, W. (2018). Master of Science in nursing and doctor of nursing practice clinical curriculum map. *Journal of Nursing Education, 57*(7), 440–445. https://doi.org/10.3928/01484834-20180618-11

Gazzardo, M. T., Kohsla, N., Adams, A. L., Bussmann, J. D., Engleman, A., Ingraham, N., Gamba, R., Jones-Bey, A., Moore, M. D., Toosi, N. R., & Taylor, S. (2021). "The ones that care make all the difference": Perspectives on student-faculty relationships. *Innovative Higher Education, 46*, 41–58. https://doi.org/10.1007/s10755-020-09522-w

Hensel, D., & Billings, D. M. (2020). Strategies to teach the National Council of State Boards of Nursing clinical judgment model. *Nurse Educator, 45*(3), 12/-132. https://doi.org/10.1097/NNE.0000000000000773

Institute of Medicine. (2003). *Health professions education: A bridge to quality*. National Academies Press.

Keating, S. B. (2018). The classic components of the curriculum: Developing a curriculum plan. In S. B. Keating & S. S. DeBoor (Eds.), *Curriculum development and evaluation in nursing education* (4th ed., pp. 81–106). Springer.

Langegård, U., Kiani, K., Nielsen, S. J., & Svensson, P-A. (2021). Nursing students' experiences of a pedagogical transition from campus learning to distance learning using digital tools. *BMC Nursing, 20*(23), 2–10. https://doi.org/10.1186/s12912-021-00542-1

Mackey, A., & Bassendowski, S. (2017). The history of evidence-based practice in nursing education and practice. *Journal of Professional Nursing, 33*(1), 51–55. https://doi.org/10.1016/j.profnurs.2016.05.009

Murrock, C. (2020). Building scholarship for evidence-based practice in undergraduate nursing students. *Nursing Education Perspectives, 41*(5). E45–E46. https://doi.org/10.1097/01.NEP.0000000000000612

National Academy of Medicine. (2021). *The future of nursing 2020–2030: Charting a path to achieve health equity. A consensus study from the national academy of medicine.* https://nam.edu/publications/the-future-of-nursing-2020-2030/

National Council of State Boards of Nursing. (2019). *NCSBN clinical judgment measurement model.* https://www.ncsbn.org/14798.htm

National Institute of Nursing Research. (n.d.). *Mission and strategic plan. NINR strategic plan 9(2022–2026) under development.* https://www.ninr.nih.gov/aboutninr/ninr-mission-and-strategic-plan

National League for Nursing. (2019). *Faculty census survey 2018–2019.* http://www.nln.org/newsroom/nursing-education-statistics/nln-faculty-census-survey-2018-2019

National League for Nursing. (2021). *Interprofessional collaboration in education and practice: A living document from the National League for Nursing* (2015). http://www.nln.org/professional-development-programs/teaching-resources/interprofessional-education-(ipe)

Office of Disease Prevention and Health Promotion. (2021). *Healthy people 2030. Building a healthier future for all.* https://health.gov/healthypeople

Omics Nursing Science & Education Network. (2021). *ONSEN resources.* https://omicsnursingnetwork.net/

Schimek, G. P. (2016). Visual expression of liberal education mission (Order No. 10137976). Available from ProQuest dissertations & theses global: The humanities and social sciences collection. (1820073299). https://search.proquest.com/docview/1820073299?accountid=13802

Seibert, D. (2020). Genomics in nursing education. *Journal of the American Association of Nurse Practitioners, 32*(12), 785–787. https://doi.org/10.1097/JXX.0000000000000529

Stamps, D. C. (2021). Nursing leadership must confront implicit bias as a barrier to diversity in health care today. *Nurse Leader.* Advanced online publication. https://doi.org/10.1016/j.mnl.2021.02.004

Titler, M. G. (2018, May). Translation research in practice: An introduction. *The Online Journal of Issues in Nursing, 23*(2), Manuscript 1. https://ojin.nursingworld.org/

Tyre, M. (2020, September). Building the brand: How the physical campus shapes student experience (even during a pandemic). *New England Journal of Higher Education.* https://nebhe.org/journal/building-the-brand-how-the-physical-campus-shapes-student-experience-even-during-a-pandemic/

U.S. Department of Health and Human Services. (2021, March last reviewed). *About the affordable care act.* https://www.hhs.gov/healthcare/about-the-law/index.html

U.S. Department of Health and Human Services. Office of Civil Rights. (2020). *Fact sheet: HHS finalizes ACA section 1557 rule.* https://www.hhs.gov/sites/default/files/1557-final-rule-factsheet.pdf

Wentworth, K. M., Dorfman, L., & Taddeo, J. (2020). Reactions of nursing students when faced with violations of the American Nurses Association Code of Ethics. *Nursing Education Perspectives, 41*(6), 364–366. https://doi.org/10.1097/01.NEP.0000000000000580

Woodward, B., Smart, D., & Benavides-Vaello, S. (2016). Modifiable factors that support political preparation by nurses. *Journal of Professional Nursing, 22*(1), 54–61. https://doi.org/10.1016/j.profnurs.2015.06.005

CHAPTER 6

Implementation of the Curriculum

Heidi A. Mennenga

CHAPTER OBJECTIVES

Upon completion of Chapter 6, the reader will be able to:

- Analyze the application of learning theories for implementing the curriculum.
- Compare learner-focused instructional strategies.
- Correlate student evaluation to the mission and goals of the curriculum.

OVERVIEW

When planning a newly developed curriculum or a major curriculum revision, educators must address many aspects of actual implementation: When will the curriculum be implemented? How will faculty members, stakeholders, and students be informed of the plan for curriculum implementation? What are the logistics of curriculum implementation that need to be addressed? Other questions may be posed if an existing curriculum is being replaced: How will the existing curriculum be phased out? How will the change impact faculty workloads and scheduling? Beyond the logistical details of curriculum implementation, educators need to consider the foundational questions of the curriculum. What are faculty member beliefs in how students learn? What is the role of the faculty member and the student? How do faculty members best facilitate student learning? What instructional strategies will be utilized in the delivery of the curriculum? How will student learning be evaluated? How does the philosophical foundation of the curriculum impact the mission, goals, and outcomes of the program?

As faculty members consider these questions, often the task of implementing the curriculum can seem overwhelming. However, many of these decisions can be supported by having early conversations and discussions regarding the philosophical underpinnings that provide the foundation of the curriculum. Making a decision about a strong theoretical foundation for learning cannot be overemphasized as it allows faculty to provide a consistent rationale for decision-making as the curriculum planning and implementation process moves forward (Dennick, 2012). The theoretical foundation provides the basis and the rationale for many other decisions, including specific instructional strategies that will be used. As educators transition from utilizing primarily teacher-centered instructional methods to more student-centered active learning strategies, this foundation may be necessary to convince hesitant faculty members to attempt new evidence-based instructional strategies to aid in achieving the mission, goals, and outcomes of the program. Furthermore, how students are evaluated needs to be discussed and adapted to be relevant to the selected instructional strategies.

For the purpose of this chapter, the following learning theories are briefly reviewed: behaviorist learning theory, cognitive learning theory, constructivist learning theory, humanistic learning theory, adult learning theory, brain-based learning, deep learning, and multiple intelligences. This chapter concludes with an overview of learner-focused instructional strategies and student evaluation.

DEFINITION OF LEARNING

To start at the beginning, we must consider the definition of *learning*. Many definitions of *learning* exist and may vary depending on the theoretical viewpoint (Frey & Popkess, 2020). One simplified definition of learning describes it as merely "a change in behavior (knowledge, attitudes, and/or skills) that can be observed or measured and that occurs… as a result of exposure to environmental stimuli" (Bastable & Alt, 2019, p. 15). Some experts, such as Crow and Crow (1963), assert that learning does not occur that simply or as a result of environment only :

> Learning involves change. It is concerned with the acquisition of habits, knowledge, and attitudes. It enables the individual to make both personal and social adjustments. Since the concept of change is inherent in the concept of learning, any change in behavior implies that learning is taking place or has taken place. Learning that occurs during the process of change can be referred to as the learning process. (p. 1)

LEARNING THEORIES

Learning theories, which provide the philosophical foundation for the curriculum, attempt to describe, explain, or anticipate how learning occurs (Braungart et al., 2019). Learning theories provide a systematic approach to curriculum planning and implementation and allow for consistency among broader program outcomes and, more narrowly, among course outcomes. Ideally, all aspects of the curriculum should be driven by an intended philosophical base that serves as the foundation of the curriculum. This decision, like many in curriculum planning, should involve all faculty members as the learning theory can provide the basis for the teaching process and direct which instructional strategies and, therefore, which evaluation methods are utilized by faculty members. As educators see more diverse learners, additional instructional strategies and sources of evaluation may be indicated in the classroom (Hunt, 2012).

Although the select learning theories discussed in this chapter are presented separately, educators should keep in mind that they are not limited to a single learning theory but, rather, may draw from several models simultaneously to inform their teaching practice. Each has its own benefits and perspectives of the teaching and learning process, which are discussed. Whichever theory or theories are selected, a clear reflection of viewpoints about the process of teaching, learning, and the internal and external influences of the educational environment should be provided (Sullivan, 2020).

As each learning theory is discussed, the reader is encouraged to consider the following questions:

◆ What influences individual learning?
◆ What is the educator's role in learning ("sage on the stage" or facilitator)?
◆ What is the learner's role in learning (passive or active)?
◆ How does the process of learning occur?

Behaviorist Learning Theory

Behavioral learning theories are based on the general assertion that behavior is learned and can be molded and rewarded to achieve desirable outcomes. Behaviorist learning theory emphasizes that behaviors, not thoughts or emotions of the learner, affect the consequences (Candela, 2020). Change in behavior occurs as a result of a stimulus or response (Warburton et al., 2016). The emphasis of learning is on the environmental stimuli versus the learner's internal thinking process. The behavior (generally a desirable behavior) is repeated when reinforcement occurs and the learner begins to form associations with either positive or negative stimuli that occur in new situations (Braungart et al., 2019; Candela, 2020).

In education, behaviorism is illustrated by including behavioral student-learning outcomes that are measurable and observable. Students are aware of what they are expected to accomplish through these outcomes (Candela, 2020). In the teaching–learning process, behaviorism focuses on the faculty member as the facilitator who is responsible for designing the learning experiences and providing ongoing feedback to the student. In this theory, the role of the educator is to provide a stimulus, manipulate the environment, and merely transfer the information to the student. The student is thereby a passive recipient of the knowledge (Aliakbari et al., 2015).

Behaviorist learning theory focuses on the notion of simple to complex when planning a curriculum. It includes positive reinforcement and rewards for achieving behavioral outcomes. Continual reinforcement with positive feedback produces desirable outcomes (Candela, 2020). Critical thinking is also a key component of this learning theory, requiring the learner to sometimes practice "trial and error" to achieve the desired outcomes (Aliakbari et al., 2015).

Behaviorism occurs in the classroom or clinical settings when rewards or punishments are offered in response to desirable or undesirable behaviors. For example, the educator offering praise or positive responses may reinforce students' likelihood of answering questions in class (Braungart et al., 2019). Conversely, the educator may set up a behavioral modification contract to change behaviors for a student who is not performing well in the clinical setting. Behavioral learning theories are easy to understand and are typically used in conjunction with other learning theories. However, a main criticism is that it is a teacher-centered learning theory and may be outdated in today's student-centered learning environment.

Cognitive Learning Theory

Cognitive learning theory focuses on learning as an internal process including thinking, understanding, information organizing, and consciousness (Aliakbari et al., 2015). Cognitive learning theories explore the deeper aspect of learning, including how information is processed and the role of memory (Warburton et al., 2016). This theory proposes that behavior does not immediately change as a result of learning. Rather, students are equipped with the skills to question and problem solve; thus, they are able to actively learn, solve, and search for new information. They focus on past experiences to inform better understanding (Aliakbari et al., 2015).

In education, cognitivism focuses on helping students develop the skills to think, not simply the transfer of knowledge. In the teaching–learning process, cognitivism focuses on the student as an active participant rather than a passive participant; however, the faculty member still maintains a majority of control over the learning process (Candela, 2020; Warburton et al., 2016). This learning theory supports many strategies for improving understanding and fostering memory and aligns well with the inquiry and analysis that occur in nursing classrooms.

Constructivist Learning Theory

Constructivist learning theories assert that learners create new knowledge when they base it on existing knowledge while attempting to find meaning in their experiences (Candela, 2020; Warburton et al., 2016). Social learning theory, sociocultural learning, and situated learning are examples of constructivist learning theories (Candela, 2020). In the teaching–learning process, faculty members assist students in learning how to become "expert learners." That is, faculty members provide encouragement to students to assess how their learning experiences or activities help them understand. This process of self-assessment helps students understand how they learn best (Brandon & All, 2010). Constructivism is viewed as a student-centered learning theory because of the emphasis on students' control over learning (Warburton et al., 2016). Learning is an active process in which the faculty member coaches and facilitates the learning of the student (Wittmann-Price & Price, 2019).

Specifically, social learning theory emphasizes the active information process that occurs during learning. Students learn by observing role models (Candela, 2020). In social learning theory, students are able to observe others, observe the outcomes they achieve or do not achieve, and then determine whether they want to emulate that behavior. This process includes four key phases: attention, retention, reproduction, and motivation. Attention requires students to identify whom they want to observe as their model; retention occurs when students observe the behavior and the outcomes; reproduction occurs when students are able to mimic the behaviors; and motivation occurs when students decide whether or not to continue the behavior based on the response they received (Warburton et al., 2016). Common teaching strategies such as simulation, clinical experiences, and role-play are often used with social learning theory as a framework (Candela, 2020).

Sociocultural learning emphasizes that learning occurs during social interaction. Students gain the ability to do some skills or tasks independently, but they must rely on others to help with other skills or tasks. As they gain knowledge, they need less and less assistance from others, eventually achieving mastery of the skill or task (Candela, 2020).

Situated learning occurs in "real-life" situations provided by educators in the academic setting, often through the use of simulation or case studies. Students use these situations to enhance their learning and development of the skills needed in the real world (Candela, 2020).

Humanistic Learning Theory

Humanistic learning theory focuses on feelings and emotions with the idea that learning is an individual process (Warburton et al., 2016). There are several assumptions about learners in humanistic learning theory, including that they are motivated to learn, they are establishing and meeting their own set of goals, and ultimately, they will achieve self-actualization (Candela, 2020).

In education, humanism emphasizes the affective aspects of learning. Caring, individual worth, and autonomy are valued in the humanistic learning theory. Faculty members are facilitators in the learning process and role models, demonstrating values, such as caring and empathy (Candela, 2020; Warburton et al., 2016). Students are in control of the learning process, are accountable for their learning, and determine their own goals and needs (Candela, 2020; Warburton et al., 2016).

Adult Learning Theory

Classified as a cognitive development theory, the adult learning theory asserts that adults are self-directed and will learn information that is useful and relevant to them.

Additionally, adults bring their own knowledge based on their life experiences and, generally, like to be actively involved in their learning. In the teaching–learning process, students are actively involved in the process and are accountable for their own learning. Students may also provide self-reflection regarding their progress. Educators, therefore, provide assistance to learning but work collaboratively with students in planning course information and experiences (Candela, 2020).

Brain-Based Learning, Deep Learning, and Multiple Intelligences

More recent learning theories focus on the idea that the brain continues to develop and change throughout life and, often, as a result of learning. These learning theories include brain-based learning, deep learning, and multiple intelligences. Although thoroughly discussing all these is not within the scope of this chapter, an overview is included. Brain-based learning asserts that learning can be enhanced by creating conditions under which the brain learns best. These conditions may include relaxed alertness, where the environment is challenging yet nonthreatening; immersion in complex, multiple experiences; and actively engaging in the regular processing of experiences, which helps develop meaning. Deep learning allows students to dig deeper into complex and challenging learning situations instead of participating in surface learning only. Deep learning is intentional and creates new meaning for the learner (Candela, 2020). Multiple intelligences present the idea of seven constructs of intellects: bodily-kinesthetic, visual-spatial, verbal-linguistic, logical-mathematical, musical-rhythmic, interpersonal, and intrapersonal (Gardner, 1983). Each person has a different and unique intellect profile, some are more high-functioning than others, and capitalizing on everyone's intellect "talents" may aid in the learning process (Candela, 2020).

STUDENT-FOCUSED INSTRUCTIONAL STRATEGIES

After identifying the learning theories that provide the foundation for the curriculum, learning outcomes need to be developed with consideration of leveling them to promote critical thinking skills. Chapter 7 discusses in detail how to utilize an educational taxonomy to promote critical thinking skills. Educators also need to consider which instructional strategies are most appropriate to use. Faculty members must consider which learning strategy meets the goals of the curriculum as well as meets the needs of the learners.

Traditionally, lectures have been used in many nursing classrooms. Students attend class and listen to the educator speak, often following along with slides or notes. The focus has been on rote memorization with little opportunity for application or engagement in course content (Thompson, 2020). Teacher-centered learning, such as lecture, occurs when the educator focuses on pouring out information in a passive learning environment. Students are passive recipients, being provided with knowledge about facts and ideas. The focus is on "teaching," and the educator is a "sage on the stage." However, as faculty members seek out evidence-based teaching strategies and look at research surrounding student learning, a pedagogical shift occurs from teacher-focused instructional strategies to more student-focused instructional strategies. In general, these strategies focus on the educator as a facilitator of learning and students as engaged participants in learning. Students are involved in the learning process, either individually or in collaboration with peers, and are able to apply facts and ideas to actually grow their knowledge and understanding (Michaelsen & Sweet, 2008). There is research supporting this transition, stating that engaged students are more likely to meet learning outcomes (National Survey of Student Engagement, 2013).

There are several active learning strategies that can be utilized in the classroom. While it is not within the scope of this chapter to cover all of them, a select few teaching strategies are briefly discussed, including problem-based learning, team-based learning (TBL), the "flipped" classroom, and simulation. This list is not exhaustive and other active learning strategies employed by faculty members may include discussion, case studies, concept maps, portfolios, and reflection, among others (Phillips, 2020). As with learning theories, the active learning strategies are discussed separately; however, the faculty member may utilize several different approaches or appropriately combine them to achieve student learning.

Problem-Based Learning

Problem-based learning focuses on clinical problems and professional issues that the nurse may face in practice as a mechanism for teaching students. This strategy is highly structured where students focus on real-life situations in order to learn. The faculty member acts as a facilitator of learning. Students cycle through five key steps in the process of problem-based learning. They analyze a problem, establish learning outcomes, collect information, summarize, and reflect. Problem-based learning can be done face-to-face in the classroom or in the online environment. Peer learning is a key aspect of problem-based learning (Phillips, 2020).

Advantages to using problem-based learning include the engagement of students in an active learning environment that fosters peer learning and evaluation. Dealing with real-life problems allows for information that can be translated to the clinical setting. Problem-based learning has disadvantages, particularly for the faculty member. As with many active learning instructional strategies, a significant amount of time is initially required to create meaningful problems. Additionally, students need to be oriented to their roles in the learning process. Problem-based learning can be difficult to use with large class sizes (Phillips, 2020).

The evidence surrounding problem-based learning indicates positive outcomes for students. While more research needs to be done, a systematic review by Kong and colleagues (2014) found that problem-based learning may enhance critical thinking skills in nursing students. Problem-based learning has shown positive outcomes in clinical education and student outcomes (Shin & Kim, 2013).

Team-Based Learning

TBL is a structured, active learning strategy involving a sequence of three key phases: preclass preparation, readiness assurance process, and application. First used in business classrooms by Larry Michaelsen, TBL has now been used in a variety of classrooms, including nursing. The structured TBL sequence occurs with each major unit or module of instruction. Ideally, the course is divided into five to seven major units or modules. Teams of students are formed at the beginning of the course and stay intact throughout the semester. Students complete the preclass preparation, which may include assigned readings or other assignments, before the module of instruction begins. When they physically attend class, they begin the readiness assurance process that includes completing the Individual Readiness Assurance Test (IRAT) and the Team Readiness Assurance Test (tRAT). These tests are based on preclass preparation and consist of the same multiple-choice questions. The students first take the IRAT and then gather in their teams to take the tRAT. While not required, it is highly recommended that teams use the Immediate Feedback Assessment Technique (IF-AT) forms (available at www.epsteineducation.com/home/about/default.aspx). The IF-AT forms provide immediate feedback by allowing the teams to scratch off their answer choices (similar to scratching off a lottery ticket). If the answer is not correct, teams continue to scratch off their answer options until the correct answer is exposed. The immediate feedback provided by the forms allows for team discussion and learning to occur. Following the completion of the readiness assurance process, the educator can utilize class time to clarify any concepts and move on to the application phase. In their teams, students complete application exercises designed to engage students and allow the application of key course concepts (Michaelsen & Sweet, 2008).

There are several advantages to using TBL. Students are able to achieve a deeper level of understanding because they are engaged in the course content. Because students work in teams, team skills are often improved and students gain insight into their own strengths and weaknesses. There are also benefits for struggling students who tend to perform better when TBL is used. Faulty members typically see a decrease in student absenteeism due to the reliance on teamwork and in-class activities. They are able to form more personal relationships with their students because of the increased interaction with students in class and the educational process is shared mutually between students and faculty (Michaelsen & Sweet, 2008). TBL can also be used successfully in very large classrooms, up to 400 students (Clark et al., 2008). However, as with problem-based learning, there are challenges including student resistance and the time commitment required by faculty when preparing for class (Mennenga, 2013).

Evidence suggests positive student outcomes with the use of TBL, including improved examination scores and enhanced student engagement (Chad, 2012; Della Ratta, 2015; Mennenga, 2013). Overall student satisfaction may be increased with TBL (Jafari, 2014). Additionally, a review of the literature by Haidet and colleagues (2014) indicated that TBL shows evidence of positive outcomes for students regarding knowledge, engagement, and team performance.

The Flipped Classroom

Similar to TBL, the flipped classroom utilizes a reversed instruction model in which students complete preclass preparation and use in-class time for active learning activities. The idea is to "maximize the time the students and faculty have during the face-to-face time in the classroom" (Hessler, 2017, p. 12). The opportunity for students to begin learning outside of class time, independently, allows the classroom to be transformed into an engaging and interactive group learning environment. The educator acts as a facilitator of learning, guiding students as they learn to apply and critically think through concepts (Hessler, 2017).

In the flipped classroom, the typical traditional lecture is viewed by students before class time as preclass preparation. While the preparation may focus on reading assignments, many faculty members opt to use technology to capture their normal lecture content for students to view. Prerecorded video lectures, called "vodcasts," can be used to engage students and can be viewed several times until students gain an understanding of the material (Berndt, 2015; Hessler, 2017). Once in the classroom setting, students actively engage in learning activities focused on applying the content from the preclass preparation.

The flipped classroom offers several advantages to faculty members and students. Faculty members can use the class time more efficiently, clarify misperceptions of students, and cater to a variety of different learning styles. Students have the opportunity to be more engaged, to use technology in the educational process, and to actively participate in the learning process. There are, however, challenges that need to be addressed. Students and faculty may be initially resistant to a change in pedagogy, technology may not always work correctly, and, again, there is a time commitment required for preparation (Hessler, 2017).

Emerging evidence supports the use of the flipped classroom as an effective active learning strategy for students. In a study by McNally and colleagues (2017), student outcomes and participation were improved in a flipped classroom. While students in the study indicated the class was more difficult, it might be due to the increased student preparation required for the flipped classroom (McNally et al., 2017). Missildine et al.'s (2013) study found that student examination scores were higher with the flipped classroom strategy, but students were less satisfied. A systematic review of the flipped classroom in nursing education found neutral or positive outcomes in academic performance and mixed results regarding student satisfaction. Student engagement was noted because of the flipped classroom strategy (Betihavas et al., 2016).

Simulation

Simulation allows students to participate in activities that mimic real-life scenarios or situations. Simulations offer students a safe place to practice and critically think through highly realistic and often complex situations they may face in the real world (Forneris, 2020). Simulation, which may include manikins, standardized patients, role-play, or virtual simulations, has been promoted by leaders in nursing education, such as the National League for Nursing (2015; Society for Simulation in Healthcare, 2021). In nursing education, simulation allows students to participate in experiences under the direction of a faculty member. Typically, simulation includes a debriefing that is essential to student learning. Simulation offers opportunities for interprofessional experiences and a strategic approach to structured clinical experiences in the simulation setting (Forneris, 2020). Faculty members are called on to integrate simulation with a clear idea of how it assists in achieving student-learning outcomes (National League for Nursing, 2015).

There is strong evidence supporting the use of simulation in nursing education. Benefits include active involvement of students in the learning process, effective use of faculty, improved student instruction, and opportunities for immediate feedback. One of the main challenges is ensuring faculty preparation to utilize simulation as an effective teaching strategy (Forneris, 2020). Based on the conclusions of a recent National Council of State Boards of Nursing study, there is evidence that simulation can replace traditional clinical experiences for up to 50% of the time in nursing education (Hayden et al., 2014).

When selecting instructional strategies, faculty members must also consider the most appropriate methods to meet the needs of diverse learners. Nursing students may vary in age, including traditional high school graduates who immediately entered college and older, more experienced learners, including some with a previous college degree. Learners may also vary in background, ethnicity, socioeconomic status, and academic abilities. These differences among students may impact their motivation to learn, how they learn, and their expectations (Candela, 2020). It is helpful if the faculty member can capture these differences to engage learners and enhance the learning environment.

There are many active learning strategies that can be used to assess and evaluate students beyond only multiple-choice tests (Tomlinson & McTighe, 2006). Nursing programs can reflect the need for ongoing assessment as early as the philosophy statement. It can be realized through the use of outcomes that are subjected to periodic assessment. This can further facilitate success in achieving intended learning outcomes.

THEORETICAL LINK TO STUDENT-FOCUSED INSTRUCTIONAL STRATEGIES

It is important to provide the theoretical link to the selected student-focused instructional strategies used. For example, when this author used TBL in theory courses, she provided an orientation for students to the teaching strategy and the rationale for using it. Included in this student orientation is the link to the adult learning theory and how the use of student-focused instructional strategies can aid in their learning overall.

STUDENT EVALUATION

Student evaluation determines whether program goals, program outcomes, and/or specific-course student-learning outcomes have been met by the learner. While often these are "end" goals for learning, educators should consider the process of how students will be evaluated early in the curriculum planning process (Dennison et al., 2015). As discussed earlier in this chapter, decisions regarding the different components of the curriculum, including student evaluation, should be based on a philosophical foundation or learning theory.

Consistency, among overall program goals, program outcomes, specific-course student-learning outcomes, and evaluation of student learning, helps achieve a robust and methodologically sound curriculum plan.

On a broader scale of evaluation, curriculum planning should include alignment of overall program goals and outcomes with benchmark performance goals. These may include graduation rates, professional placement and performance of students following graduation, and performance on the NCLEX-RN®. Additionally, student evaluation of learning will help guide faculty in determining whether the overall program goals and outcomes have been met.

In the classroom, faculty members should measure learning according to specific-course student-learning outcomes. How learning is evaluated depends on the course student-learning outcomes, the educational taxonomy level, and the instructional strategy used by the faculty member. For example, if an educator is interested in how well a learner applies information in the clinical setting, a multiple-choice exam may not be the most useful way of evaluating student learning. As the focus transitions from teacher-focused to student-focused instructional strategies, student evaluation needs to be modified. Faculty members should consider the following questions when determining how students will be evaluated:

◆ Do the cognitive level student-learning outcomes and the evaluation method match?
◆ Do the learning domain of the student-learning outcome and the evaluation method match?
◆ Are there various methods of evaluation included in the course?
◆ Are assignments group or individual?
◆ Are the course assignments and examinations manageable and realistic for the student to complete?
◆ Are the course assignments and examinations manageable and realistic for faculty? (Consider grading and providing required feedback in a timely manner.)
◆ Are the assignments and examinations weighted to show appropriate significance?
◆ Do the methods of evaluation optimize the opportunity for student success?
◆ Do the methods of evaluation provide early signs of poor student performance (Dennison et al., 2015)?

While it is recognized that students have to pass the NCLEX-RN, which is a multiple-choice examination, it is recommended that a variety of evaluation methods be utilized in nursing education (Dennison et al., 2015). In a study with schools of nursing across the United States by Eder (2014), it was found that 95% of nursing faculty members utilize examinations as a source of evaluation. Examinations are often the preferred method of evaluation because they are relatively easy to grade and do not require large amounts of faculty time (Dennison et al., 2015).

Other alternative sources of evaluation used by faculty members may include simulations, clinical performance, demonstrations, case studies, concept maps, class discussion, role-play, games, papers, posters, presentations, portfolios, and reflections (Dennison et al., 2015; Eder, 2014; Phillips, 2020). All these types of evaluation are appropriate for use in nursing education and may be considered by faculty members as forms of student evaluation. However, while examinations offer a straightforward, timely, objective method of evaluation, the suggested alternative sources of student evaluation may require more faculty time for planning and grading and introduce some subjectivity to the grading process. A proposed method for addressing subjectivity in the grading process is to use rubrics to evaluate students. A rubric is a tool used for scoring that clearly outlines the expectations of an assignment. Typically, a rubric includes levels of quality and the student is scored accordingly. To develop a rubric, the faculty member should use the course student-learning outcomes to determine how the specific form of student evaluation contributes to demonstrating achievement of the outcomes. Next, the criteria that are essential to the evaluation are listed with a description of the various levels of quality or performance. It should clearly describe what meets expectations and what does not meet expectations. It is recommended that the faculty member test the rubric to identify any items that may need to be edited before using it with students. Students should be educated as to how they can use the rubric to evaluate themselves before submitting assignments. Finally, the faculty member uses the rubric for student evaluation and, if indicated, makes any revisions necessary based on the outcomes of evaluation (Dennison et al., 2015).

SUMMARY

As healthcare rapidly becomes more complex and diverse, nurses are required to know more, critically think in stressful situations, and act quickly in response to patient needs. In response, nurse educators are required to find ways to deliver the ever-increasing amounts of content, consider appropriate student-learning outcomes, experiences, and forms of evaluation. The ability of nursing educators to design a meaningful, purposeful curriculum will aid in the development of nurses who are prepared to meet today's challenges.

This chapter outlined the importance of identifying a philosophical foundation to inform decisions made in the curriculum. Beginning with an overview of select learning theories, the chapter illustrates the linkages considered in the process of implementing the curriculum. Education is transitioning to more learner-focused instructional strategies that are applicable to specific content, specific students, and specific environments. Appropriate use of student evaluation methods needs to be considered as well. This chapter is intended as an overview and readers who are interested in gaining a more thorough understanding of the content should seek additional specific resources.

END-OF-CHAPTER RESOURCES

DISCUSSION QUESTIONS

1. What are the main differences and similarities among the learning theories that were presented?

2. How does the use of learner-centered instructional strategies promote learning?

3. What are various methods of student assessment and evaluation?

LEARNING ACTIVITIES

Student-Learning Activities

1. Write a paper identifying your personal philosophy as an educator. Describe the faculty role and the student role related to accomplishing learning outcomes.

2. Identify a nursing course that would interest you to teach in your future role as an educator. Develop four student course-learning outcomes and align them with appropriate assessment and evaluation methods.

3. From the activity in Item 2 in the Student-Learning Activities, identify which learner-centered instructional strategy would be most appropriate.

Faculty Development Activities

1. Select a course you teach and plot your assignments according to the course outcomes. Share with a colleague and discuss findings.

2. Select a course you teach that is primarily teacher-focused. Revise one module or activity using one of the learner-focused instructional strategies described in this chapter.

3. Develop a scoring rubric for an existing or new course assignment. Share with a colleague and ask them to score an assignment using the rubric. Discuss and revise as necessary.

A robust set of instructor resources designed to supplement this text is located at **http://connect.springerpub.com/content/book/978-0-8261-8686-7.** Qualifying instructors may request access by emailing **textbook@springerpub.com.**

REFERENCES

Aliakbari, F., Parvin, N., Heidari, M., & Haghani, F. (2015). Learning theories application in nursing education. *Journal of Education and Health Promotion, 4,* 2. https://doi.org/10.4103/2277-9531.151867

Bastable, S., & Gonzalez, K. (2019). Overview of education in health care. In S. Bastable (Ed.), *Nurse as educator: Principles of teaching and learning for nursing practice* (5th ed., pp. 3–34). Jones & Bartlett.

Berndt, J. (2015). Using a "flipped classroom" model to engage learners. In L. Caputi (Ed.), *Building the future of nursing* (Vol. 2, pp. 71–75). National League for Nursing.

Betihavas, V., Bridgman, H., Kornhaber, R., & Cross, M. (2016). The evidence for "flipping out": A systematic review of the flipped classroom in nursing education. *Nurse Education Today, 38,* 15–21. https://doi.org/10.1016/j.nedt.2015.12.010

Brandon, A., & All, A. (2010). Constructivism theory analysis and application to curricula. *Nursing Education Perspectives, 31*(2), 89–92. https://www.ncbi.nlm.nih.gov/pubmed/20455364

Braungart, M., Braungart, R., & Gramet, P. (2019). Applying learning theories to healthcare practice. In S. Bastable (Ed.), *Nurse as educator: Principles of teaching and learning for nursing practice* (5th ed., pp. 69–116). Jones & Bartlett.

Candela, L. (2020). Theoretical foundations of teaching and learning. In D. Billings & J. Halstead (Eds.), *Teaching in nursing: A guide for faculty* (6th ed., pp. 247–269). Elsevier Saunders.

Chad, P. (2012). The use of team-based learning as an approach to increased engagement and learning for marketing students: A case study. *Journal of Marketing Education, 34*(2), 128–139. https://doi.org/10.1177/0273475312450388

Clark, M., Nguyen, H., Bray, C., & Levine, R. (2008). Team-based learning in an undergraduate nursing course. *Journal of Nursing Education, 47*(3), 111–117. https://doi.org/10.3928/01484834-20080301-02

Crow, L., & Crow, A. (1963). *Readings in human learning.* McKay.

Della Ratta, C. (2015). Flipping the classroom with team-based learning in undergraduate nursing education. *Nurse Educator, 40*(2), 71–74. https://doi.org/10.1097/NNE.0000000000000112

Dennick, R. (2012). Twelve tips for incorporating educational theory into teaching practices. *Medical Teacher, 34*(8), 618–624. https://doi.org/10.3109/0142159X.2012.668244

Dennison, R., Rosselli, J., & Dempsey, A. (2015). *Evaluation beyond exams in nursing education: Designing assignments and evaluating with rubrics.* Springer.

Eder, D. (2014). Healthy assessment: What nursing schools can teach us about effective assessment of student learning. *Assessment Update, 26*(3), 3–4, 13. https://doi.org/10.1002/au.20005

Forneris, S. (2020). Teaching and learning using simulations. In D. Billings & J. Halstead (Eds.), *Teaching in nursing: A guide for faculty* (6th ed., pp. 353–373). Elsevier Saunders.

Frey, J., & Popkess, A. (2020). Strategies to support diverse learning needs of students. In D. Billings & J. Halstead (Eds.), *Teaching in nursing: A guide for faculty* (6th ed., pp. 15–37). Elsevier.

Gardner, H. (1983). *Frames of mind.* Basic Books.

Haidet, P., Kubitz, K., & McCormack, W. (2014). Analysis of the team-based learning literature: TBL comes of age. *Journal on Excellence in College Teaching, 25*(3–4), 303–333. https://www.ncbi.nlm.nih.gov/pmc/articles/PMC4643940

Hayden, J. K., Smiley, R. A., Alexander, M., Kardong-Edgren, S., & Jeffries, P. R. (2014). The NCSBN National Simulation Study: A longitudinal, randomized, controlled study replacing clinical hours with simulation in prelicensure nursing education. *Journal of Nursing Regulation, 5*(2 Suppl.), S1–S64. https://www.ncsbn.org/JNR_Simulation_Supplement.pdf

Hessler, K. (2017). *Flipping the nursing classroom: Where active learning meets technology.* Jones & Bartlett.

Hunt, E. (2012). Educating the developing mind: The view from cognitive psychology. *Educational Psychology Review, 24*(1), 1–7. https://doi.org/10.1007/s10648-011-9186-3

Jafari, Z. (2014). A comparison of conventional lecture and team-based learning methods in terms of student learning and teaching satisfaction. *Medical Journal of the Islamic Republic of Iran, 28*(5). https://www.ncbi.nlm.nih.gov/pmc/articles/PMC4154282/pdf/mjiri-28-5.pdf

Kong, L., Qin, B., Zhou, Y., Mou, S., & Gao, H. (2014). The effectiveness of problem-based learning on development of nursing students' critical thinking: A systematic review and meta-analysis. *International Journal of Nursing Studies, 51*, 458–469. https://doi.org/10.1016/j.ijnurstu.2013.06.009

McNally, B., Chipperfield, J., Dorsett, P., Del Fabbro, L., Frommolt, V., Goetz, S., Lewohl, J., Molineux, M., Pearson, A., Reddan, G., Roiko, A., & Rung, A. (2017). Flipped classroom experiences: Student preferences and flip strategy in a higher education context. *Higher Education, 73*(2), 281–298. https://doi.org/10.1007/s10734-016-0014-z

Mennenga, H. (2013). Student engagement and examination performance in a team-based learning course. *Journal of Nursing Education, 52*(8), 475–479. https://doi.org/10.3928/01484834-20130718-04

Michaelsen, L., & Sweet, M. (2008). Fundamental principles and practices of team-based learning. In L. Michaelsen, D. Parmelee, K. McMahon, & R. Levine (Eds.), *Team-based learning for health professions education* (pp. 9–34). Stylus.

Missildine, K., Fountain, R., Summers, L., & Gosselin, K. (2013). Flipping the classroom to improve student performance and satisfaction. *Journal of Nursing Education, 52*(10), 597–599. https://doi.org/10.3928/01484834-20130919-03

National League for Nursing. (2015). *A vision for teaching with simulation: A living document from the National League for Nursing NLN Board of Governors.* http://www.nln.org/docs/default-source/about/nln-vision-series-(position-statements)/vision-statement-a-vision-for-teaching-with-simulation.pdf?sfvrsn=2

National Survey of Student Engagement. (2013). *A fresh look at student engagement: Annual results 2013*. http://nsse.indiana.edu/NSSE_2013_Results/pdf/NSSE_2013_Annual_Results.pdf

Phillips, J. (2020). Strategies to promote student engagement and active learning. In D. Billings & J. Halstead (Eds.), *Teaching in nursing: A guide for faculty* (6th ed., pp. 286–303). Elsevier.

Shin, I., & Kim, J. (2013). The effect of problem-based learning in nursing education: A meta-analysis. *Advances in Health Science Education*, *18*(5), 1103–1120. https://doi.org/10.1007/s10459-012-9436-2

Society for Simulation in Healthcare. (2021). *About simulation*. https://www.ssih.org/About-SSH/About-Simulation

Sullivan, D. (2020). An introduction to curriculum development. In D. Billings & J. Halstead (Eds.), *Teaching in nursing: A guide for faculty* (6th ed., pp. 103–134). Elsevier Saunders.

Thompson, B. (2020). The connected classroom: Using digital technology to promote learning. In D. Billings & J. Halstead (Eds.), *Teaching in nursing: A guide for faculty* (6th ed., pp. 374–391). Elsevier Saunders.

Tomlinson, C. A., & McTighe, J. (2006). *Integrating differentiated instruction: Understanding by design*. Association for Supervision and Curriculum Development.

Warburton, T., Trish, H., & Barry, D. (2016). Facilitation of learning: Part 1. *Nursing Standard*, *30*(32), 40–47. https://doi.org/10.7748/ns.30.32.40.s43

Wittmann-Price, R., & Price, S. (2019). Educational theories, learning theories, and special concepts. In L. Wilson & R. Wittmann-Price (Eds.), *Review manual for the certified healthcare simulation educator™ (CHSE™) Exam* (2nd ed., pp. 165–196). Springer.

CHAPTER 7

Using Educational Taxonomies to Promote Critical Thinking

Heidi A. Mennenga

CHAPTER OBJECTIVES

Upon completion of Chapter 7, the reader will be able to:

- Examine the evolution of educational taxonomies in curriculum development and evaluation.
- Explore updates in and revisions to educational taxonomies.
- Analyze the development of critical thinking in the context of educational taxonomies.
- Categorize objectives to progress cognitive, affective, and psychomotor skills through nursing education levels.

OVERVIEW

According to the *Merriam-Webster* (n.d.) dictionary, *taxonomy* is the study of classification. In education, taxonomy provides educators with a systematic process for organizing the overall curriculum. Using an educational taxonomy, educators can develop goals, outcomes, and structure assignments from simple to complex or concrete to abstract concepts. Educational taxonomies have evolved since the 1950s, initially focusing on the cognitive domain. More recently, taxonomies have expanded to include the affective and psychomotor domains of learning as well.

The development of critical thinking occurs when educators utilize all levels of taxonomy. As students utilize the various levels of taxonomy, they develop critical thinking skills. All levels of taxonomy are influential in the development of critical thinking skills; however, educators must be intentional in their use to purposefully cultivate these skills. Learning to critically think does not happen by accident.

THE USEFULNESS OF EDUCATIONAL TAXONOMIES

Taxonomy provides a common language and framework for classifying, categorizing, and defining educational goals. Using educational taxonomy allows educators to develop, communicate, and evaluate expectations of what students are to learn. Educational taxonomies, such as Bloom's taxonomy, are widely used in developing outcomes at the broader program level and, more narrowly, at course or module levels. Educational taxonomies serve to provide a framework for educators to identify, develop, and evaluate learning outcomes using a standardized system. They are helpful in identifying the level at which students need to demonstrate learning to achieve the expected outcomes (Scheckel, 2020). Furthermore, the use of educational taxonomy allows educators to map the progression of student learning and easily evaluate outcomes at all levels (course, semester, or program outcomes).

OBJECTIVES AND OUTCOMES

Educational taxonomies are generally worded with a focus on what the student is expected to learn. The standardized language provides outcomes that are understandable and clear to both other educators and students. Commonly, faculty members may use educational taxonomies as a method to structure student-learning outcomes (from simple to more complex) across the curriculum.

There are several terms used to describe what students should learn. Common terms used are *learning objectives* and *learning outcomes*. These terms are often used interchangeably in many nursing programs, and some experts have determined there is no difference between the two terms (Harden, 2002). Both terms refer to what the student should learn or accomplish at the end of the module, course, or program. They both serve to describe the learner, the expected behavior, and the content (Wittmann-Price & Fasokla, 2010). The main difference, argued by Wittmann-Price and Fasokla (2010), is that objectives relate to the process and the goal of learning, therefore pertaining to both the student and the faculty member. Conversely, outcomes relate to the goal, or the end product, therefore pertaining to the student (Wittmann-Price & Fasokla, 2010). Stated simply, "outcomes relate directly to professional practice; objectives relate to instruction" (Glennon, 2006, p. 55). Since education is shifting the focus of the teaching and learning environment away from the faculty member and onto the student, the term *outcomes* is more appropriate and is used in this chapter.

EDUCATIONAL TAXONOMIES

Domains of Learning within Taxonomies

Educational taxonomies provide the terminology to focus on the three main domains of learning: cognitive, psychomotor, and affective. Developed by Benjamin Bloom in the 1950s, Bloom's Cognitive Taxonomy is probably the most familiar and most commonly used educational taxonomy used. In the process of developing Bloom's taxonomy, Bloom and his colleagues determined that evaluation of learning must be considered through the domains of learning: cognitive, which focused on knowledge; psychomotor, which focused on hands-on learning and skills; and affective, which focused on feelings, values, and beliefs (Halawi et al., 2009). While this chapter briefly outlines Bloom's work, a detailed account of the work can be found in the publication of *The Taxonomy of Educational Objectives, Handbook 1: Cognitive Domain* (Bloom, 1956). This chapter also briefly discusses other educational taxonomies, although they may be less commonly used.

The Cognitive Domain

Bloom's Cognitive Taxonomy

While attending the American Psychological Association conference in 1948, Bloom and his colleagues developed the ideas for this taxonomy (Bloom, 1994). Bloom and the group wanted to develop a common framework to promote sharing of ideas for examination materials, research on the examinations, and their connection to education. The group determined that this framework could be best achieved if it included "a system of classifying the goals of the educational process using educational objectives" (Bloom, 1994, p. 2). Bloom's original taxonomy addressed six levels of cognitive learning, including knowledge, comprehension, application, analysis, synthesis, and evaluation. The levels were ordered from simple to complex with the idea that a learner had to master the simpler level before they could progress to a more complex level (Krathwohl, 2002). The main focus of Bloom's original taxonomy was on developing tests to evaluate students (Su & Osisek, 2011).

Bloom's taxonomy has been widely used in all levels of education to both establish and evaluate learning (Athanassious et al., 2003; Cochran et al., 2007). McNeill et al. (2011) describe the use of Bloom's taxonomy in connecting course outcome indicators to program-level evaluation. Bloom's taxonomy has been used across various educational levels and disciplines and translated into at least 22 languages (Krathwohl, 2002; Manton et al., 2008). The taxonomy provides a structure for educators to consider learning and the products of learning.

Despite the popularity of Bloom's taxonomy, there are some critics, including those that think it is too simplistic (Kuhn, 2008). The hierarchal structure of the taxonomy is unidirectional and presumes that each simpler category, such as remembering, must be "achieved" before the next level can occur (Krathwohl, 2002; Paul, 1993). Many experts will argue that one level may not necessarily be more difficult than another may and that this presumption is not supported by evidence (Asim, 2011; Soozandehfar & Adeli, 2016). Additionally, some experts assert Bloom's taxonomy is outdated and irrelevant based on new knowledge about how students learn (Soozandehfar & Adeli, 2016).

The Revised Bloom's Cognitive Taxonomy

In 2001, Anderson, who was a student of Bloom's and Krathwohl's and a collaborator on the original taxonomy, substantially revised Bloom's taxonomy based on new knowledge and changes in the educational process (Bumen, 2007). The focus of the revised taxonomy was on student learning rather than only on the development of tests (Su & Osisek, 2011). Whereas the original taxonomy was one-dimensional (cognitive), the revised taxonomy was two-dimensional (cognitive processes and knowledge). Additionally, the revised taxonomy used six levels with new terminology: remembering, understanding, applying, analyzing, evaluating, and creating.

The Revised Bloom's Cognitive Taxonomy Levels

The first level of the revised Bloom's taxonomy is remembering. This is defined as memory of material or content previously learned by recalling (Anderson & Krathwohl, 2001). Some of the common verbs used to illustrate remembering include *choose, define, "list,* and *recall.* An example of a learning outcome at the remembering level is as follows: The student will define the term *auscultation.*

The second level, understanding, is defined by demonstrating an understanding of ideas. Students can begin to organize, compare, translate, and interpret at this level. Some of the common verbs used to illustrate understanding include *compare, contrast, outline,* and *summarize.* An example of a learning outcome at the understanding level is as follows: The student will compare normal and abnormal findings of the skin.

The third level is applying. This is defined by solving problems in new situations by using previous knowledge in a new way. Some of the common verbs used to illustrate applying include *apply, choose, identify,* and *solve.* An example of a learning outcome at the applying level is as follows: The student will identify appropriate placement for auscultating heart sounds.

The fourth level is analyzing, defined as examining and breaking apart information to identify causes. At this level, students can make inferences about information. Common verbs used to illustrate analyzing include *analyze, conclude, examine,* and *distinguish.* An example of a learning outcome at the analyzing level is as follows: The student will examine national statistics to convey the significance of a topic.

The fifth level is evaluating. This level is defined as presenting and defending opinions and making judgments about information. Common verbs used to illustrate evaluating include *appraise, conclude, determine,* and *evaluate.* An example of a learning outcome at the evaluating level is as follows: The student will evaluate a patient's plan of care.

The final level of Bloom's revised taxonomy is creating. This level focuses on the student's ability to compile information in a different way and possibly propose alternative solutions. Common verbs used to illustrate creating include *adapt, change, design,* and *plan.* An example of a learning outcome at the applying level is as follows: The student will plan a meal appropriate for a patient with diabetes.

The Affective Domain

The affective domain was first described in 1964 and credited to Krathwohl, who was a member of the original taxonomy group. The affective domain focuses on feelings and emotions that are expressed as values and interests. Like Bloom's Cognitive Taxonomy, the affective domain is arranged in a hierarchal format from simpler feelings to more complex. The five levels include: receiving, responding, valuing, organization, and characterization (Wilson, 2021). According to O'Neill (2010), "learners move from being aware of what they are learning to a stage of having internalized the learning so that it plays a role in guiding their actions" (p. 2).

Receiving refers to the student's consciousness of stimuli. Receiving focuses on awareness, willingness to receive, and controlled or selected attention (Krathwohl et al., 1964). Common verbs used to illustrate receiving include *feel, sense,* and *perceive.* An example of a learning outcome at the receiving level is as follows: The student will listen to others with respect.

Responding refers to the student's attention to stimuli and their motivation to learn. Responding focuses on acquiescence, willing responses, or feelings of satisfaction (Krathwohl et al., 1964). Common verbs used to illustrate responding include *allow, cooperate,* and *contribute.* An example of a learning outcome at the responding level is as follows: The student will express enjoyment when participating in extracurricular activities.

Valuing refers to the student's beliefs and attitudes. Valuing refers to acceptance, preference, or commitment to a value satisfaction (Krathwohl et al., 1964). Common verbs used to illustrate valuing include *believe, seek,* and *persuade.* An example of a learning outcome at the valuing level is as follows: The student will show sensitivity toward individuals with cultural differences.

Organization refers to the internalization of values and beliefs. As the student internalizes values and beliefs, they organize them according to priority satisfaction (Krathwohl et al., 1964). Common verbs used to illustrate organization include *examine, clarify,* and *integrate.* An example of a learning outcome at the organization level is as follows: The student will accept professional nursing standards for practice.

Characterization refers to the highest level of internalization at which the internalized values and beliefs now translate into actions, which follow the student's values and beliefs satisfaction (Krathwohl et al., 1964). By the time a person reaches the highest level of the affective domain, they have internalized values and placed them into an internal organized system. Behaviors are consistent and in tune with those values. This process is gradual and may take a lifetime to achieve. Common verbs used to illustrate characterization include *internalize, review,* and *judge.* An example of a learning outcome at the characterization level is as follows: The student will value others for who they are rather than base their value on their appearance.

The Psychomotor Domain

The psychomotor domain focuses on physically doing things (Wilson, 2021). In the 1970s, there were three different psychomotor domains described. The most referred to domain is credited to Anita Harrow (1972) however; Simpson (1972) and Dave (1970) also developed psychomotor taxonomies as well. For the purpose of this chapter, Harrow's (1972) work is discussed.

Harrow (1972) proposed six categories of the psychomotor domain: reflex movements, fundamental movements, perceptual abilities, physical abilities, skilled movements, and nondiscursive communication. Reflex movements are the very foundation of this domain and focus on automatic reactions, such as reflexes. Fundamental movements include simple movements, such as running or jumping, that then can provide the foundation for more complex movements. Perceptual abilities refer to the ability to consider environmental cues and adjust movements accordingly. Physical abilities focus on endurance, flexibility, agility, strength, or dexterity. Skilled movements are activities that must be learned for specific performances or games. Nondiscursive communication refers to expressive movements, just as those used in body language or expressive dance. Educators can write more simplistic learning outcomes to focus on one single category or meld multiple categories into more complex learning outcomes.

The Holistic Taxonomy of Hauenstein

In 1998, Hauenstein proposed a taxonomy that synthesized cognitive, affective, and psychomotor learning into a fourth domain he called "behavior domain." Hauenstein (1998) felt the need for an integrated and connected taxonomy to achieve a holistic curriculum that focused on student understanding, skills, and dispositions. The cognitive domain focuses on the process of knowing and the development of intellectual abilities and skills. The affective domain is directed toward developing dispositions in relation to feelings, values, and beliefs, and the psychomotor domain is focused on the development of physical abilities and skills.

Additionally, the behavioral domain, which includes acquisition, assimilation, adaptation, performance, and aspiration, is the "tempered demeanor" one displays as a reaction to a social stimulus, an inner need, or both. The acquisition objective is the process of understanding, perceiving, and conceptualizing new information. Assimilation involves comprehending concepts in relation to prior knowledge and explaining it in their own terms. Adaptation involves the ability to modify knowledge, skills, or dispositions to conform to an established standard or criterion. Performance is the ability to analyze, qualify, evaluate, and integrate information with personal values and beliefs so that it becomes ingrained and able to be repeated in either new or routine situations (Hauenstein, 1998).

Fink Taxonomy of Significant Learning

The Fink (2003) taxonomy grew from the work of Bloom but added major considerations in the areas of motivation and human interaction. Rather than hierarchical, the taxonomy is circular and is composed of six categories: foundational knowledge, application, integration (making connections), human dimension (student learning about themselves and others—why one does what one does), caring, and learning how to learn. The taxonomy sees learning as multidirectional and asserts significant learning requires alignment among learning goals, learning activities, and learning assessment (Levine et al., 2008).

A New Taxonomy

In 2007, Marzano and Kendall published *The New Taxonomy of Educational Objectives*, providing a detailed description of the theories behind and the use of a two-dimensional taxonomy: levels of processing and domains of knowledge. The new taxonomy builds on the work of Bloom's original taxonomy and Anderson's revised taxonomy.

A common criticism of Bloom's taxonomy is the hierarchical nature of the levels, thereby indicating increased difficulty with each ascending level. The authors of the new taxonomy disagreed, asserting that even the most difficult mental processes become simple as they become more familiar. The number of steps needed to carry out the mental process and the relationships between steps may not change but the speed at which one can perform them does change. For example, a student nurse may take 15 minutes or more to match medications to a medication administration record and administer the medications. That same nurse would likely be able to carry out the task in less than 2 minutes if they had performed it several times.

The new taxonomy features six horizontal levels of processing and three vertical rows of knowledge domains. The first four levels of processing are within the cognitive system: retrieval (recognizing, recalling, executing), comprehension (integrating, symbolizing), analysis (matching, classifying, analyzing errors, generating, specifying), and knowledge utilization (decision-making, problem-solving, experimenting, investigating). The next level is the metacognitive system, which specifies and monitors knowledge in terms of goals, processes, clarity, and accuracy. Self-system thinking is the sixth level of processing. This level is concerned with how motivated a person is in learning a new task given the importance, efficacy, and emotional responses attached to it. Emotions can hinder or facilitate learning (Sousa, 2011). Shulman (2002) discussed the influence of engagement and motivation as both a purpose of education and a "proxy" for subsequent learning.

The self-system decides whether to engage in a new learning task. The following are examples of internal questions that affect motivation to learn: How important is this to learn? How much do I believe I can learn it? How positive or negative do I feel about this new task? Once the self-system decides to engage, activation of the metacognitive system occurs, followed by the cognitive system (Marzano & Kendall, 2007).

The three domains of knowledge are information, mental procedures, and psychomotor procedures. The information domain (declarative knowledge) is represented as hierarchical. The lower three are described as details (vocabulary terms, facts, time sequences), while the higher levels are organizing ideas (principles, generalizations). The mental procedures domain (procedural knowledge) contains two categories: a skills category that uses algorithms, tactics, and single rules, and a processes category of macroprocedures. Unlike the procedures in the skills category that learned so well requires little or no conscious thought, macroprocedures are highly complex and require conscious control. The psychomotor domain involves a skill category of simple combination and foundational procedures as well as a process level of complex combination procedures.

According to the authors, the new taxonomy differs because it (a) addresses cognitive, affective, and psychomotor learning domains very specifically; (b) places the metacognitive system above the cognitive system; and (c) considers the self-system at the top of the six processing levels. For a more detailed discussion of the new taxonomy, readers are encouraged to consult the Marzano and Kendall (2007) book.

Bloom's Digital Taxonomy

There continue to be revisions to Bloom's taxonomy based on new research and information discoveries. One example is the work of Andrew Churches (2007, 2008), an educator in an elementary/secondary school in New Zealand. Using the revised taxonomy, he created "Bloom's Digital Taxonomy." The taxonomy depicts each increasingly complex level of cognitive ability with technology to ascending levels of higher order thinking—from accessing and finding information to using and analyzing it to designing it. This all occurs within the context of developing communication by using technology (Churches, 2007, 2008).

While Churches did not work with college-level students, there is relevance to nursing in his work. Technology is a key component in many nursing programs, specifically related to locating and utilizing resources as well as the use of technology in patient care. Both the Accreditation Commission for Education in Nursing (ACEN, 2020) and the American Association of Colleges of Nursing (AACN, 2008) contain verbiage regarding the use of technology as a competence for students in prelicensure nursing programs. Creative uses of taxonomy such, as the one proposed by Churches may be helpful in progressing the competence level of students in using technology throughout the curriculum.

CURRICULUM ALIGNMENT USING A TAXONOMY TABLE

Educational taxonomies provide educators the framework to develop outcomes that are structured from simple to complex or concrete to abstract concepts. When developing a curriculum, using a taxonomy table may be beneficial to ensure there is an alignment among curricular objectives, instruction, and assessment (Anderson, 2002). Misalignment of the curriculum may result in assessments and/or outcomes that do not reflect instruction (Airasian & Miranda, 2002).

It is helpful to visually depict, or plot, outcomes, class activities, and assessment/evaluation methods into a taxonomy table. By having this information mapped, educators can review and update it regularly to ensure curriculum alignment and students learned current and important information. Exhibit 7.1 illustrates the application of the new taxonomy of educational objectives to align program outcomes, course outcomes, learning content and experiences, and assessments and evaluations.

The use of a taxonomy table also helps educators ensure activities and assessment or evaluation methods incorporate the various levels and domains of taxonomy. For example, if an educator is having students complete a concept map, the taxonomy level would be analysis and the domain is cognitive. An examination might integrate all levels of taxonomy in the cognitive domain. Having all this information in one table allows the educator to clearly and quickly identify any gaps in levels and/or domains or taxonomy.

CRITICAL THINKING AND TAXONOMY

The use of educational taxonomies directly relates to the role of critical thinking in nursing education. By utilizing all levels of taxonomy, educators can ensure that students develop the skills needed to critically think through situations. This requires well-thought-out learning outcomes as well as structured, strategically developed activities and appropriate student evaluation of learning.

Educators are faced with the challenge of preparing graduates who are equipped with the skills necessary to care for patients in an ever-changing, highly complex environment. Patients are sicker and more complex than ever before (Finkelman & Kenner,

EXHIBIT 7.1: Alignment of Taxonomy and Educational Outcomes

Course: _____

Date Developed: _____ Date Reviewed: _____

Related Program Outcome	Related Course Outcome	Related Learning Activity	Related Assessment or Evaluation	Taxonomy Level	Domain

2012; Spector et al., 2015). While educators are constantly changing and updating content within the curriculum to keep up with the evolving demands of nurses in practice, the reality is that time with students is limited. There is only so much information that can be provided within the curriculum. Additionally, some of the content currently taught will be obsolete by the time students are practicing nurses. These challenges illustrate how important it is to teach students how to use critical thinking skills, clinical reasoning skills, and clinical judgment skills. While these terms are often used interchangeably, there are notable differences as defined here.

Critical thinking is defined by the AACN (2008) as, "all or part of the process of questioning, analysis, synthesis, interpretation, inference, inductive and deductive reasoning, intuition, application, and creativity. Critical thinking underlies independent and interdependent decision making" (p. 37). *Clinical reasoning* is defined as the process used to acquire information, analyze data, and make decisions regarding patient care (Simmons et al., 2003). *Clinical judgment* is defined as the outcomes of critical thinking in practice, a process that begins with the end in mind. Clinical judgment is based on evidence and looks at meaning and outcomes achieved (Pesut, 2001). To state another way, critical thinking and clinical reasoning are processes that occur and result in clinical judgment (Alfaro-LeFevre, 2019). The ability to critically think through situations is crucial in the provision of safe, quality care in any setting.

In a scoping review of the literature, Zuriguel Pérez et al. (2015) concluded that critical thinking in the nursing profession is very different from critical thinking in other professions. In the literature, *critical thinking* is defined as "controlled, useful thinking that requires strategies in order to obtain the desired results … the process of searching, obtaining, evaluating, analyzing, synthesizing and conceptualizing information … its attributes are reflection, context, dialogue and time" (p. 824).

While *critical thinking* is often an umbrella term that includes a complex list of aspects necessary for nurses to possess both in and out of the clinical setting, experts conclude that engaging students and using active learning strategies is an effective approach in teaching students to "think like a nurse" (Alfaro-LeFevre, 2019; Ward & Morris, 2016). Students must be equipped with well-developed critical thinking skills to gain licensure as a nurse and provide safe, quality care to patients. The National Council Licensure Examination for Registered Nurses (NCLEX-RN®) assesses the candidate's ability to critically think by utilizing higher levels of educational taxonomies. Critical thinking skills are even more essential with the introduction of the Next Generation NCLEX examination, which will require students to use clinical judgment skills in real-world situations (National Council of State Boards of Nursing, 2021). Additionally, the sheer complexity of care required in today's nursing world mandates the ability of new nurses to critically think through situations (Alfaro-LeFevre, 2019).

Ward-Smith (2020) discusses the need for nurses to be expert critical thinkers. Educators have a key role in developing critical thinkers. The move toward using active learning strategies allows educators to act as a facilitator of learning and allows students to engage in the learning process. This approach allows educators to see how students use their knowledge in situations that can then be assessed (Mayer, 2002).

Students may come from backgrounds in which learning has been largely passive. This may lead to students who may come to class unprepared and resist active learning through disengagement or disruption; therefore, educators need to be persistent and clear about engaging students and maintaining expectations about class preparation.

Critical thinking is complex (Frey & Popkess, 2020) and takes time to develop. Being intentional can assist educators in cultivating this skill. Bloom (1994) acknowledged that problem-solving associated with critical thinking is based on knowledge and the ability to apply the knowledge "to new situations and problems" (Bloom, 1994, p. 16). Bissell and Lemons (2006) assert that critical thinking is apparent at the higher levels of the taxonomy while Friedman et al. (2010) argued that elements of critical thinking exist at every level. Educators can use the levels of educational taxonomy to ensure the development of critical thinking.

SUMMARY

Today's nurses today need to be equipped to think and act quickly in diverse healthcare settings that are increasingly complex. Nurse educators are challenged to find ways to sift through ever-growing amounts of information and decide what to include as content, all the while considering course outcomes, learning experiences, and assessment/evaluation. The use of an educational taxonomy provides a framework for developing, implementing, and evaluating course, semester, and program outcomes. A particular benefit of the use of taxonomy is attention to the development of critical thinking at all levels. Critical thinking may be facilitated using active learning strategies, as discussed in the previous chapter that both motivate and engage students. Educators' attention to alignment throughout the process of curriculum development and ongoing revisions help facilitate the education and development of students.

END-OF-CHAPTER RESOURCES

DISCUSSION QUESTIONS

1. What drove the need for the original Bloom's taxonomy to evolve, and what changes resulted?

2. How can taxonomy be used to align student learning to program outcomes?

3. Identify one criticism associated with the use of taxonomy and how it could be overcome.

4. How can the use of an educational taxonomy facilitate the development and evaluation of critical thinking?

LEARNING ACTIVITIES

Student-Learning Activities

1. Select any two, accredited BSN programs that identify program outcomes on their internet sites. Next, review the most recent literature from the AACN, the National League for Nursing, the ACEN, the Commission on Collegiate Nursing Education, and the Institute of Medicine. Analyze the outcomes for both programs considering what abilities are needed (as articulated in the literature you reviewed). Explain the fit of each of the programs to what these professional organizations call for.

2. From the activity in Item 1, develop a brief paper showing how the outcomes from the program could be modified to better reflect the abilities needed by nurse graduates for entry into practice.

3. Take one of the program outcomes from Item 2 and develop a measurable objective from two of the taxonomy domains (affective, psychomotor, cognitive) for first- or second-semester students in a medical–surgical or professional development course.

Faculty Development Activities

1. How can a taxonomy table illustrate progression toward learning outcomes at the program, year/semester, and course levels?

2. Using a taxonomy table, plot one of your multiple-choice tests (by item number) into a taxonomy table (cognitive level and knowledge domains). Then exchange your test with a colleague and repeat. Now share the results with your colleague and discuss results. In areas where you differ, review the question and determine whether to revise.

3. Conceptualize your course by aligning it to the program outcomes or end of program objectives. Try using a table or schematic to visualize your course in delivering course outcomes.

 A robust set of instructor resources designed to supplement this text is located at **http://connect.springerpub.com/content/book/978-0-8261-8686-7.** Qualifying instructors may request access by emailing **textbook@springerpub.com.**

REFERENCES

Accreditation Commission for Education in Nursing. (2020). *ACEN accreditation manual 2017 standards and criteria.* https://www.acenursing.org/acen-accreditation-manual/

Airasian, P. W., & Miranda, H. (2002). The role of assessment in the revised taxonomy. *Theory into Practice, 41*(4), 249–254. https://doi.org/10.1207/s15430421tip4104_8

Alfaro-LeFevre, R. (2019). *Critical thinking, clinical reasoning, and clinical judgment: A practical approach* (7th ed.). Elsevier.

American Association of Colleges of Nursing. (2008). *The essentials of baccalaureate education for professional nursing practice.* https://www.aacnnursing.org/portals/42/publications/baccessentials08.pdf

Anderson, L., & Krathwohl, D. (2001). *A taxonomy for learning, teaching and assessing: A revision of Bloom's taxonomy of educational objectives.* Longman.

Anderson, L. W. (2002). Curricular realignment: A re-examination. *Theory Into Practice, 41*(4), 255–260. https://doi.org/10.1207/s15430421tip4104_9

Asim, A. (2011). Finding acceptance of Bloom's revised cognitive taxonomy on the international stage in Turkey. *Educational Sciences: Theory & Practice, 11*(2), 767–772. http://www.kuyeb.com/pdf/en/263fdbeb0076bbb9a65734ffeb534f82TAMEN.pdf

Athanassious, N., McNett, J. M., & Harvey, C. (2003). Critical thinking in the management classroom: Bloom's taxonomy as a learning tool. *Journal of Management Education, 27*(5), 533–555. https://doi.org/10.1177/1052562903252515

Bissell, A. N., & Lemons, P. P. (2006). A new method for assessing critical thinking in the classroom. *BioScience, 56*, 66–72. https://doi.org/10.1641/0006-3568(2006)056[0066:ANMFAC]2.0.CO;2

Bloom, B. S. (1956). *Taxonomy of educational objectives, handbook 1: The cognitive domain.* Longmans.

Bloom, B. S. (1994). Reflections on the development and use of the taxonomy. In L. W. Anderson & L. A. Sosniak (Eds.), *Bloom's taxonomy: A forty-year retrospective* (pp. 1–8). The National Society for the Study of Education.

Bumen, N. T. (2007). Effects of the original versus revised Bloom's taxonomy on lesson planning skills: A Turkish study among pre-service teachers. *International Review of Education, 53*(4), 439–455. https://doi.org/10.1007/s11159-007-9052-1

Churches, A. (2007). *Educational origami: Bloom's digital taxonomy.* http://edorigami.wikispaces.com/Bloom%27s+Digital+Taxonomy

Churches, A. (2008). *Bloom's taxonomy blooms digitally.* Tech & Learning. www.techlearning.com/artcile/8670

Cochran, D., Conklin, J., & Modin, S. (2007). A new Bloom: Transforming learning. *Learning & Leading with Technology*, 34(5), 22–25.

Dave, R. H. (1970). Psychomotor levels. In R. J. Armstrong (Ed.), *Developing and writing behavioral objectives*. Educational Innovators Press.

Fink, L. D. (2003). *Creating significant learning experiences: An integrated approach to designing college courses*. Jossey-Bass.

Finkelman, A., & Kenner, C. (2012). *Learning IOM: Implications of the Institute of Medicine reports for nursing education*. American Nurses Association.

Frey, J., & Popkess, A. (2020). Strategies to support diverse learning needs of students. In D. M. Billings & J. A. Halstead (Eds.), *Teaching in nursing: A guide for faculty* (6th ed., pp. 15–37). Saunders Elsevier.

Friedman, D. B., Crews, T. B., Caicedo, J. M., Besley, J. C., Weinberg, J., & Freeman, M. L. (2010). An exploration into inquiry-based learning by a multidisciplinary group of higher education faculty. *Higher Education*, 59, 765–783. https://www.jstor.org/stable/40602433

Glennon, C. D. (2006). Reconceptualizing program outcomes. *Journal of Nursing Education*, 45(2), 55–58. https://doi.org/10.3928/01484834-20060201-03

Halawi, L. A., McCarthy, R. V., & Pires, J. (2009). An evaluation of e-learning on the basis of Bloom's taxonomy: An exploratory study. *Journal of Education for Business*, 84(6), 274–380. https://eric.ed.gov/?id=EJ844509

Harden, R. M. (2002). Learning outcomes and instructional objectives: Is there a difference? *Medical Teacher*, 24(2), 151–155. https://doi.org/10.1080/0142159022020687

Harrow, A. J. (1972). *A taxonomy of the psychomotor domain*. David McKay Company.

Hauenstein, A. D. (1998). *A conceptual framework for educational objectives: A holistic approach to traditional taxonomies*. University Press of America.

Krathwohl, D. R. (2002). A revision of Bloom's taxonomy: An overview. *Theory Into Practice*, 41(4), 212–218. http://www.depauw.edu/files/resources/krathwohl.pdf

Krathwohl, D. R., & Anderson, L. W. (2010). Merlin C. Whitlock and the revision of Bloom's taxonomy. *Educational Psychologist*, 45, 64–65. https://doi.org/10.1080/00461520903433562

Kuhn, M. S. (2008). Connecting depth and balance in class. *Learning and Leading with Technology*, 36(1), 18–21.

Levine, L. E., Fallahi, C. R., Nicoll-Senft, J. M., Tessier, J. T., Watson, C. L., & Wood, R. M. (2008). Creating significant learning experiences across disciplines. *College Teaching*, 56(4), 247–254. https://doi.org/10.3200/CTCH.56.4.247-254

Manton, E. J., English, D. E., & Kernek, C. R. (2008). Evaluating knowledge and critical thinking in international marketing courses. *College Student Journal*, 42(4), 1037–1044.

Marzano, R. J., & Kendall, J. S. (2007). *The new taxonomy of educational objectives* (2nd ed.). Corwin.

Mayer, R. E. (2002). A taxonomy for computer-based assessment of problem solving. *Computers in Human Behavior*, 18, 623–632. https://doi.org/10.1016/S0747-5632(02)00020-1

McNeill, M., Gosper, M., & Hedberg, J. (2011). Academic practice in aligning curriculum and technologies. *International Journal of Computer Information Systems and Industrial Management Applications*, 3, 679–686.

Merriam-Webster. (n.d.). *Taxonomy*. In *Merriam-Webster.com dictionary*. https://www.merriam-webster.com/dictionary/taxonomy

National Council of State Boards of Nursing. (2021). *Next generation NCLEX project*. https://www.ncsbn.org/next-generation-nclex.htm

O'Neill, G. (2010). *Assessment: guide to taxonomies of learning*. www.ucd.ie/teaching

Paul, R. (1993). *Critical thinking: How to prepare students for a rapidly changing world*. Foundation for Critical Thinking Press.

Pesut, J. (2001). Clinical judgment: Foreground/background. *Journal of Professional Nursing*, 17(5), 25. https://doi.org/10.1053/jpnu.2001.26303

Scheckel, M. (2020). Designing courses and learning experiences. In D. Billings & J. Halstead (Eds.), *Teaching in nursing: A guide for faculty* (6th ed., pp. 181–201). Elsevier.

Shulman, L. S. (2002). Making differences: A table of learning. *Change, 34*(6), 36–44. https://doi.org/10.1080/00091380209605567

Simmons, B., Lanuza, D., Fonteyn, M., & Hicks, F. (2003). Clinical reasoning in experienced nurses. *Western Journal of Nursing Research, 25*(6), 701–719. https://doi.org/10.1177/0193945903253092

Simpson, E. J. (1972). *The classification of educational objectives in the psychomotor domain.* Gryphon House.

Soozandehfar, S., & Adeli, M. (2016). A critical appraisal of Bloom's taxonomy. *American Research Journal of English and Literature, 2*(2016), 1–9. https://doi.org/10.21694/2378-9026.16014

Sousa, D. A. (2011). *How the brain learns* (4th ed.). Corwin.

Spector, N., Blegen, M., Silvestre, J., Barnsteiner, J., Lynn, M., Ulrich, B., Fogg, L., & Alexander, M. (2015). Transition to practice study in hospital settings. *Journal of Nursing Regulation, 5*(4), 24–38. https://doi.org/10.1016/S2155-8256(15)30031-4

Su, W., & Osisek, P. (2011). The revised Bloom's taxonomy: Implications for educating nurses. *Journal of Continuing Education in Nursing, 42*(7), 321–327. https://doi.org/10.3928/00220124-20110621-05

Ward-Smith, P. (2020). The nurse as a critical thinking expert. *Urologic Nursing, 40*(1), 5, 49. https://doi.org/10.7257/1053-816X.2020.40.1.5

Ward, T., & Morris, T. (2016). Think like a nurse: A critical thinking initiative. *Association of Black Nursing Faculty in Higher Education Journal, 27*(3), 64–66. http://excelsior.sdstate.edu/login?url=http://search.ebscohost.com/login.aspx?direct=true&db=keh&AN=116990911&site=ehost-live

Wilson, L. (2021). *Three domains of learning—Cognitive, affective, psychomotor.* https://thesecondprinciple.com/instructional-design/threedomainsoflearning/

Wittmann-Price, R., & Fasolka, B. (2010). Objectives and outcomes: The fundamental difference. *Nursing Education Perspectives, 31*(4), 233–236. http://excelsior.sdstate.edu/login?url=http://search.ebscohost.com/login.aspx?direct=true&db=keh&AN=57511435&site=ehost-live

Zuriguel Pérez, E., Lluch Canut, M., Falcó Pegueroles, A., Puig Llobet, M., Moreno Arroyo, C., & Roldán Merino, J. (2015). Critical thinking in nursing: Scoping review of the literature. *International Journal of Nursing Practice, 21*(6), 820–830. https://doi.org/10.1111/ijn.12347

CHAPTER 8

Curriculum Planning for Undergraduate Nursing Programs

Kimberly Baxter

CHAPTER OBJECTIVES

Upon completion of Chapter 8, the reader will be able to:

- Summarize current trends in prelicensure nursing education.
- Analyze current regulatory, accreditation, political, and social factors that affect the development and revision of associate and baccalaureate degree pre- and postlicensure nursing education.
- Describe the integration of the *Essentials: Core Competencies for Professional Nursing Education* as a foundation for developing a BSN curriculum.
- Analyze the relationship among generic, ABSN, and RN-to-BSN programs.
- Evaluate the strengths and challenges for baccalaureate graduate residency programs that facilitate transition into practice.
- Design a curriculum plan and program of study for a baccalaureate program.

OVERVIEW

This chapter provides an overview of the process of curriculum development for associate degree (ADN) and baccalaureate/BSN programs. It reviews the utilization of *The Essentials: Core Competencies for Professional Nursing Education* (American Association of Colleges of Nursing [AACN], 2021) in curriculum development and discusses accelerated programs and RN-to-BSN programs. The chapter summarizes the advantages and challenges related to residency/externship programs for the new graduate.

WHEN IS IT TIME FOR A CURRICULUM CHANGE?

The nature of today's complex healthcare environment, overwhelmed with changes in healthcare reform, advancing technology, and educational accountability led to an urgent call for transformation in nursing education (Institute of Medicine [IOM], 2010, 2015; National Academy of Medicine [NAM], 2021). The population of the United States is becoming more diverse, the income gap is widening, and baby boomers are aging.

Veterans are continuing to struggle with mental health issues and the prevalence of chronic illness is at an all-time high (Centers for Disease Control and Prevention [CDC], 2021). A diverse, dynamic nursing workforce is needed to fulfill these increasingly sophisticated and expanded roles in direct and indirect patient care. All of these factors affect the kinds of programs that are offered at schools of nursing, the content of the curricula, and the way that faculty teach in nursing education.

In order to prepare graduates of prelicensure nursing education programs for practice in an ever-changing healthcare environment, nursing curricula must be revised or updated on a regular basis. Oermann (2021) acknowledges recognition of the need for change as a primary factor in launching a formal revision. Nursing schools rely on a robust evaluation plan to provide information that guides curriculum revision. In addition, there are compelling factors external to individual nursing programs that influence the need for curricular change within baccalaureate nursing programs across the country. These are reflected in the *Essentials: Core Competencies for Professional Nursing Education* (AACN, 2021).

Nursing is the largest sector of the nation's healthcare workforce, with estimates of greater than 3.8 million RNs (AACN, 2019a; Smiley et al., 2018). Today's nursing workforce in the United States consists of four levels of prelicensure nursing preparation: diploma, associate degree, baccalaureate, and entry-level master's. According to the National Council of State Boards of Nursing (NCSBN, 2020a), in 2019 out of the 171, 374 U.S.-educated first-time NCLEX-RN® test takers, 49.18% had graduated from accredited BSN programs versus 49.48% who had graduated from ADN programs, with 1.31% graduating from diploma programs. Examining the data 5 years prior, ADN programs provided the majority of prelicensure nursing education at 58%, while BSN programs provided 38%, and diploma programs at 4% (National League of Nursing [NLN], 2014). The IOM in 2010 called for 80% of nurses to hold a BSN by 2020. The increase in RN-to-BSN graduates grew by 236% between 2010 and 2020, which showed great promise, but the call fell short (NAM, 2021). Healthcare organizations continue to express concern with the quality of prelicensure nursing education and echo the need for advances in education, health technology, and educational research that identifies more effective teaching–learning strategies. *The Future of Nursing 2020–2030 Report* recognizes the importance of "robust nursing education, supportive work environments and autonomy" (NAM, 2021, p. 1).

A more educated nursing workforce is needed in the current healthcare environment because nurses are expected to fill roles that are increasingly complex, sophisticated, and expanded (AACN, 2019b). Leaders within the nursing profession call for an increase in the number of nurses prepared at the baccalaureate level due to the need to advance the profession. Currently, employers demonstrate a preference for baccalaureate-prepared nurses, with 46% requiring a BSN and 88% with a strong preference for BSN-prepared nurses (AACN, 2020). The Tri-Council for Nursing (2021), an alliance of five autonomous nursing organizations including the AACN, American Nurses Association (ANA), American Organization for Nursing Leadership (AONL), the NCSBN, and the National League for Nursing (NLN) issued a policy statement calling for a more highly educated nursing workforce as a means to meet the nation's need for safe and effective patient care. Spetz (2018) identified the positive impact of BSN-prepared nurses on patients in acute care facilities, specifically those with diagnoses of heart failure, decubitus ulcers, postoperative deep vein thrombosis, and pulmonary emboli. Through extensive effort and support of academic progression at both associate and baccalaureate degree institutions, access to and enrollment in RN-to-BSN degree completion programs have increased by 56%, greatly improving the percentage of baccalaureate-prepared nurses in many states (AACN, 2019b; NAM, 2021). These achievements, combined with continued collaboration between leaders in nursing education and practice sectors, support a highly educated nursing workforce with both clinical competency and excellence in care delivery (AACN, 2019a, 2019b).

COMPONENTS OF CURRICULUM DESIGN

Nursing programs exist within a context of regulation, accreditation, professional standards, and an educational milieu. Any nursing program that educates prelicensure candidates for registered nursing must adhere to regulations and standards. In 2015, the Tri-Council for Nursing developed a framework that offered guiding principles to be used by state boards of nursing, facilities, and nurses for regulating education and scope practice. This algorithm is regularly reviewed by representatives from the ANA, NLN, state boards of nursing, along with the NCSBN staff, to support a uniform tool used across states (NCSBN, 2021). Nursing programs that exist within a public or private educational institution also meet regional accreditation standards through the parent institution, such as the Northwest Commission on Colleges and Universities or other national accrediting agencies, such as the Accreditation Commission for Independent Colleges and Schools.

ASSOCIATE DEGREE PROGRAMS

The current model of ADN education providing entry into practice began after World War II when there was a nursing shortage. Haase (1990), in describing the sequence of events leading to the development of associate degree programs, states that in 1948, the Committee on the Functions of Nursing made a recommendation that nursing practice consists of two tiers of nurses, one professional and the other technical. An educational model for the community college setting was developed intended to educate a technical nurse with a more limited scope of practice than a professional nurse but broader than that of a practical nurse. This model was piloted in an expanding number of community colleges, and graduates were found to have similar knowledge and qualities as compared with university and diploma nursing graduates (Haase, 1990). Although the model was subsequently implemented, the practice issue of technical versus professional nurse was not addressed. The model did, however, provide an evolutionary educational step by moving nursing education from the type of apprentice program (diploma) that was controlled by hospitals and physicians to the college and university system (Orsilini-Hain & Waters, 2009).

Part of the attraction of ADN programs is that they are affordable and provide streamlined access to the nursing profession. For students living in a rural or underserved area and too far from access to a 4-year, BSN program, the community college option of an ADN provides a viable option. These community or junior college programs have the largest number of minorities and preparation of rural nurses in underserved areas and support the supply of the nursing workforce (AACN, 2017; Organization for Associate Degree Nursing [OADN], 2021). The NLN (2016) states that there continues to be an increase in the percentage of underrepresented students enrolled in prelicensure programs, specifically African American, Spanish/Hispanic/Latino, and Asian. ADN programs educate greater numbers of African American, Spanish/Hispanic/Latino, and Indigenous American RNs than any other prelicensure program (OADN, 2021).

Healthcare reform continues to be the driving force associated with the need for a changed nursing education model as care moves from the hospital to different practice settings. This was particularly seen during the pandemic and how and where patients were cared for during and between surges. These changes demand that nursing students be competent in such areas as health policy, financing, leadership, quality improvement, and systems thinking since graduates are called on to work within teams and lead care coordination efforts. Reduction in credit requirements no longer supports the ability of nursing students to learn everything they need to know about the content areas of maternity, mental health, pediatrics, and medical–surgical nursing. The AACN (2016) identified greater than 50% of employers were requiring new hires to have a bachelor's degree in nursing. In an era pushing for increased education, these combined forces have the potential to negatively impact associate degree nursing education

Currently, ADN programs receive accreditation status through the Accreditation Commission for Education in Nursing (ACEN).

The ACEN (2020) has six standard categories:

1. Mission and Administrative Capacity
2. Faculty and Staff
3. Students
4. Curriculum
5. Resources
6. Outcomes

Mission or Vision and Philosophy Statements

ACEN (2020) accreditation standards for ADN programs require that the nursing program's mission and/or philosophy reflect the governing organization's core values and be congruent with the outcomes, strategic goals, and objectives. When developing or revising the mission and philosophy statements, the faculty and leaders of the nursing program should develop the program's mission in relation to those of the institution. Recommended sources of guidance are other programs within a system or programs that are similar or have good reputations. An ongoing program evaluation process ensures that the mission statement is continuously evaluated for both congruence and currency. The philosophy flows from the mission statement and reflects the beliefs of the program's faculty and staff about nursing, nursing education, students, teaching and learning, critical thinking, and evidence-based practice. These are generally longer statements that help guide curricular development and content.

Student-Learning Outcomes

Establishing learner outcomes and assessing whether students achieve those outcomes are required by all accrediting agencies. According to the ACEN (2020), student-learning outcomes (SLOs) are used to organize the curriculum, guide the delivery of instruction, direct learning activities, and evaluate student progress. SLO statements are broad and describe desired and expected behaviors of the program's graduates and differ from program outcomes such as first-time NCLEX-RN graduate pass rates, retention rates, employment rates, and program satisfaction. The SLOs should be reflected in level and course objectives.

Quality and Safety Education for Nurses (QSEN) provides an example of competencies that can be used to embed safety and quality outcomes within a curriculum for nurses (Pauly-O'Neill et al., 2016). QSEN developed a comprehensive listing of the knowledge, skills, and attitudes necessary to continuously improve the quality and safety of the care that nurses provide (QSEN, 2020).

Program of Study

There are many practical matters to consider in developing and revising nursing programs of study. Course sequencing, program length, credit totals, prerequisite and corequisite courses, and admission criteria should be based on national and regional standards, as well as any respective state board of nursing regulations. The ACEN (2020) standards require that the nursing program length must meet state and national standards and best practices. The parent college or university establishes requirements for credit totals, corequisite, and general education courses that must be included within the program of study.

ADN programs were designed at inception to require only 2 years of instruction (Orsilini-Hain & Waters, 2009). However, additive curricula and the increasing complexity of nursing practice expanded the curricula, which now must be reevaluated in order to serve graduates. In revising a curriculum, each program needs to determine what students need in order to be successful in their program's nursing curriculum, and course SLOs need to flow from the program SLOs.

Assessment

The achievement of SLOs must be evaluated by the faculty as a means of determining the quality of instruction and identify any overall improvement needs (ACEN, 2020). Through regular and systematic assessment, each program must demonstrate that students who complete their programs, no matter where or how they are offered, achieved these outcomes. For nursing programs, this means that each course within a nursing curriculum must have course and content learning outcomes or objectives that guide the delivery of content. These are the important and measurable behaviors or competencies for students in the course.

Level objectives for each semester or year are developed to assess the expected performance at specific points. All objectives and program learning outcomes are measurable so that they can be assessed at each step within the program. If results are less than expected, curriculum and instructional changes should be made that are based on evidence. ACEN (2020) standards and criteria can be used to establish a method of curriculum review that offers an evaluation of both student learning and the curriculum itself.

BACCALAUREATE PROGRAMS

There is significant concern with the preparedness of entry-level nurses to provide quality care within the complex and changing healthcare environments in which they practice. In addition, the shortage of nursing faculty and reduced capacity of clinical sites compel nursing educators to reconsider more traditional models of prelicensure clinical education. The IOM, now known as the NAM, has, over the last two decades, put forward recommended changes in healthcare education, compelling schools of nursing to focus on patient-centered quality and safety in the healthcare system. Those who develop and revise curriculum must be aware of changes in practice that create an educational gap for current nursing students. Billings (2019) identified making clinical judgments and implementing quality and safety education for nurses as the two gaps that need immediate attention. Closing these gaps has tremendous potential to contribute to reducing patient errors. Since the pandemic, many national organizations have joined together to support changes in nursing education based on lessons learned over the last year from COVID-19 (AONL, 2021; Tri-Council for Nursing, 2021). These lessons provide opportunities for transforming current curriculum.

Baccalaureate Essentials

The *Essentials: Core Competencies for Professional Nursing Education* provides a framework for nursing education across the educational and experiential spectrum, including all degree levels (AACN, 2021). The evolution of *the Essentials* series, from 1986 to this most recent version, demonstrates the advancement of nursing as a profession with the goal of preparing the nursing workforce of the future. The accompanying domains, competencies, and concepts provide the foundation for baccalaureate curricular design and program assessment (AACN, 2021, p. 18). The new *Essentials* are based on the underpinnings of "nursing as a discipline, the foundation of a liberal education, and the principles of competency-based education" (AACN, 2021, p. 3). The 10 domains include both entry- and advanced-level competencies and subcompetencies (see Table 8.2 for entry-level domains and competencies).

Past IOM reports and QSEN (2020) competencies for patient-centered care, teamwork and collaboration, evidence-based practice, quality improvement, safety, and informatics provided groundwork in the development of the new *Essentials*. Along with the *Essentials*, other <u>influential documents</u> impacting nursing curricula include *Healthy People 2030* (U.S. Department of Health and Human Services, 2020), the *Future of Nursing 2020-2030: Charting a Path to Achieve Health Equity* (NAM, 2021), and numerous research and position papers authored by a variety of key healthcare and educational organizations. The reenvisioned AACN *Essentials: Core Competencies for Professional Nursing Education*, with a focus on the entry-level competencies, are the foundation for BSN curriculum development and are referenced frequently throughout the discussion in this chapter.

Entry-level competencies and subcompetencies have been linked to each domain and were developed to be used in pre- and postlicensure baccalaureate programs that prepare the student to become a generalist for practice across the life span. Although 10 distinct domains have been identified, the *Essentials* acknowledge that "the expert practice of nursing requires integration of most domains in every practice situation or patient encounter" (AACN, 2021, p. 11). The teaching and evaluation of a competency and subcompetency are not one-and-done processes. Competency development is an ongoing process that builds on multiple opportunities for practice, feedback, and evaluation.

The following provides an example of the application of the *Essentials* domains, competencies, and subcompetencies to a traditional BSN student. Exhibit 8.1 focuses on a first-semester health assessment course (Tables 8.1 and 8.2).

EXHIBIT 8.1: Application of Domains, Competencies and Subcompetencies: Health Assessment

---

Upon completion of this course, students will be able to:

1. Perform a competent, comprehensive physical exam on the adult individual according to skill laboratory guidelines (Domain 2: Person-Centered Care, Competency 2.3, Subcompetency 2.3b, Concepts: Clinical Judgment, Communication, Diversity, Equity, and Inclusion)

Assignment(s):

Formative Assessment

Using a systems approach, the students will work in dyads weekly applying content learned in their health assessment course to assessments of their partners. Check-off and feedback will be provided by faculty at each encounter. Students must achieve a score of 75% or better to successfully pass the activity. If a student is struggling with any part of the assessment, they may be assigned additional time in open lab for supervised practice and ongoing feedback.

TABLE 8.1: Example of Rubric

Test Item	Point Value	Points Earned	Faculty Comments
COMMUNICATION	11 PT		

(continued)

TABLE 8.1: Example of Rubric (*continued*)

Test Item	Point Value	Points Earned	Faculty Comments
◆ Introduces self to client ◆ Identifies patient using two forms of patient identification ◆ Washing/foaming in and out	3		
◆ Explains procedures before performing them	2		
◆ Professionalism (focused vs. casual demeanor; points can be deducted for patient partner who offers verbal, facial, or other hints to examiner)	2		
◆ Terminology: uses correct anatomical and healthcare terms to describe landmarks	2		
◆ Organization (logical progression, organized, minimal disorganization, not bouncing from one system or body area to next), head-to-toe format, **completes exam in 12 minutes**.	2		

(*continued*)

TABLE 8.1: Example of Rubric (*continued*)

Test Item	Point Value	Points Earned	Faculty Comments
GENERAL ASSESSMENT/ QUESTIONING	8 PT		
◆ **General appearance:** Hygiene, body posture, demeanor, appears stated age, level of consciousness, facial expression, signs of comfort, pain or distress, appropriately dressed for weather/situation, no pallor, or cyanosis, and other pertinent objective observations related to systems on exam	3		
◆ **Subjective:** Regarding the systems covered come up with at least 2 for each system (skin, respiratory, CV). Remember to be age-appropriate.	5		
TOTAL POINTS	19	/19	

CV, cardiovascular.

Summative Assessment

During the final class meeting, the student will demonstrate a head-to-toe physical assessment based on a skills checklist within a given timeframe. Students must achieve a score of 75% or better to successfully pass the activity.

Students will also have the opportunity to apply these skills in their fundamental's clinical practicum with real patients and have feedback provided by their clinical faculty (per clinical grading rubric). In each clinical course throughout the program, students will revisit this specific domain, competencies, and subcompetencies with the expectation of applying these skills to new and increasingly complex patient care situations. These assessment skills will be applied to varied populations, such as pediatric patients, laboring and postpartum mothers, general medical/surgical patients, and critically ill patients. By the end of the program, the successful meeting of the competency identifies a student possessing well-honed, competent physical assessment skills that can be applied throughout the life span in multiple patient care situations.

The Essentials: Core Competencies for Professional Nursing Education

TABLE 8.2: Entry-Level Essential Domains and Core Competencies

Domain	Entry-Level Competencies	
Domain 1: Knowledge for Nursing Practice	1.1	Demonstrate an understanding of the discipline of nursing's distinct perspective and where shared perspectives exist with other disciplines
	1.2	Apply theory and research-based knowledge from nursing, the arts, and other sciences
	1.3	Demonstrate clinical judgment founded on a broad knowledge base
Domain 2: Person-Centered Care	2.1	Engage with the individual in establishing a caring relationship
	2.2	Communicate effectively with individuals
	2.3	Integrate assessment skills in practice
	2.4	Diagnose actual or potential health problems and needs
	2.5	Develop a plan of care
	2.6	Demonstrate accountability for care delivery
	2.7	Evaluate outcomes of care
	2.8	Promote self-care management
	2.9	Provide care coordination
Domain 3: Population Health	3.1	Manage population health
	3.2	Engage in effective partnerships
	3.3	Consider the socioeconomic impact of the delivery of healthcare
	3.4	Advance equitable population health policy
	3.5	Demonstrate advocacy strategies
	3.6	Advance preparedness to protect population health during disasters and public health emergencies
Domain 4: Scholarship for the Nursing Discipline	4.1	Advance the scholarship of nursing
	4.2	Integrate best evidence into nursing practice
	4.3	Promote the ethical conduct of scholarly activities
Domain 5: Quality and Safety	5.1	Apply quality improvement principles in care delivery
	5.2	Contribute to a culture of patient safety
	5.3	Contribute to a culture of provider and work environment safety
Domain 6: Interprofessional Partnerships	6.1	Communicate in a manner that facilitates a partnership approach to quality care delivery
	6.2	Perform effectively in different team roles, using principles and values of team dynamics
	6.3	Use knowledge of nursing and other professions to address healthcare needs
	6.4	Work with other professions to maintain a climate of mutual learning, respect, and shared values

(continued)

TABLE 8.2: Entry-Level Essential Domains and Core Competencies (*continued*)

Domain	Entry-Level Competencies	
Domain 7: Systems-Based Practice	**7.1**	Apply knowledge of systems to work effectively across the continuum of care
	7.2	Incorporate consider of cost-effectiveness of care
	7.3	Optimize system effectiveness through application of innovation and evidence-based practice
Domain 8: Informatics and Healthcare Technologies	**8.1**	Describe the various information and communication technology tools used in the care of patients, communities, and populations
	8.2	Use information and communication technology to gather data, create information, and generate knowledge
	8.3	Use information and communication technologies and informatics processes to deliver safe nursing care to diverse populations in a variety of settings
	8.4	Use information and communication technology to support documentation of care and communication among providers, patients, and all system levels
	8.5	Use information and communication technologies in accordance with ethical, legal, professional, and regulatory standards, and workplace policies in the delivery of care
Domain 9: Professionalism	**9.1**	Demonstrate an ethical comportment in one's practice reflective of nursing's mission to society
	9.2	Employ participatory approach to nursing care
	9.3	Demonstrate accountability to the individual, society, and the profession
	9.4	Comply with relevant laws, policies, and regulations
	9.5	Demonstrate the professional identity of nursing
	9.6	Integrate diversity, equity, and inclusion as core to one's professional identity
Domain 10: Personal, Professional, and Leadership Development	**10.1**	Demonstrate a commitment to personal health and well-being
	10.2	Demonstrate a spirit of inquiry that fosters flexibility and professional maturity
	10.3	Develop capacity for leadership

Source: American Association of Colleges of Nursing. (2021). The essentials: Core competencies for professional nursing education (pp. 29–62). https://www.aacnnursing.org/Portals/42/AcademicNursing/pdf/Essentials-2021.pdf

Curriculum Development

The curriculum reflects the commitment and dedication of a nursing faculty member. For each school, at least some of the current faculty members were most likely involved in developing the existing curriculum and are invested in its success. The curriculum expresses the faculty members' values and beliefs about nursing and education and reflects their professional identities. In most schools of nursing, the curriculum is familiar and comforting. These factors mean that curriculum change is one of the most challenging undertakings. It may prove difficult to build consensus about a new program based on different values and priorities among a diverse group of faculty members. Some faculty members keep up with best practices and innovation in nursing education, while others are content with the status quo. Ideally, curriculum revision is driven by the faculty and begins with an agreement by the faculty as a whole to enter into the process. The approval of the AACN (2021) *Essentials: Core Competencies for Professional Nursing Education* provides an impetus to reimagine curriculum with a goal of competency-based implementation.

Once a decision has been made to revise an existing curriculum or develop a new curriculum, next steps include selecting a work group or committee, developing a plan, and exploring best practices in nursing education. The composition of the group that will be leading the work is of primary importance to the success of the endeavor, and the members should be selected with intention. A strong team includes a collaborative group that has various areas of expertise and backgrounds, tenured and nontenured, clinical faculty and members from both undergraduate and graduate programs. Graduate faculty can provide insight into undergraduate curriculum that lays the foundation for future advanced registered nurse practitioners, educators, and nursing leaders. Members should be those who are committed to the goal and motivated to do the difficult work of curriculum development. In addition to faculty with a passion for curriculum, a balanced group includes both faculty members with current practice experience and those with expertise by virtue of their long teaching careers. Nursing students bring a unique and practical perspective to the work and their participation enriches the curriculum development process. As the group organizes, a discussion about roles within the committee and ground rules facilitates the process. An early discussion of bias, territoriality concerns, and "sacred cows" contributes to the process. Other suggestions include a tentative plan and timeline to help the group stay on schedule, a plan for communicating the progress of the curriculum revision, and points for feedback from the faculty as a whole.

The initial preparatory work of the curriculum development group is to review national consensus frameworks, such as the AACN Essentials (2021), and program evaluation data and plan a variety of strategies to identify best practices in nursing education. The extent of this effort will depend on the time elapsed since the last curriculum revision and the extent of the planned revision. The following information and documents will inform the committee and provide data for difficult discussions and decision-making:

◆ The *Essentials* (AACN, 2021) document is foundational and should be made available to all members from the beginning. The document includes core competencies, rationale, competency-based indicators, and sample content for each essential that are helpful in understanding the scope of each statement for application to a particular program of study. If your program is being accredited by the Commission on Collegiate Nursing Education (CCNE, 2019), it is important to determine which Essentials will be used for evaluating the program. If a prior version to the new 2021 Essentials is being used, it is recommended that all members have a copy of this document. The CCNE will determine when the expectation is to fully integrate the 2021 Essentials during its regular review of accreditation standards.

◆ A comprehensive search of the literature identifies best practices and innovation in nursing education; synthesizing the information for the faculty as a whole facilitates shared understanding.

◆ A review of professional standards such as the ANA *Code of Ethics* (2015) and various published competencies for BSN graduates is important. Based on current issues and priorities in nursing practice, specific baccalaureate-level competencies for quality and safety (QSEN, 2020), cultural competency (AACN, 2019c; National League for Nursing Center for Diversity and Global Initiatives, 2017), genetics and genomics (ANA and International Society of Nurses in Genetics, 2016), geriatric nursing care (AACN & John A. Hartford Foundation, 2010), equity and health equity (NAM, 2021; Tri-Council for Nursing, 2021), and palliative and end-of-life care (AACN, 2016; NLN, 2021).

◆ A survey of other regional and national programs provides examples of model programs of study. Programs that have been recently updated and incorporate innovation, have similar missions, and have been recently accredited may be of most value.

◆ Focus groups or surveys of stakeholders including students, faculty, and clinical or community partners provide invaluable information regarding expectations and priorities and create an inclusive process. These surveys provide meaningful local information about what was working and not working in the old curriculum, suggested changes or direction, new information and trends to be aware of, and priority knowledge and skills to include in the new curriculum.

Information in this chapter is relevant to the development or revision of curricula for several types of baccalaureate programs that are addressed, including 4-year traditional collegiate nursing programs, transfer programs in which students' complete prerequisites and general education courses before entering the nursing program, accelerated (second baccalaureate or fast-track) bachelor's degree programs, and RN completion programs. If a school has more than one type of program, there must be consistency and congruency among programs. The suggested approach is to start with the development of the generic prelicensure program and then develop modifications based on the core curriculum model.

Concept-Based Curriculum Development

The concept-based model for curriculum development is one strategy to reduce content saturation brought about by faculty's penchant for overloading courses with "need to know" content. The conceptual framework (theoretical or organizational model) guides the development of the program of study and makes it unique; it unifies the curriculum and creates a coherent approach across courses and levels to better prepare students for complex healthcare environments. In this approach, nursing faculty identifies, classifies, and defines concepts that subsequently provide the organizational framework for the curriculum and are threaded through courses (Harrison, 2020; Hendricks & Wangerin, 2017). While nursing faculty members are using many active learning strategies in their content delivery, lengthy lectures continue to be a mainstay in prelicensure nursing education (Hendricks & Wangerin, 2017; Solheim et al., 2021). Faculty barriers to implementation of the concept-based model include lack of administrative buy-in, a lack of knowledge, role identify struggles, and a resistance to change (Hendricks & Wangerin, 2017). Strategies to support faculty and program success in the implementation of a concept-based curriculum include detailed planning, training, and the availability of resources with supportive feedback (Patterson et al., 2021). Nielsen et al. (2020) demonstrated that structured concept-based learning in the clinical setting fosters deep learning and promotes clinical judgment in prelicensure nursing students. Often, conceptual integration and chosen exemplars take on a disease-based and acute care nursing focus. The effective integration of concepts encompassing population health, such as social determinants of health, is vital to the integrity of all baccalaureate nursing curriculum (Jordan et al., 2021; Porter et al., 2020).

Curriculum Outcomes

The next step in the BSN curriculum development process is to identify the level and terminal or end-of-program outcomes/SLOs (objectives or competencies), which must be directly related to the *Essentials* (AACN, 2008, 2021) in the context of the school's philosophy. Mapping or creating cross-tables are strategies for ensuring that all elements of the *Essentials* (AACN, 2021) are included. Whether a school uses *outcomes, objectives,* or *competencies* to create the curricular structure, the term must be defined, used consistently, and leveled across the program. The outcomes form the backbone of the curriculum and will be the foundation for program evaluation. SLOs (end-of-program outcomes) are developed by reviewing each essential and writing outcome statements that address the key concepts. This task can be completed either by the curriculum development group or can be more inclusive and involve the faculty as a whole by assigning a small group of individuals to write outcomes for specific *Essentials* (AACN, 2021). When all outcome statements are reviewed and analyzed as a package, there will most likely be overlap and areas that need to be strengthened in preparing the final document. As the outcomes statements are combined and synthesized, some may address more than one essential, but all *Essentials* (AACN, 2021) must be addressed somewhere within the program. When the terminal outcomes are identified, the level outcomes are developed and stepped to show students' progression through the program.

ADVANCES IN EDUCATIONAL TECHNOLOGY

Advances in educational technology and web-based learning radically altered the process of prelicensure nursing education delivery and impacted the structure of the curriculum and how nurses are taught (NLN, 2015). In late 2019, the majority of prelicensure nursing programs were delivered in an in-person format with relatively few courses offered completely online. By March 2020, the CDC and the World Health Organization (WHO) had declared COVID-19 a global pandemic. In many cases, faculty rapidly transitioned content to an online course delivery model for most didactic information. In the United States, prelicensure nursing clinical practicum was tremendously impacted due to clinical agency and institute of higher education (IHE) policies (CDC, 2020). Schools of nursing scrambled to integrate the use of technologies to provide digital alternatives for clinical learning. In response to the limiting of clinical experiences, the NCSBN streamlined a list of regulatory updates on a state-by-state basis that would facilitate the completion of nursing programs (NCSBN, 2020b). As digital natives, nursing students are often more technologically competent than faculty; however, faculty need to have the ability to support meaningful use of emerging technologies to support student success (Foronda et al., 2020). Computer-based or virtual simulations, such as the virtual neighborhood or community, virtual ward, vSim for Nursing Practice, or I-Human, are examples of innovations woven throughout the structure of the curriculum (Foronda et al., 2020). Applications are also available for teaching students to use electronic health records (Foronda et al., 2017, 2020). Distance education, virtual simulation platforms, and high-fidelity simulation learning strategies have been expanded and integrated into BSN programs, even more so following the COVID-19 global pandemic. Exciting new technologies are under development, as well as research surrounding their use with the potential to identify how students best learn and adapt accordingly Foronda et al., 2020; Kubin et al., 2021).

Distance Education

Online learning is increasingly integrated into nursing education, although the application of web-based approaches varies widely between nursing programs. Lessons learned from the COVID-19 pandemic necessitate innovation and a vision for nursing education that looks beyond fully in-person programs (Tri-Council for Nursing, 2021). Quality standards, such as Quality Matters (www.qualitymatter.org), have been developed for online education and faculty development and instructional design support are essential to ensure the effective delivery of online coursework (Authement & Dormire, 2020). While specific nonclinical courses may be taught online or offered as an alternative method of delivery, most prelicensure programs continued to be offered in a face-to-face format prior to the COVID global pandemic in 2020. The rapid transition to remote learning proved stressful to both faculty and students. One qualitative descriptive study interviewed baccalaureate students during this time and found themes of technological challenges, academic relationship changes, role stress and strain, and resilience (Wallace et.al., 2021). Distance learning–related stress emerged as a global phenomenon and has been recognized as an important challenge to nursing student success (Masha'al et al., 2020). As COVID-19 numbers decrease and we return to increasing in-person teaching, lessons learned have great potential to allow an increased use of distance education in prelicensure nursing programs.

Distance education is increasingly becoming the primary pedagogy for baccalaureate completion programs (Hensley et al., 2020). Distance applications include electronic classrooms and videoconferencing that facilitate inclusion of rural students and teaching across college campuses, or facilitate supervision for students involved in off-site practicum experiences. The availability of distance education technologies and the related philosophy of an academic institution toward their use as a teaching–learning methodology have significant implications for curriculum development. The use of cloud-based platforms for video- and audio conference, such as Zoom, has skyrocketed and greatly increased the opportunity for student engagement (Serembus & Kemery, 2020). As with all technology use in nursing education, the expertise and support of educators using these modalities are vital to student success.

High-Fidelity Simulation

Nursing education focuses on integrating theoretical knowledge with experiential learning. In the traditional nursing education model, the opportunities to apply knowledge may be limited. Even in an optimal clinical setting, a lack of predictable experiences and potential risk to patients impacted the ability to provide consistent, guaranteed experiences. While nursing educators have long employed low- and mid-fidelity simulation in nursing skills labs, high-fidelity simulation has become the "gold standard" as schools of nursing incorporate this teaching strategy into curricula to prepare students for clinical experiences and to supplement or replace clinical hours. Simulated learning experiences can be developed to support the progressive achievement of curriculum outcomes by intentionally spiraling core concepts and skills throughout the curriculum in increasingly more complex scenarios (Hanshaw & Dickerson, 2020). The NLN Institute for Simulation and Technology (2021) supports nurse educators in staying up-to-date on best practices in simulation and develops simulation scenarios to meet curricular needs across the curriculum. Interprofessional simulations can provide an opportunity for students to learn about teamwork and collaboration and the roles of other healthcare professions (Lee et al., 2021). Although students routinely report high stress in the simulated learning environment, the human patient simulation experiences were found to be a valuable learning tool (Cantrell et al., 2017; Hanshaw & Dickerson, 2020). Simulation has been shown as a powerful teaching strategy for improving cultural awareness and understanding social determinants of health (O'Brien et al., 2021).

According to Hayden et al. (2014), the landmark NCSBN National Simulation Study of 2014 highlighted the positive role of simulation as a substantive clinical opportunity. This landmark national multisite randomized control trial concluded that simulation could be substituted for up to 50% of traditional clinical experiences. Additionally, faculty supporting these simulation experiences should be formally trained with subject matter experts conducting any debriefing experiences. There is also the opportunity to integrate lower fidelity and task trainers as an alternative, depending on the goal of instruction and competency outcome that faculty wish to achieve with students. Simulation using live actors as standardized patients, in virtual, telehealth, and face-to-face formats, is also a powerful strategy with the potential to change attitudes, beliefs, and behaviors among student participants (Powers et al., 2020; Wynn, 2020).

The focus on simulation in nursing education has been primarily on learning, including prebriefing and debriefing, with less emphasis on more high-stakes summative evaluation (Cantrell et al., 2017). In planning for use of simulation in a curriculum, schools are advised to check with their state boards of nursing regarding regulations for the percentage or replacement of clinical hours with high-fidelity simulation. Up to 50% of total clinical hours may be completed using simulation in an increasing number of states. Limited availability of clinical experiences, in specialty areas, such as maternal and child, pediatrics, and mental health, has led to increased utilization of high-fidelity simulation to support student learning (Peterson et al., 2021; Reid et al., 2020). The importance of evidence-based faculty training and support cannot be underestimated and supports positive student and program outcomes (Hanshaw & Dickerson, 2020). In order to make the best use of this technology, simulation must be approached with vision and intention in the curriculum development process. All aspects of simulation within a given curriculum should be guided by evidence-based approaches, such as the Standards of Best Practice: Simulation (Becker et al., 2020; International Nursing Association for Clinical Simulation and Learning, 2016).

TRANSFORMATIVE APPROACHES TO CLINICAL EDUCATION

One of the most challenging aspects of curriculum revision is designing an approach to students' clinical experiences that reflects the school's theoretical model and integrates new learning pedagogies in the context of local realities regarding the availability of qualified clinical faculty and clinical sites. While clinical experience is essential in preparation for practice, what constitutes clinical experience? What kinds of clinical learning activities and how much time in what kind of healthcare settings are most effective for BSN students to meet generalist competencies and transition successfully into practice? The NCSBN (2016) reinforces that it is not the number of hours but rather the quality of the experiences that is most important to student success and patient outcomes. The AACN Vision for Nursing Education Task Force (AACN, 2019d) made recommendations for a broad reenvisioning of baccalaureate nursing education to encompass a competency-based model that was tied to integrative experiences, including cross-disciplinary experiences; new relationships within learning communities framed by innovative formalized academic-practice partnerships; and reconceptualized learning experiences in which all students do not have clinical experiences in traditional rotations. These transformative approaches thread seamlessly into a rich transition to practice programs (AACN, 2019d). As discussed previously, the disruption caused by the COVID-19 global pandemic provided an opportunity for innovation and transformation that forced the evaluation of novel learning environments and allowed us to step closer to these recommendations (Carolan, 2020). The Tri-Council for Nursing (2021) utilizing lessons learned from the COVID-19 pandemic recommends expansion of nursing curricula to include public health, crisis management, health equity, mental health, and social determinants of health.

The landmark NCSBN National Simulation Study of 2014 highlighted the positive role of simulation as a substantive clinical opportunity. These researchers broke through barriers and changed the landscape in what learning experiences can constitute nursing clinical experiences. While there are scarce data about the effectiveness of either traditional or other new clinical models, it is incumbent on nurse educators to develop and test models and approaches and contribute to the database. Each school of nursing needs to develop an approach that best utilizes its resources and fits its theoretical model. Discuss the vital role of discourse and clinical supervisor–student relationship and coaching in intentional learning (Lee, 2021). Frameworks and tools support clinical faculty and preceptors in providing feedback and evaluating clinical development (Jessee & Tanner, 2016; Nielsen et al., 2016). Despite the innovative potential for transforming clinical nursing education, most schools of nursing continue to deliver clinical using the traditional apprenticeship model (Leighton et al., 2018).

COMPLETING THE CURRICULUM DEVELOPMENT PROCESS

Concurrent with the development of the program of study, additional work must be completed as part of the comprehensive curriculum package. A glossary defines terms that have special meaning within the mission, vision, and philosophy; theoretical model; and curriculum plan, including concepts that provide the organizational framework for the curriculum. Prerequisites including humanities, science, and social science courses that serve as the foundation for the nursing coursework must be identified and negotiated with various other departments. These include college-wide requirements such as general education. Progression issues must be considered, including criteria for admission into the school of nursing, a description of how students will progress from semester to semester, and prerequisites and corequisites for each course. The curriculum development group will need to work with the administrative team to cost out the curriculum, including faculty and other resources that will be needed to manage the new curriculum. Often old and new curricula will be offered simultaneously for a time until the students in the original program graduate, which may require additional resources. The curriculum package must be approved by the nursing faculty and be directed through broader academic channels for approval. The new curriculum must be submitted to the state board of nursing, regional accrediting bodies, and the national accrediting body for formal approval.

THE INCLUSIVE CURRICULUM: PAYING ATTENTION TO DIVERSITY, EQUITY, AND INCLUSION

There is a national call to increase the enrollment of students from underrepresented populations in schools of nursing, and recent reports show that some progress is being made (AACN, 2019c; Association of American Colleges and Universities [AACU], 2020). Relf (2016) described the need for academic nursing to increase its efforts to ensure the nursing workforce matches the demographics of the U.S. population. The uniqueness of each individual includes recognition of differences in race, ethnicity, gender, sexual orientation, gender identity, socioeconomic status, age, physical abilities, religious beliefs, political beliefs, and other attributes (AACU, 2020; NLN, 2016). Schools of nursing typically have not considered the needs of students who are minorities; low-income students; first in family to attend college; multilingual, nonnative English speakers; or disabled in developing the plan of study or the curriculum structure. Further complicating the goal of meaningful inclusion is the lack of nursing educators from underrepresented and diverse populations (AACN, 2017; NLN, 2016).

It is logical to assume that diversity and inclusion should be threaded throughout the curriculum, including the mission statement, as well as course, level, and program outcomes (AACU, 2020). Ideally, the curriculum should be creative, flexible, and reflect culturally informed care, determinants of health, and the multicultural perspectives of the pluralistic society (Moore & Clark, 2016; Tri-Council for Nursing, 2021). The AACU (2020) promotes *inclusive excellence*, a commitment to making equity a pervading focus of educational reform. This philosophy presupposes a broad definition of *diversity* and compels faculty members to facilitate the success of all students, including those with diverse backgrounds and learning styles. Faculty may not be aware of how programmatic organization affects students differentially. These learners best achieve academically in a curriculum model that more closely integrates theory and clinical experience. All students should be ensured an education that allows them as the nursing leaders of the future to meet the needs of an increasingly diverse society and bring civic readiness and engagement to their positions as nursing leaders (AACN, 2017).

Other ways of demonstrating inclusiveness in curriculum planning include preentry nursing courses, parallel academic support courses, culture-focused or special interest general education courses or electives, and international experiences as part of the program of study. The co-curriculum can play an important role in supporting and validating underrepresented students on the campus. Other ideas include developing clinical models that facilitate clinical experiences with diverse populations and intentionally threading exemplars throughout the curriculum that address healthcare issues experienced by particular ethnic, cultural, or minority groups. And finally, admission and progression requirements for incoming students that support or, conversely, disadvantage those who were educated in another country or are multilingual nonnative English speakers will shape the student body and affect the quality of learning for all the students. A diverse student body has been shown to be associated with improved outcomes among all students (AACU, 2020; Murray et al., 2016).

INTERPROFESSIONAL EDUCATION: PREPARING FOR COLLABORATIVE PRACTICE

In response to safety and quality standards in healthcare and a vision for accessible, patient-centered care, AACN collaborated with leadership from other professional organizations to develop competencies that promote team-based, interprofessional healthcare (Interprofessional Education Collaborative, 2016). The WHO (2010) stated that interprofessional education (IPE) "occurs when students from two or more professions learn about, from and with each other to enable effective collaboration and improve health" (p. 7). Health professions schools are developing models for IPE in classroom, simulation, and, more recently, clinical and community settings. IPE models have been studied in undergraduate nursing programs (Ross et al., 2020). IPE can include multiple disciplines within, as well as those outside, the healthcare field. How interesting and innovative to have a group of computer science, engineering, business, and nursing students all together to discuss the feasibility of creating a care program for spinal cord rehabilitation. It is more of a "think tank" to identify innovative ideas of care and the complexities involved in that creation.

Although there are significant logistical, cultural, and historical barriers to IPE and practice, the benefits of IPE for prelicensure students are many, including a greater understanding of roles and contributions of other healthcare professionals and dynamics within the healthcare team, development of professional pride and identity, importance of effective interprofessional communication and reflective practice, knowledge of patient conditions and increased comfort with targeted patient populations, improved cultural sensitivity, building of professional networks, and an improved sense of collaboration and cooperation (Kostoff et al., 2016; Lee et al., 2020; Ross et al., 2020; Rutledge et al., 2020; Swift et al., 2020). Each school has unique opportunities, and moving forward,

IPE/interprofessional collaborative practice must be considered as an integral element of every baccalaureate curriculum.

TRANSITION TO PRACTICE

The transition of new BSN graduates io clinical practice is recognized as an issue since *Reality Shock* was first published (Kramer, 1974). A variety of rich clinical experiences with engaged faculty prior to beginning work in the professional role have been shown as one curriculum strategy that contributes to graduate nurses prepared to step into practice (Patterson et al., 2021). Recommendations from national reports about the transition from the academic environment to the nursing practice environment showed significant support for the formation of academic and service partnerships to develop standardized residency programs (AACN, 2012; Benner et al., 2010; CCNE, 2019; IOM, 2010). The CCNE (2019) revised the accreditation standards for entry-to-practice nurse residency programs. The standards for accreditation focus on entry-to-practice nurse residency programs course faculty, institutional commitment and resources, program curriculum, and program effectiveness.

The goal of transition programs is primarily to facilitate professional formation and socialization into the culture of the healthcare organization, assist the new graduate to develop clinical competency, improve recruitment retention, and reduce orientation costs for the employer. Programs may be situated prior to graduation or following, and include educational and psychosocial support strategies such as mentoring, preceptor training, clinical coaching, expanded orientation, clinical and professional skill development, classes, and other learning and support activities targeted at the needs of the developing professional (Chan & Burns, 2021).

Published in 2019, a model residency program that promotes point-of-care leadership was developed and evaluated by AACN and Vizient. This curriculum focuses on three content areas: leadership, patient safety, and professional role. Among other findings, an evaluation demonstrated that the residents' perceptions of confidence and competence, capacity to organize and prioritize, and ability to communicate and provide leadership improved significantly.

One major challenge in residency program management is preparing and maintaining committed and effective mentor/preceptors. Additional barriers to a successful transition to practice include a lack of understanding of existing gaps in knowledge and skills, limited orientations, and a lack of respect from coworkers (Charette et al., 2019). In the current climate of scarce resources, hiring institutions must evaluate their return on investment in relation to transition programs for new nursing graduates. One might include performance evaluation of nursing graduates/residents against national benchmarks. The National Database of Nursing Quality Indicators or accreditation standards (Get with the Guidelines for Stroke and Heart Failure centers) provide an evaluation of patient outcomes. This content is important to include in the nursing curriculum. Transitioning to practice should not be the first time the new graduate nurse hears this information.

ALTERNATIVE BACCALAUREATE PATHWAYS

ABSN Programs

The first ABSN programs were initiated in the early 1970s and grew rapidly in number since the 1990s. A 2018 survey found 23,354 students enrolled in accelerated baccalaureate programs, a 16% increase in enrollment compared with 2017 (AACN, 2019e). Accelerated programs are geared to students who have demonstrated success in previous baccalaureate education and are generally offered as intensive full-time courses of study with no breaks between semesters or terms. Most programs are 11 to 18 months in length (AACN, 2019e). Graduates from ABSN programs are highly valued by employers because of their maturity, their ability to learn quickly, and their clinical skills (AACN, 2019e).

Having successfully completed a prior baccalaureate, students in accelerated programs are experienced learners who understand the challenges of college and have learned how to effectively navigate the system. These skills, grounded in their previous college experiences, help them cope with the rigors of a professional program. As mature and motivated as ABSN students might be, they have reported high levels of stress when challenged by the expectations of the student role and balancing the demands of family, work, and finances (Abshire et al., 2018; Kramlich et al., 2020; Wiersma et al., 2020).

Brandt et al. (2017) found that ABSN graduates were motivated to find a job and felt the rigor of the accelerated program prepared them well for professional practice. ABSN programs are producing graduates who remain in the workplace and also pursue advanced degrees soon after graduation (AACN, 2019e). As engaged and motivated adult learners, ABSN students and graduates can offer important insights as part of the planning group during curriculum redesign initiatives.

Baccalaureate Completion Programs

Baccalaureate completion programs, also called "RN-to-BSN" programs, are designed for RNs who are graduates of accredited associate degree or hospital-based diploma programs and who seek a BSN degree. Based on research demonstrating improved performance on quality and safety outcomes when nurses are educated at the baccalaureate level or higher, AACN maintains that the BSN degree should be the minimum educational requirement for professional nursing practice (Tri-Council for Nursing, 2021). The BSN has become the preferred preparation for practice in healthcare settings, including Magnet hospitals and organizations that require the baccalaureate for specific nursing roles. Nurses who seek positions in case management, public health and community-based settings, and leadership find that the BSN is an essential requirement for employment.

Nurses who enroll in RN-to-BSN programs have a variety of life and work experiences, in addition to experiences in previous educational programs. They are often motivated to enroll in RN-to-BSN programs and achieve the higher degree in order to secure employment, advance their careers, or fulfill their personal goals (Wojnar & Whelan, 2017). The BSN degree is the gateway to graduate education and subsequent roles in advanced practice, nursing education, and research. The purpose of the completion program is to assist students to develop higher level critical thinking skills, broaden their scope of practice, and understand the social, cultural, economic, and geopolitical context of healthcare in order to assume expanded professional roles (AACN, 2017). Clinical partnerships prove to be a valuable partner in identifying and implementing rich didactic content and securing diverse clinical opportunities for this population of students (Wojnar & Whelan, 2017).

Academic Progression for Nurses

Based on increasing demands in healthcare and the need for high-quality health outcomes across all care settings, the IOM (2010) recommended that the nursing education system be improved to support nurses' achievement of higher levels of education. Subsequently, the IOM challenged nurse leaders to work together to increase the number of baccalaureate-prepared nurses from 50% to 80% by 2020. As a result, academic nurse leaders recognized the need to develop collaborative relationships between community colleges and higher degree programs (AACN, 2019f). Certain states have mandated articulation agreement requirements that facilitate academic progression for nurses.

Articulation agreements are renewable agreements negotiated to ensure equivalency between college and university courses, support educational mobility, and facilitate the seamless transfer of academic credit between associate degree (ADN) and baccalaureate (BSN) programs (AACN, 2019f). Articulation agreements address the needs of students and programs by facilitating a more streamlined progression experience. Students benefit from transferring credit between institutions, making informed decisions about course selection, and experiencing collaboration across nursing programs (AACN, 2019f; Wojnar & Whelan, 2017). Some agreements have been as specific as offering dual enrollment in the associate and baccalaureate programs upon admission to the associate degree program, while others look to establish competency during the first year in an ADN curriculum prior to beginning baccalaureate-level coursework. Dual enrollment provides students with additional benefits such as academic advising and support as well as more diverse course offerings. For healthcare agencies looking to provide preference to students pursuing a BSN, this dual enrollment can open employment opportunities not seen by the traditional ADN-seeking student.

Other models for academic progression for the ADN-prepared nurse include the conferral of BSN degrees at the community college level (Farmer et al., 2017). Researchers found potential in the use of a competency-based curriculum that allows the RN-to-BSN student to demonstrate competency in program-designated clinical and professional outcomes (Sitzman et al., 2020; Wagner et al., 2020). This model has the potential to reduce redundancy and identify significant content; however, it is challenged by the lack of a unified set of competencies for BSN degree completion. Master's or graduate entry programs are a popular option that allows progression and expedites the journey to advanced degrees (AACN, 2021c).

Well-known major barriers to BSN degree completion are time and cost. More recently, the absence of mentoring/guidance and a lack of exposure to evidence supporting the importance of a BSN or higher degree have been identified (Sitzman et al., 2020). Academic partnerships with clinical agencies that employ ADN-prepared nurses, coupled with regulatory support, have the potential to address these important issues. There is no shortage of RN-to-BSN completion programs with their numbers exceeding current 4-year and ASBN programs (AACN, 2019g).

RN-to-BSN Program of Study

The mission, vision, philosophy, theoretical model, and SLOs for an RN-to-BSN program are often the same as the generic BSN program at a particular school, although the program of study may look very different. Program credits and length are variable between schools, and the design of the curriculum often offers part-time and online options in order to meet the needs of working nurses.

Credit for Prior Learning

As the nursing workforce is challenged to meet the increasingly complex needs of the current and future healthcare system, nursing programs across the country are challenged to encourage RNs to return to school for BSN completion. Nursing programs responded to this challenge by acknowledging that the RN holds knowledge, skills, and abilities related to prior work experience that can be applied to the current degree they are seeking. It is typical for RN-to-BSN completion programs to require introductory courses that are designed to validate this prior knowledge and to "bridge" or "transition" the RN from diploma or associate degree preparation. In addition to providing an opportunity to validate prior knowledge and skills, these introductory courses offer learning experiences, such as professional portfolio activities, that assist with the role transition and socialization to the BSN level of preparation. The nurse is granted credit for selected prelicensure courses offered at the upper division level once the transition course is successfully completed.

Curriculum Strategies

The RN-to-BSN curriculum addresses nurses' need for socialization, preparation for a broader scope of practice, preparation for graduate study, career growth, and leadership development (AACN, 2019g; Sitzman et al., 2020; Wojnar & Whelan, 2017). In the typical RN-to-BSN curriculum, the nurse is prepared for an expanded professional role through coursework focused on enhancing professional communication, theoretical perspectives, community and population-based nursing care, health promotion, and leadership. The senior practicum hours are spent working with nurse preceptors in acute care settings as well as in community-based settings where the nurses build on previous knowledge and enhance their effectiveness across the continuum of care. Many programs incorporate professional projects designed to meet the needs of the clinical agency from an evidence-based perspective, while other activities include projects related to nursing leadership, health promotion, disease prevention, and the care of vulnerable populations.

With a growing awareness about the positive outcomes associated with advancing to higher levels of education and increasing encouragement from employers who provide tuition support for RN-to-BSN programs, more and more nurses are returning to school to complete a baccalaureate degree (AACN, 2019g). In order to meet the demand for BSN completion, nursing programs responded by offering curricula delivered through online and distance learning and the traditional classroom setting or by using combined methods such as hybrid or web-enhanced approaches (AACN, 2019g). Distance education provides RN-to-BSN students, who are usually employed and juggling multiple roles, with greater accessibility to attend class at times of the day that meet their needs. Nurses attending online completion programs also benefit from geographic flexibility, self-directed learning and motivation, professional socialization, and peer support.

Clinical Experiences

The increasing enrollment in RN-to-BSN programs creates additional strain on scarce clinical practicum sites and faculty. However, the fact that RN-to-BSN students are licensed, as compared to BSN students, allows for placement of licensed nurses in a variety of traditional and nontraditional clinical sites. This ability generates opportunities for students to provide nursing care in settings in which they can begin to view caring in new ways, awakening a sense of advocacy, civic responsibility, and concern for political action (AACN, 2019g). A sense of responsibility is gained from various types of experiential and service-learning experiences that extend beyond the singular nurse–client relationship to embrace the client's family, community, and society. Clinical experiences designed for service in community-based settings assist the nurse in adopting a broader, global view of nursing practice (Goliat et al., 2020).

RN-to-BSN students benefit from being able to explore areas of interest for their clinical experiences, as well as collaborating with faculty to identify creative ways to meet their goals for learning. There is the potential for deep engagement and mutuality for preceptors and staff in clinical sites within the student's community. RN-to-BSN students often choose experiences in public and community health, school-based health settings, correctional nursing, mental and behavioral health centers, addiction treatment and homeless shelters, geriatric settings, and home health and hospice settings. In addition,

RN-to-BSN students are uniquely suited for participation in global healthcare delivery when interested in opportunities for international travel and meeting the needs of the vulnerable and underserved.

International clinical placements and studies abroad are recognized as broadening students' cultural understanding and preparing them for authentic relationships in the professional clinical setting (Jansen et al., 2021; Morrison-Beedy et al., 2021). Students have the opportunity to explore diverse cultures and communities as well as gain knowledge of different healthcare systems. RN-to-BSN students who complete international clinical experiences have described meaningful learning related to awareness of diversity and cultural competence in nursing, enhanced skills in intercultural communication, an increased awareness of social and political injustices, and a greater understanding of poverty.

Inexperienced RN-to-BSN Students

As the trend toward hiring "BSN preferred" nurses continues, it is anticipated that more nurses will enter RN-to-BSN completion programs immediately following graduation from associate degree and diploma programs. In order to meet admission requirements for RN-to-BSN completion programs, applicants must pass the NCLEX examination for licensure and obtain an RN license. Since the RN-to-BSN curriculum builds on the prior work experience of the RN, nurses just beginning nursing practice require special consideration related to their relative lack of clinical experience. There may be new graduate nurses who have not found nursing jobs following completion of their initial degree and have no work experience, which challenges some of the assumptions of many RN-to-BSN programs. Depending on the structure of the curriculum, inexperienced RN-to-BSN students may have difficulty engaging in classroom activities designed for experienced RNs to apply new knowledge and insights to their current practice. In the clinical setting, the less experienced RN requires additional oversight and support by faculty and preceptors beyond what is usually provided for licensed students.

Despite some of the challenges for new graduate nurses who enter completion programs, RN-to-BSN programs provide valuable experiences for students. Students benefit from learning collaboratively with nurses who have varied years and types of clinical experiences. Research suggests that RN students, in their quest for higher education, seek to attain professional credibility, career mobility, personal achievement, and longevity in nursing (Goliat et al., 2020). The RN-to-BSN completion programs provide a rich and supportive environment for nurses returning to school. Nursing faculty members have the opportunity to mentor and model professional behaviors that assist in building positive connections and influence the learning of their students.

SUMMARY

Robust baccalaureate nursing education programs are foundational to the health of the profession and the population and as preparation for graduate nursing education. Curriculum development and revision are both a challenge and an opportunity to shape the future. Collaboration with stakeholders including other healthcare professionals, consumers of healthcare, and healthcare service organizations is essential in order to innovate and find local solutions in a new age of healthcare reform. It is incumbent on nursing educators to try new curricular approaches, evaluate their efficacy, and share the results with the professional community.

END-OF-CHAPTER RESOURCES

DISCUSSION QUESTIONS

1. Identify your primary partners in service or education. What is the nature of those relationships and how could they be expanded to create innovative clinical experiences for both prelicensure and RN-to-BSN nursing students?

2. What are the most common groups of underrepresented students in your region? How could your admission process and curriculum be changed to be more inclusive of these groups?

3. What are the barriers to prelicensure graduates' successful transition into practice? Describe strategies in your curriculum that help mediate "reality shock." What are some new ideas that could be developed? Do any clinical agencies in your area have a new graduate residency program?

4. How will or has the new reenvisioned Baccalaureate Essentials affect your prelicensure program? Interview the chair of the undergraduate curriculum committee at your school to determine if there is a plan for curriculum revision.

5. Create an innovative clinical educational model and describe how this would integrate and meet learning outcomes within a given curriculum.

6. Describe IPE activities that could be integrated into the curriculum at each of the various levels at your college or university. Think about different professions with whom you could partner.

LEARNING ACTIVITIES

Faculty Development Activities

1. Map your curriculum outcomes according to the AACN *Essentials: Core Competencies for Professional Nursing Education* (2021). What changes need to be made to update your program?

2. Create a visual representation of your school's theoretical/conceptual model.

3. Invite a colleague to coffee and discuss the "sacred cows" at your institution that could be barriers to innovative curriculum revision.

A robust set of instructor resources designed to supplement this text is located at **http://connect.springerpub.com/content/book/978-0-8261-8686-7.** Qualifying instructors may request access by emailing **textbook@springerpub.com.**

REFERENCES

Abshire, D. A., Graves, J. M., Roberts, M. L., Katz, J., Barbosa-Leiker, C., & Corbett, C. F. (2018). Student support in accelerated nursing programs: Gender-based perspectives and impact on academic outcomes. *Nursing Outlook, 66*(1), 84–93. https://doi.org/10.1016/j.outlook.2017.08.010

Accreditation Commission for Education in Nursing. (2020). *ACEN 2020 standards and criteria associate.* https://www.acenursing.org/acen-accreditation-manual-standards-a/

American Association of Colleges of Nursing. (2008). *The essentials of baccalaureate education for professional nursing practice*. http://www.aacnnursing.org/Portals/42/Publications/BaccEssentials08.pdf

American Association of Colleges of Nursing. (2012). *AACN-AONE Task Force on Academic-Practice Partnerships: Guiding principles*. https://www.aacnnursing.org/Academic-Practice-Partnerships/The-Guiding-Principles

American Association of Colleges of Nursing. (2016). *CARES: Competencies and recommendations for educating undergraduate nursing students. Preparing nurses to care for the seriously ill and their families*. https://www.aacnnursing.org/Portals/42/ELNEC/PDF/New-Palliative-Care-Competencies.pdf

American Association of Colleges of Nursing. (2017). *Diversity, equity, and inclusion in academic nursing*. https://www.aacnnursing.org/Portals/42/News/Position-Statements/Diversity-Inclusion.pdf

American Association of Colleges of Nursing. (2019a). *Fact sheet: Creating a more highly qualified nursing workforce*. https://www.aacnnursing.org/Portals/42/News/Factsheets/Nursing-Workforce-Fact-Sheet.pdf

American Association of Colleges of Nursing. (2019b). *Fact sheet: The impact of education on nursing practice*. https://www.aacnnursing.org/Portals/42/News/Factsheets/Education-Impact-Fact-Sheet.pdf

American Association of Colleges of Nursing. (2019c). *Fact Sheet: Enhancing diversity in the nursing workforce*. https://www.aacnnursing.org/Portals/42/News/Factsheets/Enhancing-Diversity-Factsheet.pdf

American Association of Colleges of Nursing. (2019d). *AACN vision for academic nursing*. https://www.aacnnursing.org/Portals/42/News/White-Papers/Vision-Academic-Nursing.pdf

American Association of Colleges of Nursing. (2019e). *Fact sheet: Accelerated baccalaureate and master's degrees in nursing*. https://www.aacnnursing.org/Portals/42/News/Factsheets/Accelerate-Programs-Fact-Sheet.pdf

American Association of Colleges of Nursing. (2019f). *Articulation agreements among nursing education programs*. https://www.aacnnursing.org/Portals/42/News/Factsheets/Articulation-Agreements-Fact-Sheet.pdf

American Association of Colleges of Nursing. (2019g). *Degree completion programs for registered nurses: RN to master's degree and RN to baccalaureate programs*. https://www.aacnnursing.org/Portals/42/News/Factsheets/Degree-Completion-Factsheet.pdf

American Association of Colleges of Nursing. (2020). *Employment of new nurse graduates and employer preferences for baccalaureate-prepared nurses*. https://www.aacnnursing.org/Portals/42/News/Surveys-Data/Research-Brief-12-20.pdf

American Association of Colleges of Nursing. (2021). *The essentials: Core competencies for professional nursing education*. https://www.aacnnursing.org/Portals/42/AcademicNursing/pdf/Essentials-2021.pdf

American Association of Colleges of Nursing & the John A. Hartford Foundation Institute for Geriatric Nursing. (2010). *Recommended baccalaureate competencies and curricular guidelines for the nursing care of older adults*. https://www.aacnnursing.org/Portals/42/AcademicNursing/CurriculumGuidelines/AACN-Gero-Competencies-2010.pdf

American Association of Colleges of Nursing & Vizient. (2019). *Vizient/AACN nurse residency program*. https://www.vizientinc.com/our-solutions/clinical-solutions/vizient-aacn-nurse-residency-program

American Nurses Association. (2015). *Code of ethics for nurses with interpretive statements*.

American Nurses Association and International Society of Nurses in Genetics. (2016). *Genetics/genomics nursing: Scope and standards of practice* (2nd ed.). American Nurses Association.

American Organization of Nursing Leadership. (2021). *Key stakeholders examine lessons learned from COVID-19 pandemic and issue report on current and future challenges and opportunities*. https://www.aonl.org/press-releases/tricouncil-for-nursing-calls-for-transformation-in-nursing-education

Association of American Colleges and Universities. (2020). *What liberal education looks like: What it is, who it's for, & where it happens*.

Authement, R. S., & Dormire, S. L. (2020). *Introduction to the online nursing education best practices guide*. https://journals.sagepub.com/doi/10.1177/2377960820937290

Becker, D., Collazo, M., Garrison, C. M., & Sandahl, S. S. (2020). Finding your way with the INACSL standards of best practice: Simulation[SM]: Development of an interactive web-based guide and roadmap. *Clinical Simulation in Nursing, 48*, 75–79. https://doi.org/10.1016/j.ecns.2020.08.005

Benner, P., Sutphen, M., Leonard, V., & Day, L. (2010). *Educating nurses: A call for radical transformation*. Jossey-Bass.

Billings, D. M. (2019). *Closing the education–practice gap*. https://www.wolterskluwer.com/en/expert-insights/closing-the-educationpractice-gap

Brandt, C. L., Boellaard, M. R., & Wilberding, K. M. (2017). Accelerated second-degree bachelor of science in nursing graduates' transition to professional practice. *Journal of Continuing Education in Nursing, 48*(1), 14–19. https://doi.org/10.3928/00220124-20170110-05

Cantrell, M. L., Meyer, S. L., & Mosack, V. (2017). Effects of simulation on nursing student stress: An integrative review. *Journal of Nursing Education, 56*(3), 139–144. https://doi.org/10.3928/01484834-20170222-04

Carolan, C. (2020). COVID-19: Disruptive impacts and transformative opportunities in undergraduate nurse education. *Nurse Education in Practice, 46*, 102807. https://doi.org/10.1016/j.nepr.2020.102807

Center for Disease Control and Prevention. (2020). *Considerations for institutions of higher education*. https://www.cdc.gov/coronavirus/2019-ncov/community/colleges-universities/considerations.html

Centers for Disease Control and Prevention. (2021). *National center for chronic disease prevention and health promotion*. https://www.cdc.gov/chronicdisease/index.htm

Chan, G. K., & Burns, E. M. (2021). Quantifying and remediating the new graduate nurse resident academic-practice gap using online patient simulation. *The Journal of Continuing Education in Nursing, 52*(5), 240–247. https://doi.org/10.3928/00220124-20210414-08

Charette, M., Gourdreau, J., & Bourbonnais, A. (2019). Factors influencing the practice of new graduate nurses: A focused ethnography of acute care settings. *Journal of Clinical Nursing, 28*, 3618–3631. https://doi.org/10.1111/jocn.14959

Commission on Collegiate Nursing Education. (2019). *Procedures for accreditation of baccalaureate and graduate nursing programs*. https://www.aacnnursing.org/Portals/42/CCNE/PDF/Procedures.pdf

Farmer, P., Meyer, D., Sroczynski, Close, L, Gorski, M. S., & Wortock, J. (2017). RN to BSN at the community college: A promising practice for nursing education transformation. *Teaching and Learning in Nursing, 12*(2), 103–108. https://doi.org/10.1016/j.teln.2016.12.003

Foronda, C., Alfes, C. M., Dev, P., Kleinheksel, A. J., Nelson, D. A., O'Donnell, J. M., & Samosky, J. T. (2017). Virtually nursing: Emerging technologies in Nursing. *Nurse Educator, 42*(1), 14–17. https://doi.org/10.1097/NNE.0000000000000295

Foronda, C. L., Fernandez-Burgos, M., Nadeau, C., Kelley, C. N., & Henry, M. N. (2020). Virtual simulation in nursing education: A systematic review spanning 1996 to 2018. *Simulation in Healthcare, 15*(1), 46–54. https://doi.org/10.1097/SIH.0000000000000411

Goliat, L., Gravens, K. A., Bonnett, P. L., Schrull, P. L., Bowler, C., Prosser, R., Vitantonio, D. A., Batch-Wilson, W., Szweda, C., Kavanagh, J. M., Mau, K. A., Sharpnack, P. A., Dillon-Bleich, K., & Drennen, C. (2020). Reducing barriers for RN-BSN education. *Nursing Education Perspectives, 41*(5), 309–311. https://doi.org/10.1097/01.NEP.0000000000000719

Haase, P. T. (1990). *The origins and rise of associate degree nursing education*. Duke University Press.

Hanshaw, S. L., & Dickerson, S. S. (2020). High fidelity simulation evaluation studies in nursing education: A review of the literature. *Nurse Education in Practice, 46*, 102818. https://doi.org/10.1016/j.nepr.2020.102818

Harrison, C. V. (2020). Concept-based curriculum: Design and implementation strategies. *International Journal of Nursing Scholarship, 17*(1), 20190066. https://doi.org/10.1515/ijnes-2019-0066

Hayden, J. K., Smiley, R. A., Alexander, M., Kardong-Edgren, S., & Jeffries, P. R. (2014). The NCSBN National Simulation Study: A longitudinal, randomized, controlled study replacing clinical hours with simulation in prelicensure nursing education. *Journal of Nursing Regulation, 5*(2 Suppl.), S1–S64. https://doi.org/10.1016/S2155-8256(15)30062-4

Hendricks, S. M., & Wangerin, V. (2017). Concept-based curriculum: Changing attitudes and overcoming barriers. *Nurse Educator*, *42*(3), 138–142. https://doi.org/10.1097/NNE.0000000000000335

Hensley, A., Wilson, J. L., Culp-Roche, A., Hampton, D., Hardin-Fanning, F., Cheshire, M., & Wiggins, A. T. (2020). Characteristics of RN to BSN students in online programs. *Nurse Education Today*, *89*, 104399. https://doi.org/10.1016/j.nedt.2020.104399

Institute of Medicine. (2010). *The future of nursing: Leading change, advancing health*. National Academies Press.

Institute of Medicine. (2015). *Assessing progress on the IOM report. The future of nursing*. http://nationalacademies.org/hmd/reports/2015/assessing-progress-on-the-iom-report-the-future-of-nursing.aspx

International Nursing Association for Clinical Simulation and Learning Standards Committee. (2016). *Standards of best practice: Simulation*. https://ctl.sinclair.edu/ctlevents/assets/File/16C-INACSL%20Standards%20of%20Best%20Practice%20-%20Simulation.pdf

Interprofessional Education Collaborative. (2016). *Core competencies for interprofessional collaborative practice: 2016 update*. https://ipec.memberclicks.net/assets/2016-Update.pdf

Jansen, M. B., Lund, S. W., Baume, K., Lillyman, S., Rooney, K., & Nielsen, S. S. (2021). International clinical placement-Experiences of nursing students' cultural, personal, and professional development; a qualitative study. *Nurse Education in Practice*, *51*, 102987. https://doi.org/10.1016/j.nepr.2021.102987

Jessee, M. A., & Tanner, C. A. (2016). Pursuing improvement in clinical reasoning: Development of the clinical coaching interactions inventory. *Journal of Nursing Education*, *55*(9), 495–504. https://doi.org/10.3928/01484834-20160816-03

Jordan, K., Lofton, S., & Richards, E. A. (2021). Strategies for embedding population health concepts into nursing education. *Nursing Forum*, *56*, 208–213. https://doi.org/10.1111/nuf.12498

Kostoff, M., Burkhardt, C., Winter, A., & Shrader, S. (2016). An interprofessional simulation using the SBAR communication tool. *American Journal of Pharmaceutical Education*, *80*(9), 1–8. https://doi.org/10.5688/ajpe809157

Kramer, M. (1974). *Reality shock: Why nurses leave nursing*. Mosby.

Kramlich, D., Holt, K., & Law-Ham, D. (2020). Strategies to promote the success of academically at-risk accelerated bachelor of science in nursing students. *Nurse Educator*, *45*(4), 193–197. https://doi.org/10.1097/NNE.0000000000000748

Kubin, L., Fogg, N., & Trinka, M. (2021). Transitioning child health clinical content from direct care to online instruction. *Journal of Nursing Education*, *60*(3), 177–179. https://doi.org/10.3928/01484834-20210222-11

Lee, C., Milbury, B., Movius, M., & Zhuang, J. (2021). The effect of high-fidelity, interprofessional simulation on teamwork skills and attitudes toward interprofessional education. *Nursing Education Perspectives*, *42*(2), 101–103. https://doi.org/10.1097/01.NEP.0000000000000620

Lee, K. C. (2021). The Lasater clinical judgment rubric: Implications for evaluating teaching effectiveness. *Journal of Nursing Education*, *60*(2), 67–73. https://doi.org/10.3928/01484834-20210120-03

Leighton, K., Kardong-Edgren, S. K., McNelis, A. M., Foisy-Doll, C., & Sullo, E. (2021). Traditional clinical outcomes in prelicensure nursing education: An empty systematic review. *Journal of Nursing Education*, *60*(3), 136–142. https://doi.org/10.3928/01484834-20210222-03

Masha'al, D., Rababa, M., & Shahrour, G. (2020). Distance learning–Related stress among undergraduate nursing students during the COVID-19 pandemic. *Journal of Nursing Education*, *59*(12), 666–674. https://doi.org/10.3928/01484834-20201118-03

Moore, B. S., & Clark, M. C. (2016). The role of linguistic modification in nursing education. *Journal of Nursing Education*, *55*(6), 309–315. https://doi.org/10.3928/01484834-20160516-02

Morrison-Beedy, D., Jenssen, U., Bochenek, J., Bowles, W., King, T. S., & Mathisen, L. (2021). Building global nursing citizens through curricular integration of sustainable development goals within an international clinical experience. *Nurse Educator*, *46*(1), 10–12. https://doi.org/10.1097/NNE.0000000000000831

Murray, T. A., Pole, D. C., Ciarlo, E. M., & Holmes, S. (2016). A nursing workforce diversity project: Strategies for recruitment, retention, graduation, and NCLEX-RN success. *Nursing Education Perspectives*, *37*(3), 138–144. https://doi.org/10.5480/14-1480

National Academy of Medicine. (2021). *The future of nursing 2020–2030: Charting a path to achieve health equity*. https://www.nationalacademies.org/our-work/the-future-of-nursing-2020-2030

National Council of State Boards of Nursing. (2016). *NCSBN simulation guidelines for prelicensure nursing programs*. https://www.ncsbn.org/16_Simulation_Guidelines.pdf

National Council of State Boards of Nursing. (2020a). *2019 nurse license volume and NCLEX examination statistics*. https://www.ncsbn.org/2019_NCLEXExamStats.pdf

National Council of State Boards of Nursing. (2020b). *Changes in education for nursing programs during COVID-19*. https://www.ncsbn.org/Education-Requirement-Changes_COVID-19.pdf

National League for Nursing. (2014). *Annual survey of schools of nursing, 2014*. http://www.nln.org/docs/default-source/newsroom/nursing-education-statistics/percentage-of-basic-rn-programs-by-program-type-1994-to-1995-and-2003-to-2012-and-2014-(pdf).pdf?sfvrsn=0

National League for Nursing. (2015). *A vision for the changing faculty role: Preparing students for the technological world of health care*. http://nln.org/docs/default-source/about/nln-vision-series-%28position-statements%29/nlnvision_8.pdf?sfvrsn=4

National League for Nursing. (2016). *Achieving diversity and meaningful inclusion in nursing education*. http://www.nln.org/docs/default-source/about/vision-statement-achieving-diversity.pdf?sfvrsn=2

National League for Nursing. (2021). *End-of-life decision making for older adults: Competent and compassionate care*. http://www.nln.org/professional-development-programs/teaching-resources/ace-s/teaching-strategies/aces-knowledge-domains/vulnerability-during-life-transitions/end-of-life-decision-making-for-older-adults-competent-and-compassionate-care

National League for Nursing Center for Diversity and Global Initiatives. (2017). *NLN diversity and inclusion toolkit*. http://www.nln.org/docs/default-source/default-document-library/diversity-toolkit.pdf?sfvrsn=2

National League for Nursing Institute for Simulation and Technology. (2021). *Institute for simulation and technology*. http://www.nln.org/enterprise-development/nln-center-for-innovation-in-education-excellence/institute-for-simulation-and-technology

Nielsen, A., Lanciotti, K., Garner, A., & Brown, L. (2020). Concept-based learning for capstone clinical experiences in hospital and community settings. *Nurse Educator, 46*(6), 381–385. https://doi.org/10.1097/NNE.0000000000000964

Nielsen, A., Lasater, K., & Stock, M. (2016). A framework to support preceptors' evaluation and development of new nurses' clinical judgment. *Nurse Education in Practice, 19*, 84–90. https://doi.org/10.1016/j.nepr.2016.03.012

O'Brien, E-M., O'Donnell, C., Murphy, J., O'Brien, B., & Markey, K. (2021). Intercultural readiness of nursing students: An integrative review of evidence examining cultural competence educational interventions. *Nurse Education in Practice, 50*, 102966. https://doi.org/10.1016/j.nepr.2021.102966

Oermann, M. H. (2021). COVID-19 disruptions to clinical education. *Nurse Educator, 46*(1), 1. https://doi.org/10.1097/NNE.0000000000000947

Organization for Associate Degree Nursing. (2021). *OADN's response to the NH legislature*. https://oadn.org/wp-content/uploads/2021/03/210209-NH-Letter-Final-CC-Nursing-Programs.pdf

Orsilini-Hain, L., & Waters, V. (2009). Education evolution: A historical perspective of associate degree nursing. *Journal of Nursing Education, 48*(5), 266–271.

Patterson, J. A., Chrisman, M., Skarbek, A., Martin-Stricklin, S., & Patel, S. E. (2021). Challenges of preparing nursing students for practice: The faculty perspective. (2021). *Journal of Nursing Education, 60*(4), 225–228. https://doi.org/10.3928/01484834-20210322-08

Pauly-O'Neill, S., Cooper, E., & Prion, S. (2016). Student QSEN participation during an adult medical–surgical rotation. *Nursing Education Perspectives, 37*(3), 165–172.

Peterson, E., Morgan, R., & Calhoun, A. (2021). Improving patient- and family-centered communication in pediatrics: A review of simulation-based learning. *Pediatric Annals, 50*(1), e32–e38. https://doi.org/10.3928/19382359-20201211-02

Porter, K., Jackson, G., Clark, R., Waller, M., & Ansley, G. S. (2020). Applying social determinants of health to nursing education using a concept-based approach. *Journal of Nursing Education, 59*(5), 293–296. https://doi.org/10.3928/01484834-20200422-12

Powers, K., Neustrup, W., Thomas, C., Saine, A., Sossoman, L. B., Ferrante-Fussili, F. A., Ross, T. C., Clark, K., & Dexter, A. (2020). Baccalaureate nursing students' experiences with multi-patient, standardized patient simulations using telehealth to collaborate. *Journal of Professional Nursing, 36*(5), 292–300. https://doi.org/10.1016/j.profnurs.2020.03.013

Quality and Safety Education for Nurses. (2020). *QSEN competencies.* https://qsen.org/competencies/pre-licensure-ksas/

Reid, C. A., Ralph, J. L., El-Masri, M., Ziefle, K. (2020). High-fidelity simulation and clinical judgment of nursing students in a maternal–newborn course. *Western Journal of Nursing Research, 42*(10), 829–837. https://doi.org/10.1177/0193945920907395

Relf, M. V. (2016). Advancing diversity in academic nursing. *Journal of Professional Nursing, 32*(5), S42–S47. https://doi.org/10.1016/j.profnurs.2016.02.010

Ross, J. G., Meakim, C., & Stacy, G. H. (2020). Outcomes of Team STEPPS training in prelicensure health care practitioner programs: An integrative review. *Journal of Nursing Education, 59*(11), 610–616. https://doi.org/10.3928/01484834-20201020-03

Rutledge, C., Hawkins, E. J., Bordelon, M., & Tina, S. G. (2020). Telehealth education: An interprofessional online immersion experience in response to COVID-19. *Journal of Nursing Education, 59*(10), 570–576. https://doi.org/10.3928/01484834-20200921-06

Serembus, J. F., & Kemery, D. C. (2020). Creating dynamic learning with Zoom. *Nurse Educator, 45*(6), 291–293. https://doi.org/10.1097/NNE.0000000000000915

Sitzman, K., Carpenter, T., & Cherry, K. (2020). Student perceptions related to immediate workplace usefulness of RN-to-BSN program content. *Nurse Educator, 45*(5), 265–268. https://doi.org/10.1097/NNE.0000000000000775

Smiley, R. A., Lauer, P., Bienemy, C., Berg, J. G., Shireman, E., Reneau, K. A., & Alexander, M. (2018). The 2017 national nursing workforce survey. *Journal of Nursing Regulation, 9*(3), S1–S54. https://doi.org/10.1016/S2155-8256(18)30131-5

Solheim, K., Mittelstadt, K., Muehrer, R., Pinekenstein, B., & Willis, D. (2021). Sustaining a concept-based curriculum: beyond the launch. *Nurse Educator.* Advanced online publication. https://doi.org/10.1097/NNE.0000000000001016

Spetz, J. (2018). Projections of progress toward the 80% bachelor of science in nursing recommendation and strategies to accelerate change. *Nursing Outlook, 66*(4), 394–400. https://doi.org/https://doi.org/ 10.1016/j.outlook.2018.04.012.

Swift, M. C., Stosberg, T., Foley, A., & Brocksmith, E. (2020). Nursing program outcome improves with interprofessional simulation. *Journal of Allied Health, 49*(3), 157–163, 163A.

Tri-Council for Nursing. (2021). *Transforming together: Implications and opportunities from the COVID-19 pandemic for nursing education, practice and regulation.* https://img1.wsimg.com/blobby/go/3d8c2b58-0c32-4b54-adbd-efe8f931b2df/downloads/Tri-Council-COVID-19-Report-5-2021.pdf?ver=1620247943137

U.S. Department of Health and Human Services. (2020). *Healthy People 2030.* U.S. Government Printing Office. https://health.gov/healthypeople

Wagner, J., Foster, B., & O'Sullivan, R. (2020). Measuring learning outcomes in a RN-to-BSN program. *Teaching and Learning in Nursing, 15*(1), 19–24. https://doi.org/10.1016/j.teln.2019.07.006

Wiersma, G., Pintz, C., & Karen, F. W. (2020). Transition to practice experiences of new graduate nurses from an accelerated bachelor of science in nursing program: Implications for academic and clinical partners. *The Journal of Continuing Education in Nursing, 51*(9), 433–440. https://doi.org/10.3928/00220124-20200812-09

Wojnar, S. M., & Whelan, E. M. (2017). Preparing nursing students for enhanced roles in primary care: The current state of prelicensure and RN-to-BSN education. *Nursing Outlook, 65*(2), 222–232. https://doi.org/10.1016/j.outlook.2016.10.006

World Health Organization. (2010). *WHO framework for action on interprofessional education and collaborative practice.* WHO Press.

Wynn, S. T. (2020). Using virtual standardized patients in behavioral health interprofessional education. *Journal of Nursing Education, 59*(10), 599–600. https://doi.org/10.3928/01484834-20200921-14

CHAPTER 9

Curriculum Planning for Specialty Master's Nursing Degrees and Entry-Level Graduate Degrees

Stephanie Stimac DeBoor

CHAPTER OBJECTIVES

Upon completion of Chapter 9, the reader will be able to:

- Discuss the process of curriculum development for master's programs in nursing, including

  - RN-to-MSN programs
  - Entry-level MSN
  - Clinical nurse leader
  - Advanced practice programs
  - Functional roles, for example, case management, nursing administration/leadership, and nurse educator

- Review recommendations from accrediting, professional specialty and educational organizations, and certification agencies for master's degrees in nursing

- Analyze issues surrounding graduate-level nursing at the master's level:

  - Entry into practice
  - Terminal degrees and advanced practice
  - Postmaster's certificates
  - Certification, licensure, and regulation

OVERVIEW

In the 20th century, as nursing education matured in the academic world and the profession grappled with the issue of defining itself as a discipline, graduate education in nursing evolved. Nursing leaders recognized the need for additional education to be prepared for faculty and administrator roles. As Ervin (2018, 2021) identified earlier in Chapter 1, the latter half of the 20th century, found graduate nursing education more established with the rapid growth and development of master's and doctoral programs throughout the country. Despite the pandemic and financial burden of the country, we continue to see those seeking to advance their nursing education within graduate educational programs.

Nurses in practice focus their services on clinical specialties such as pediatrics, obstetrics, psychiatric/mental health, medical/surgical nursing, and intensive care, and they, too, felt the need for additional specialty training, many seeking nondegree certification. In community settings, it was recognized that public health nurses (PHNs) needed knowledge in epidemiology and the public health sciences, and the specialty roles of nurse midwives and nurse anesthetists required advanced educational preparation and clinical practice. Many of these programs were first offered in baccalaureate programs or as certificate programs to expand on knowledge and skills from basic nursing programs; however, all eventually moved into the graduate level.

The first master's degree in a clinical nursing specialty was awarded in 1956 from Columbia University School of Nursing (2021). In the 1970s, schools of nursing in higher degree institutions developed master's degree programs that focused on the preparation of nursing faculty, administrators, and some of the classic specialties such as pediatrics, maternity, community health, and psychiatric/mental health nursing. These latter specialties became clinical nurse specialties, and as they were developing, the advent of the nursing role in primary care began with the introduction of nurse practitioners. With acute care rising in complexity, it became apparent that nurses with blended specialty role preparation were needed, such as the acute care nurse practitioner. More recently, the pandemic provided us with an opportunity to examine outdated regulations as the demand for advanced practice nurses has increased exponentially.

See Chapter 1 for a history of graduate nursing education to gain an appreciation for how nursing evolved in its role in healthcare to match the needs of the healthcare system with its growing demands for well-educated providers of care. Out of all these changes and demands came master's degrees that focused on the specialties, primary care, management/administration, and education. The opportunity to advance one's education brings additional opportunities for employment within nursing. There is a continued movement to advance entrance to practice for those seeking a degree in advanced clinical practice toward the practice doctorate (DNP; National Organization of Nurse Practitioner Faculty [NONPF], 2018). Nursing's history, as well as that of the other healthcare professions, traditionally took place in silos of education such as schools of medicine, nursing, physical therapy, psychology, and so forth with few opportunities for combined theory courses and clinical practice, yet the complex healthcare system calls for interprofessional collaboration to meet the needs of the population and improve outcomes of care. Recently, many academic medical centers are promoting and developing interprofessional educational programs to meet these challenges (Gerard et al., 2015).

This chapter discusses the various types of master's-level programs offered in today's nursing educational system. In April 2021, there are approximately 645 master's-level nursing programs in the United States accredited by the Accreditation Commission for Education in Nursing (2020) and the Commission on Collegiate Nursing Education (2021). The chapter breaks the various master's-level programs into groups from the RN to MSN, entry-level master's (generic), advanced generalist (CNL), and, finally, to the advanced practice specialty and functional roles available in today's graduate programs. Each group is reviewed and its role in graduate nursing, and the profession is discussed. Some of the major issues related to master's-level nursing education are discussed throughout.

RN-TO-MSN PROGRAMS

With the National Academy of Medicine's (previously known as the Institute of Medicine [IOM]) consensus study *The Future of Nursing 2020–2030: Charting a Path to Achieve Health Equity* expanding on *The Future of Nursing* (IOM, 2010) and the *Assessing Progress on the Institute of Medicine Report on the Future of Nursing* (IOM, 2015) to meet the needs of the U.S. healthcare system, there is renewed interest in advancing nursing education. One way for those seeking to return to school to advance their nursing education is through accelerated RN-to-MSN programs. According to the American Association of Colleges of Nursing (AACN, 2019) in 2019, there were, then, 219 RN-to-MSN programs available across the United States with an additional 24 in the planning stages. The shortage of nursing faculty adds to this need for nurses with clinical work experience to gain higher education in order to assume faculty roles.

There are several variations of curricula for accelerating RNs who have a diploma or associate degree to the master's degree. One format awards the baccalaureate along the way as the RN completes courses equivalent to the upper division–level BSN. The other format is to not award the BSN but, rather, have the RN complete both upper division baccalaureate and master's-level courses and receive the MSN on completion of the program. Sometimes, both the BSN and MSN are awarded upon completion of the program. Factors that determine the type of program of study include regional accreditation issues, parent institution standards, and the faculty's philosophy. For example, awarding the BSN along the way of the program gives students a baccalaureate whose circumstances prohibit them from completing the master's portion of the program.

The typical patterns for the curricula consist of a 2- to 3-year program of study, with an accelerated first-year plan to complete the baccalaureate upper division–level equivalent courses. Following completion of these courses, students enter graduate-level courses and, depending on the program, may take another 1 to 2 years of master's-level courses depending on the type of master's degree, with advanced practice degrees spending more theory courses and clinical hours specific to that branch of advanced practice. Some courses are developed to match the experience of the RNs to the level of education indicated and double count toward both the higher level of the baccalaureate and the introductory-level master's courses. Since the large majority of RN students are working, the usual platforms for delivery of the programs are web-based, online, evenings, and/or weekend classes to accommodate their needs.

There remains a gap in the literature that compares RN-to-MSN graduates to post-BSN and entry-level master's programs. The types of master's program (advanced practice or functional role) and the platform for delivery of the program (online, nontraditional, or traditional) should be studied for their effectiveness and student, faculty, and employer satisfaction.

ENTRY-LEVEL MASTER'S DEGREE PROGRAMS IN NURSING (GENERIC, ACCELERATED MASTER'S FOR NONNURSES, SECOND-DEGREE MASTER'S)

When planning an entry-level master's program, it is wise to consult with the regional accrediting body and the state board of nursing to identify any possible barriers to offering the degree. For example, some regional or state accrediting bodies and boards of nursing may require a baccalaureate in nursing prior to earning a master's degree in the same discipline, even if the person has a baccalaureate in another discipline. There are two major pathways or programs of study for nonnursing college graduates to reach licensure (RN) requirements and a graduate degree in nursing. They are described as follows.

The first program provides basic nursing knowledge and skills courses specifically designed for college graduates and taught at the postbaccalaureate level. Included in the program or required as prerequisites are the usual sciences, social sciences, and liberal arts courses. Examples of classic prerequisites for any entry-level nursing program (associate degree, baccalaureate, and master's) are anatomy, chemistry, English, genetics, human development, mathematics/statistics, microbiology, nutrition, physiology, psychology, sociology, and speech/communications. Students in the entry-level master's complete nursing theory and clinical courses at the upper division level, advanced nursing theory and clinical courses at the graduate level, and a capstone experience that can be a thesis, project, and/or comprehensive examination. (Fewer master's programs are requiring a thesis because of the increase in research-focused/translational science doctoral-level education.) Schools of nursing differ in their preparation of these graduates by offering either an advanced generalist master's degree for entry into practice or a specialist track to prepare graduates for advanced levels of nursing practice or roles.

The other entry-level curriculum requires students to complete courses equivalent to or the same as existing courses in baccalaureate-level nursing programs. They are not necessarily specifically revised for college graduates. As with the first program, students either must have the prerequisite sciences and liberal arts courses or complete them in the program. After completion of the baccalaureate-level courses, students enter into the master's program to complete either an advanced generalist role such as the CNL or a specialty, such as clinical nurse specialist (CNS), nurse anesthetist, nurse midwife, or nurse practitioner; acute care practitioner; or a role specialty such as case management, nursing educator, or administrator. The track record for the graduates of entry-level master's programs is excellent. Students in the programs bring life experience, a previously earned higher degree, and academic achievement as most programs require at least a 3.0 grade point average in the undergraduate program for admission.

According to the AACN (2016), there were 69 entry-level master's programs in the United States. Descriptions of the programs and the student and graduate characteristics may be found in the accelerated BSN and MSN programs AACN website (www.aacn-nursing.org/Nursing-Education-Programs/Accelerated-Programs). Downey and Assein (2015) conducted an integrative literature review pertaining to the students' and faculty members' perceptions regarding accelerated master's programs for nonnursing graduates of baccalaureate or higher degree programs. They found that students entering the programs did so based on their beliefs about nursing as a caring profession. The majority were female, older, and above average academically. The students were surprised at the rigor of the nursing education program. The authors noted the lack of studies and the need for investigating to the perceptions of students and faculty as they experience the educational program. This remains a limited topic of research.

THE CLINICAL NURSE LEADER

The CNL program was developed by the AACN in response to the need for healthcare providers to manage clients or groups of clients at the point of care. AACN (2007, 2013, 2021a) provides the following description of the role of the CNL:

> The Clinical Nurse Leader[SM] or CNL® is a master's educated nurse, prepared for practice across the continuum of care within any health care setting. The CNL was developed by AACN in collaboration with leaders from health care practice and education to address the critical need to improve the quality of patient care outcomes. The CNL is a clinical leader—at the point of care—who focuses on: Care Coordination, Outcomes Measurement, Transitions of Care, Interprofessional Communication & Team Leadership, Risk Assessment, Implementation of Best Practices Based on Evidence, and Quality Improvement.

In April of 2021, there were 153 accredited nursing programs that provided the CNL major at the master's level (www.aacnnursing.org/Portals/42/CNL/eligible-CNL-programs.pdf). The AACN (2021b) document on the *Competencies and Curricular Expectations for CNL Education and Practice* provides specific information for curricular planning for programs wishing to offer this degree. Certification for the CNL is overseen and awarded by an autonomous branch of AACN, the Commission on Nurse Certification (CNC; AACN, 2021c).

Miltner et al. (2020) examined the role of the CNL within the Veterans Administration (VA) systems over the last 10 years. The use of CNL within the VA was to provide strong leadership across all clinical settings. Results indicate that while all intuitive goals had not been met, the CNL remains a valuable resource and must be allowed to practice to the full extent of their education to impact quality patient outcomes. Noles and James (2019) studied the CNL role regarding innovations within the healthcare setting. Once again results indicate if educated properly, the CNL has the ability to impact healthcare delivery and improve patient outcomes through innovative practice change. Hoffman et al. (2020) identify the capabilities of the CNL within and outside of the acute care settings during the COVID-19 pandemic. Based on the CNL skill set, the authors identify how customized the role is for challenges like the pandemic. A 2016 job analysis was conducted by the CNC and Schroeder Measurement Technologies, Inc., to examine the relationship between the knowledge, skills, and abilities of the CNL and the content of the certification examination (Commission on Collegiate Nursing Education, 2016). Based on this analysis, content specifications are reflected in the certification examination that began in April 2017. This examination blueprint is a supportive guide in curriculum development and evaluation. Establishing practice partners or academic partnerships is one strategy for arranging clinical experiences for the CNL. The U.S. Department of Veterans Affairs (VA) hospitals are frequent sites of these academic partnerships. VA medical centers have been participants of the CNL Initiative since 2013 (U.S. Department of Veterans Affairs, 2016).

ADVANCED PRACTICE MASTER'S DEGREE PROGRAMS IN NURSING

The classic advanced practice roles encompass the CNS, nurse anesthetist, nurse midwife, and nurse practitioner. As discussed in Chapter 1 on the history of master's education, the advanced practice roles emerged in the 1960s and 1970s. Nurse anesthetists (certified registered nurse anesthetists [CRNAs]) and nurse midwives predated these programs by many years (centuries for midwives and 150-plus years for CRNAs); however, their move into higher education/graduate education occurred about the same time the CNS and nurse practitioner roles did. A few advanced practice nurses still have a certificate to practice depending on state licensure laws, although most states now require a master's degree for entry into advanced practice. With the advent of the DNP degree, many of these nurses are continuing their education to earn a DNP. See Chapter 10 for a discussion of the DNP. There is a continued movement to advance entrance to practice for those seeking a degree in advanced clinical practice toward the practice doctorate (DNP; NONPF, 2018).

All master's degree programs that prepare advanced practice nurses require a baccalaureate in nursing or, in rare cases, its equivalent, and some have additional prerequisites, for example, CRNA programs often require more than one or two chemistry courses. Both the CNS and nurse practitioner programs have subspecialties, for example, adult, cardiovascular, family, geriatric, pediatrics, psychiatric/mental health, women's health, and so on.

When considering the implementation of an APRN program of study, or revising the current program, the American Association of Nurse Practitioners (AANP), the AACN, the National Council of State Boards of Nursing (NCSBN), and the NONPF provide criteria for consideration in the development of curricula. On April 6, 2021, the AACN approved *The Essentials: Core Competencies for Professional Nursing Education* (AACN, 2021d). The competencies of the new Essentials "provides a framework for preparing individuals as members of the discipline of nursing, reflecting expectations across the trajectory of nursing education and applied experience" (AACN, 2021d, p. 3). The Essentials newly developed 10 domains outline the expected competencies at the prescribed level of education. Each domain provides a defining descriptor and contextual statement. Faculty involved in the development of the curricula must then identify the components through student-learning outcomes, assignments, and measures to ensure the student is successful in meeting each competency. The following provides an example: Upon completion of this course, students will be able to:

1. Utilize knowledge and skills from previous courses to assess and diagnose acute primary care issues across the life span. (**Domain 1: Knowledge for Nursing Practice, Concept-Clinical Judgment,** NTF criterion III.B, VI. B, IV.B.2, IV.B.3, VI.A.4.)

   Assignment: Virtual Patient Encounter/SOAP (subjective, objective, assessment, and plan) Note. The purpose of this assignment is to bridge theory knowledge and your virtual clinical experience. The student will view the virtual encounter and complete a SOAP Note based on assessment, development of a problem list, development of differential diagnoses, and treatment plan. **Competency:** Students must achieve an 83% for this 25-point assignment based on the following rubric components. Chief Complaint (1 point), History of Present Illness (4 points), Past Medical History (2 points), Review of Systems (2 points), Patient Exam (4 points), Labs & Diagnostics (1 point), Problem list/Primary Diagnosis with ICD 10 code(s) (4 points), Treatment Plan (4 points), Professionalism—on-time, scholarly submission (3 points).

   Another consideration in the development of curriculum includes the 2008 Consensus Report for APRN Regulation (AACN, 2008) which limits the blended role of primary and acute care foci to adult-geriatric and pediatric roles only and specifies that graduates must be nationally certified for population foci within the primary (practitioner) and acute care (practitioner, CNS) roles. The consensus model was a product of meetings with the leading professional nursing organizations, specialty organizations, accrediting bodies, nursing education organizations, certification agencies, and the National Council of State Boards. It was the intention of the group to clarify advanced practice roles for the profession and the public and to begin an initiative for consistent regulation encompassing licensing, accreditation, certification, and education (LACE) across the various states in the nation. The APRN Regulatory Model depicting the APRN roles, population foci, and specialties is accessible at www.aacnnursing.org/Portals/42/AcademicNursing/pdf/APRNReport.pdf (p. 10). As the healthcare system evolves in the United States, the consensus model will continue to move forward in response to increased demands for well qualified and educated APRNs.

   The National Council of State Boards presents updates regarding the Consensus Report for APRN Regulation on its website. The site identifies and provides information about the major elements of APRN regulations that includes, but is not limited to, the following:

◆ **Titling:** APRN
◆ **Roles of APRNs and recognition of each follow:** certified nurse practitioner (CNP), CNS, CRNA, certified nurse midwife (CNM)
◆ **Licensure:** APRNs hold both an RN and APRN license.
◆ **Education:** Graduate education is required for APRNs regardless of role.

◆ **Certification:** Every APRN is required to meet advanced certification requirements.

◆ **Independent Practice:** The APRN shall be granted full authority to practice independently without physician oversight or a written collaborative agreement. As of April 2021, there were 35 states, including the District of Columbia, that allowed for independent-practice authority for APRNs (NCSBN, 2021).

◆ **Full Prescriptive Authority:** The APRN shall be granted full prescriptive author without physician oversight or a written collaborative agreement.

The NONPF provides additional core competencies, the National Task Force (NTF, 2016) *Criteria for Evaluation of Nurse Practitioner Programs*, as well as the scope and standards of primary and acute care practitioners. In addition, NONPF (2021) released an update to their *Statement on Acute Care and Primary Care Nurse Practitioner Practice*. This update delineates information related to education, certification, and differentiation of the scope of practice. Developing and implementing curriculum require considering this information and be reflected in the student-learning outcomes, assignments, and assessments.

The educational preparation of advanced practice nurses is important as they have a key role not only in the delivery of quality care but also at the table in the creation of policy and legislative regulations affecting healthcare. An estimated 32 million adults in the United States visit an advanced practice clinician (APC) yearly, yet insurers reimburse APCs at lower rates than their physician counterparts (Davis et al., 2017). With the ever-growing shortages in providers and reform of healthcare, Phillips (2020) identified legislative and regulatory updates that positively impact the APRN's ability to provide quality care. Some are addressing the inequity of reimbursement for services.

To provide further evidence of the impact the APRN has on the healthcare delivery system, the following reports from the literature verify this statement. Kurtzman et al. (2017) examined whether state-granted APRN independence had an effect on patient-level quality, service utilization, and referrals. Data were analyzed using propensity score matching and multivariate regression for each outcome. Results identified that outcomes were unaffected by states' APRN independence status. Similarly, Moldestad et al. (2020), conducted a qualitative student to examine the perceptions of MDs, NPs, and patients within the VA system in relation to primary care provided in full and restrictive states. Results indicated that perceptions found MDs and NPs to be comparable. There was a difference in relation to patient satisfaction and preference toward the NPs. Identified were the "preference for the holistic, interpersonal care provided by NPs" and the "more important determinant of their proficiency with delivering effective primary care than their credentials" (p. 3099). Additionally, Kapu (2021) identifies the value of the adult-gerontology acute care nurse practitioner (AGACNP, formerly known as acute care NP [ACNP]) role in caring for acutely and critically ill patients. For two decades, these practitioners have served as valued members of the team by reducing the length of stay and readmissions, preventing nosocomial infections, and increasing patient satisfaction, to name a few. This article serves as a reminder to nurse executives of the impact the AGACNP has on financial and patient outcomes of the organization.

Since the American Nurses Association published a white paper in 2012 describing the value of the APRN in improving the delivery of healthcare through care coordination, much has continued to be published identifying the benefits of APRNs in delivering primary care (American Nurses Association, 2012; Gregory et al., 2021; Tracy et al., 2020; Vogelsmeier et al., 2020). All these authors clearly identify the impact that an APRN can have on access to care, satisfaction of care, and the overall quality of care provided.

To further ensure patient safety and quality care, the scope of practice decision-making framework was developed by the Tri-Council for Nursing in collaboration with the

NCSBN in 2015. After reviewing the literature for algorithms related to decision-making, a tool was developed to assist the nurses in identifying what safely falls within their role based on each nurse's level of education, licensure, certification, and state board regulations (Ballard et al., 2016; NCSBN, 2016).

In summary, the traditional role for advanced practice continues to play an important role in the delivery of high-quality, safe, and cost-effective care. Nursing continues to find it necessary to illustrate this to not only the healthcare industry but the public as well. As advanced practice roles become more delineated, knowledge of one's scope is more important than ever in ensuring the best patient outcomes.

COMMUNITY/PUBLIC HEALTH NURSING

Community/public health nursing (C/PHN) master's programs prepare nurses for advanced practice roles in community settings. There are some schools of nursing that offer a joint degree awarding both the MSN and the MPH. Others have community health nursing as a clinical specialty.

The transformation of healthcare legislated by the American Counseling Association (ACA) has required the relationship between public health and healthcare systems to strengthen their collaborative efforts in order to meet the changes in our national healthcare landscape. In 2018, the Quad Council Coalition (made up of the Alliance of Nurses for Healthy Environments [ANHE], the Association of Community Health Nursing Educators [ACHNE], the Association of Public Health Nurses [APHN], and the American Public Health Association–Public Health Nursing Section [APHA-PHN]) updated and put forward the new C/PHN competencies. These competencies provide guidance in the development of curricula, standards of nursing practice, research, and policy at multiple levels (Campbell et al., 2020). The Council of Public Health Nursing Organizations (CPHNO, formerly the Quad Council Coalition of Public Health Nursing Organizations) continues to provide a face and voice for those who work as PHNs. This organization sets the agenda that will affect national policy related to PHNs in addition to being an advocate for excellence in PHN education, practice, leadership, and research (CPNHO, 2021).

Edmonds et al. (2016) explored the knowledge, perceptions, and practices of PHNs under the ACA. They identified the significant contributions PHNs were making based on their reported areas of involvement. Edmonds et al. (2020) continue to identify the significance of the role of the PHN especially in the face of the COVID-19 pandemic. Their educational preparation makes them one of the most valuable responders in this type of crisis, yet funding continues to be cut, reducing the number of PHNs.

The dual MSN–MPH has been in existence for quite some time and continues to be offered at universities throughout the United States. The launch of the ACA in 2010 resulted in a complex healthcare environment requiring a higher level of skills, knowledge, and expertise to ensure quality care. Shaw et al. (2016) discuss the DNP/MPH dual degree as an educational option to better prepare PHNs. Going forward, McElroy et al. (2020), propose research priorities that will set the agenda for faculty responsibilities resulting scientific knowledge that impacts student proficiencies as well as the populations and communities served.

The American Nurses Credentialing Center (ANCC, 2021a) no longer offers a PHN-Advanced specialty certification. This certification has been retired. Those who were previously certified can continue to renew as long as they continue to meet eligibility requirements. There are other certifications for the PHN, but they are not specific to the advanced practitioner.

MASTER'S DEGREES IN NURSING FOR FUNCTIONAL ROLES

There are other roles and specialties for nurses with master's degrees not included in the advanced practice and advanced generalist roles. They include case management, nursing administration, nurse educator, staff development/patient education, and other leadership roles. Nurses prepared for these roles usually have nursing theory, healthcare policy, and research as core courses along with the courses that focus them into a specific function within the healthcare system. The following discussion presents a few examples of the programs that prepare nurses for specific roles.

Case Management

The educational preparation for roles in case management in nursing usually requires at least a baccalaureate in nursing, with a master's preferred. Case managers provide coordination of services for aggregates in many healthcare settings. They work closely with other healthcare professionals. The role began in the 1970s, with its purpose to work with patients to individualize care, avoid duplication of services, enhance the quality of care, and promote cost-effectiveness (White & Hall, 2006). A Google search revealed that fewer than 20 schools of nursing offer case management master's degrees. The ANCC (2021b) offers certification, which requires 2,000 hours of clinical practice in case management, RN licensure, practice as an RN for 2 years, and 30 hours of continuing education in case management in the past 3 years.

Nursing Administration

The most common master's degrees in nursing to prepare nurse leaders are the master's in nursing administration or leadership. Some programs offer joint master's degrees with nursing, such as business administration (MBA) or healthcare administration. The graduates of these programs are not prepared for advanced practice roles such as CNSs and nurse practitioners but rather have education in the management of healthcare systems including staffing, human resources, finances, budgeting, and administration. There are several ways for nurse administrators to receive national certification through the American Organization of Nurse Leaders (2021) for executive nursing or as a nurse manager and leader. The latter requires only a baccalaureate in nursing, while the executive certification requires a master's. The ANCC (2021c, 2021d) also has two national certification exams for nurse executives. In addition to these roles in management and administration, there are other leadership certifications for infection control nurses, legal nurse consultants, quality control nurses, and risk managers. These certifications occur through specialty organizations and, for the most part, require or prefer that nurses have a master's degree as well as continuing education and experience for the specific role.

Nursing Educator

The role of the nursing educator in healthcare agencies includes staff development and patient education. Chapter 12 discusses curriculum design and evaluation for this specialty of nurse educator, known as the professional nursing development specialist (PNDS). There are programs in schools of nursing that specifically prepare nurses for this role at the master's level. The Association for Nursing Professional Development (2021) recommends that staff developers become credentialed by the ANCC (2021e) for the nursing clinical specialty in which they are prepared.

With the recent growth of nursing education programs to help relieve the shortage of nursing faculty, many of the programs offer a track for nurse educators in schools of nursing and some offer postmaster's certificates in nursing education. According to the AACN (2021e) 2020 report on enrollments, 80,521 qualified applications applicants to nursing schools were turned away due a lack of clinical sites, faculty, and budgetary resource constraints. Of this total, 8,987 master's degree applicants and 3,884 doctoral candidates were denied admission. The denial of over 12,000 graduate candidates contributes to the limitation of potential faculty pool. One must consider the effect of COVID-19 on the financial resources of prospective students, but these data continue to identify there are applicants not being admitted despite financial shortfalls. In the AACN 2019 *Special Survey on Faculty Vacancies*, it was reported that there were 1,637 faculty vacancies. Schools that participated in the survey identified that there was a need to create an additional 134 positions to meet the ongoing demand of applicants (AACN, 2020). Owing to the shortage, there remains underfilled master's and post-master's certificate programs that prepare nurses for faculty roles.

It is recommended that faculty members have at least the same degree level for the type of program in which they teach, and it is highly recommended that they have one degree higher. Therefore, faculty teaching in associate degree programs should have at the very least a baccalaureate, but most boards of nursing require the master's degree for program approval, while those teaching in baccalaureate and higher degree programs should have a doctorate. However, with the shortage in nursing, it is not uncommon for master's-prepared nurses to teach clinical courses in specialties that match their expertise, and in some states, boards of nursing allow nurses with baccalaureates in nursing to teach under the supervision of an experienced educator.

There is continuing debate about whether nursing faculty need to have special courses in education since they are specialists in their fields. There is no question that there is a separate body of knowledge related to curriculum development, instructional design and strategies, instructional technology, and program and student evaluation. Without this knowledge, many instructors in nursing do not have the background in learning theories that support best practices in education for meeting the needs of learners, nor do they have the curriculum planning and evaluation background to connect the program to the actual implementation (teaching) of the program. Such knowledge ensures the quality of the program so that learning experiences are linked to the mission and goals of the program. The same is true for evaluation for program review to measure outcomes and student evaluation to measure students' progress in the program. At the same time, it is equally important that nursing faculty members have the content knowledge and theory on the material that they are teaching. To further support these statements the National League for Nursing (2021a) offers two national certifications options (certified nurse educator and certified academic clinical nurse educator) for nurse educators. Eligibility qualifications vary between the two certifications but share some similarities; licensure, education, and, in some cases, experience. Transcripts are reviewed for specialty courses (e.g., curriculum development and evaluation, instructional design, principles of adult learning, assessment/measurement and evaluation, principles of teaching and learning, instructional technology; National League for Nursing, 2021b, 2021c).

SUMMARY

This chapter reviewed common master's degree programs in nursing and the differences among the majors available in nursing at that level. Roles for master's degree–prepared nurses were discussed and postgraduate certification possibilities were reviewed. Some issues were raised such as the advent of the DNP and its impact on advanced practice master's programs, entry into practice at the master's level, expectations of the educational preparation for nursing faculty, and the place for the advanced generalist master's degree graduate in the healthcare system.

END-OF-CHAPTER RESOURCES

DISCUSSION QUESTIONS

1. How should nursing differentiate between advanced practice roles and advanced knowledge roles such as administrators, case managers, risk managers, and so on?

2. Is it important for nursing educators in the practice setting and in schools of nursing to have graduate degrees, and what levels of advanced education are necessary? Why or why not?

LEARNING ACTIVITIES

Student-Learning Activities

1. Review the literature and websites for nursing education to identify how many possible majors there are for master's degrees in nursing. Compare the majors to the job market for these specialties in your region. Discuss the pros and cons of the continuation or discontinuation of some of the programs.

2. Go to the websites of various credentialing and certification organizations for nursing and identify how many require at least a master's degree in nursing. Discuss why or why not certification for advanced roles should continue.

Faculty Development Activities

1. Review the latest follow-up survey of the graduates of your master's program for data on the employment of the graduates in settings where they use the focus of their graduate degrees. Determine if your program prepared graduates for the needs of the healthcare system and why or why not. Consider the effect of your findings on curriculum revision or, possibly, discontinuance of a program or development of new programs.

2. Discuss among yourselves your beliefs about master's education for advanced practice or roles in leadership and if the master's degree serves your graduates as a terminal degree and/or pathway to doctoral studies.

 A robust set of instructor resources designed to supplement this text is located at **http://connect.springerpub.com/content/book/978-0-8261-8686-7.** Qualifying instructors may request access by emailing **textbook@springerpub.com.**

REFERENCES

Accreditation Commission for Education in Nursing. (2020). *Accredited programs*. https://www. acenursing.com/accreditedprograms/programsearch.htm

American Association of Colleges of Nursing. (2007). *White paper on the education and role of the clinical nurse leader*. https://nursing.uiowa.edu/sites/default/files/documents/academic-programs/graduate/msn-cnl/CNL_White_Paper.pdf

American Association of Colleges of Nursing. (2008). *Consensus model for APRN regulation: Licensure, accreditation, certification, & education*. https://www.aacn.org/~/media/aacn-website/nursing-excellence/standards/aprnregulation.pdf?la=en

American Association of Colleges of Nursing. (2013). *Competencies and curricular expectations for clinical nurse leader education and practice.* https://www.aacnnursing.org/Portals/42/News/White-Papers/CNL-Competencies-October-2013.pdf

American Association of Colleges of Nursing. (2016). *Schools offering entry-level or 2nd degree master's programs, Fall 2016 (N = 69).* https://hpa.ucdavis.edu/sites/g/files/dgvnsk4121/files/inline-files/AACN_MastersProgramsList_2016.pdf

American Association of Colleges of Nursing. (2019). *Degree completion programs for registered nurses: RN to master's degree and RN to baccalaureate programs.* https://www.aacnnursing.org/News-Information/Fact-Sheets/Degree-Completion-Programs

American Association of Colleges of Nursing. (2020). *Nursing faculty shortage.* https://www.aacnnursing.org/news-information/fact-sheets/nursing-faculty-shortage

American Association of Colleges of Nursing. (2021a). *Clinical nurse leader (CNL).* https://www.aacnnursing.org/CNL

American Association of Colleges of Nursing. (2021b). *Competencies and curricular expectations for clinical nurse leader education and practice.* https://www.aacnnursing.org/News-Information/Position-Statements-White-Papers/CNL

American Association of Colleges of Nursing. (2021c). *CNL certification.* https://www.aacnnursing.org/cnl-certification

American Association of Colleges of Nursing. (2021d). *The essentials: Core competencies for professional nursing education.* https://www.aacnnursing.org/Portals/42/AcademicNursing/pdf/Essentials-2021.pdf

American Association of Colleges of Nursing. (2021e). *Highlights for AACN's 2020 annual survey.* https://www.aacnnursing.org/Portals/42/Data/Survey-Data-Highlights-2020.pdf

American Nurses Association. (2012). *The value of nursing care coordination: A white paper of the American Nurses Association.* https://www.nursingworld.org/~4afc0d/globalassets/practiceandpolicy/health-policy/care-coordination-white-paper-3.pdf

American Nurses Credentialing Center. (2021a). *Advanced public health nursing certification.* https://www.nursingworld.org/our-certifications/advanced-public-health-nurse/

American Nurses Credentialing Center. (2021b). *Nursing case management certification (CMGT-BC).* https://www.nursingworld.org/our-certifications/nursing-case-management/

American Nurses Credentialing Center. (2021c). *Nurse executive certification.* https://www.nursingworld.org/our-certifications/nurse-executive/

American Nurses Credentialing Center. (2021d). *Nurse executive, advanced certification.* https://www.nursingworld.org/our-certifications/nurse-executive-advanced/

American Nurses Credentialing Center. (2021e). *Nursing professional development certification (NPD-BC).* https://www.nursingworld.org/our-certifications/nursing-professional-development/

American Organization of Nurse Leaders. (2021). *Certified nurse manager and leader certification.* https://www.aonl.org/initiatives/cnml

Association for Nursing Professional Development. (2021). *Become a staff educator.* https://www.anpd.org

Ballard, K., Haagenson, D., Christiansen, L., Damgaard, G., Halstead, J. A., Jason, R. R., Joyner, J. C., O'Sullivan, A. M., Silvestre, J., Cahill, M., Radtke, B., & Alexander, M. (2016). *Scope of nursing practice decision-making framework.* https://www.ncsbn.org/2016JNR_Decision-Making-Framework.pdf

Campbell, L. A., Harmon, M. J., Joyce, B. L., & Little S. H. (2020). Quad Council Coalition community/public health nursing competencies: Building consensus through collaboration. *Public Health Nursing, 37,* 96–112. https://doi.org/10.1111/phn.12666

Columbia University School of Nursing. (2021). *Our history.* https://www.nursing.columbia.edu/about-us/our-culture/our-history

Commission on Collegiate Nursing Education. (2016). *Clinical nurse leader (CNL®) 2016 job analysis summary & certification examination blueprint.* https://www.aacnnursing.org/Portals/42/CNL/2016-CNL-Job-Analysis-Final-Report.pdf

Commission on Collegiate Nursing Education. (2021). *CCNE-accredited baccalaureate and graduate nursing degree programs*. https://directory.ccnecommunity.org/reports/accprog.asp

Council of Public Health Nursing Organizations. (2021). *The council of public health nursing organizations*. https://www.cphno.org/

Davis, M. A., Guo, C., Titler, M. G., & Friese, C. R. (2017). Advanced practice clinicians as a usual source of care for adults in the United States. *Nursing Outlook, 65*(1), 41–49. https://doi.org/10.1016/j.outlook.2016.07.006

Downey, K., & Assein, M. (2015). Accelerated master's programs in nursing for non-nurses: An integrative review of students' and faculty's perceptions. *Journal of Professional Nursing, 3*(3), 215–225. https://doi.org/10.1016/j.profnurs.2014.10.002

Edmonds, J. K., Campbell, L. A., & Gilder, R. E. (2016). Public health nursing practice in the Affordable Care Act era: A national survey. *Public Health Nursing, 34*(1), 50–58. https://doi.org/10.1111/phn.12286

Edmonds, J. K., Kneipp, S. M., & Campbell, L. A. (2020). A call to action for public health nurses during the COVID-19 pandemic. *Public Health Nursing, 37*(33), 323–324. https://doi.org/10.1111/phn.12733

Ervin, S. (2018, 2021). History of nursing education in the United States. In S. Keating & S. DeBoor (Eds.), *Curriculum development and evaluation in nursing education* (pp. 5–22). Springer.

Gerard, S., Kazer, M., Babington, L., & Quell, T. (2015). Past, present, and future trends in master's education in nursing. *Journal of Professional Nursing, 30*(4), 326–332. https://doi.org/10.1016/j.profnurs.2014.01.005

Gregory, L., Doucette, J., Duffy, L., & Maniion, A. (2021). Improving access to care for pediatric patients with hypertension. *The Journal for Nurse Practitioners, 17*(3), 283–288. https://doi.org/10.1016/j.nurpra.2020.11.013

Hoffman, R. L., Battaglia, A., Perpetua, A., Wojtaszek, K., Campbell, G. (2020). The clinical nurse leader and COVID-19: Leadership and quality at the point of care. *Journal of Professional Nursing, 36*(4), 178–180. https://doi.org/10.1016/j.profnurs.2020.06.008

Institute of Medicine. (2010). *The future of nursing. Leading change, advancing health*. https://nacns.org/wp-content/uploads/2016/11/5-IOM-Report.pdf

Institute of Medicine. (2015). *Assessing progress of the Institute of Medicine Report: The future of nursing*. https://www.jonascenter.org/docs/Assessing-Progress-on-the-Institute-of-Medicine-Report-The-Future-of-Nursing_Dec2015.pdf

Kapu, A. (2021). Origin and outcomes of acute care nurse practitioner practice. *JONA, 51*(1), 4–5. https://doi.org/10.1097/NNA.0000000000000957

Kurtzman, E. T., Barnow, B. S., Johnson, J. E., Simmens, S. J., Lind Infeld, D., & Mullan, F. (2017). Does the regulatory environment affect nurse practitioner's patterns of practice or quality of care in health centers? *Health Services Research, 52*(51), 437–458. https://doi.org/10.1111/1475-6773.12643z

McElroy, K. G., Stalter, A. M., & Smith, S. D. (2020). Association of Community Health Nursing Educators 2020 research priorities and research in action model. *Public Health Nursing, 37*(6), 909–924. https://doi.org/10.1111/phn.12790

Miltner, R. S., Haddock, K. S., Patrician, P. A., & Williams, M. (2020). Implementation of the clinical nurse leader role in the Veterans Health Administration. *Nursing Administration Quarterly, 44*(3), 257–267. https://doi.org/10.1097/NAQ.0000000000000428

Moldestad, M., Greene, P. A., Sayre, G. G., Neely, E. L., Sulc, C.A., Sales, A. E., Reddy, A., Wong, E. S., & Liu, C-F. (2020). Comparable, but distinct: Perceptions of primary care provided by physicians and nurse practitioners in full and restricted practice authority states. *Journal of Advanced Nursing, 75*, 3092–3113. https://doi.org/10.1111/jan.14501

National Academy of Medicine. (2021). *The future of nursing 2020–2030*. https://nam.edu/publications/the-future-of-nursing-2020–2030/

National Council of State Boards of Nursing. (2016). *Scope of practice decision-making framework*. https://www.ncsbn.org/2016_Decision-Making-Framework.pdf

National Council of State Boards of Nursing. (2021). *CNP independent practice map*. https://www.ncsbn.org/5407.htm

National League for Nursing. (2021a). *Certification for nurse educators*. https://www.nln.org/Certification-for-Nurse-Educators

National League for Nursing. (2021b). *Certified Nurse Educator (CNE®) 2021 candidate handbook*. https://www.nln.org/docs/default-source/default-document-library/cne-handbook-2021.pdf?sfvrsn=2

National League for Nursing. (2021c).*Certified Academic Clinical Nurse Educator (CNE®cl) 2021 candidate handbook*. https://www.nln.org/docs/default-source/default-document-library/cnecl-handbook-2021.pdf?sfvrsn=2

National Organization of Nurse Practitioner Faculty. (2018). *The doctor of nursing practice degree: Entry to nurse practitioner practice by 2025*. https://cdn.ymaws.com/www.nonpf.org/resource/resmgr/dnp/v3_05.2018_NONPF_DNP_Stateme.pdf

National Organization of Nurse Practitioner Faculty. (2021). *Statement on acute care and primary care nurse practitioner practice*. https://www.nonpf.org/

The National Task Force on Quality Nurse Practitioner Education. (2016). *Criteria for evaluation of nurse practitioner programs* (5th ed.). Washington, DC: Author. https://cdn.ymaws.com/www.nonpf.org/resource/resmgr/Docs/EvalCriteria2016Final.pdf

Noles, K., & James, D. (2019). Driving innovation in health care. *Journal of Nursing Care Quality*, 34(4), 307–311. https://doi.org/10.1097/NCQ.0000000000000394

Phillips, S. (2020). 32nd Annual APRN legislative update: Improving access to high-quality, safe, and effective healthcare. *The Nurse Practitioner*, 45(1), 28–55. https://doi.org/10.1097/01.NPR.0000615560.11798.5f

Quad Council Coalition. (2018). *Community/Public health nurse (C/PHN) competencies*. https://www.cphno.org/wp-content/uploads/2020/08/QCC-C-PHN-COMPETENCIES-Approved_2018.05.04_Final-002.pdf

Shaw, K., Harpin, S., Steinke, G., Stember, M., & Krijicek, M. (2016). The DNP/MPH dual degree: An innovative graduate education program for advanced public health nursing. *Public Health Nursing*, 34(2), 185–193.

Tracy, M. F., Oerther, S., Arsianisn-Engoren, C., Girouard, S., Minarik, P., Parrician, P., Vollman, K., Sanders, N., McCausland, M., Antai-Otong, D., & Talsma, A. (2020). Improving the care and health of populations through optimal use of clinical nurse specialists. *Nursing Outlook*, 68(4), 523–527. https://doi.org/10.1016/j.outlook.2020.06.004

U.S. Department of Veterans Affairs. (2016). *Clinical nurse leader (CNL)*. https://www.va.gov/NURSING/practice/cnl.asp

Vogelsmeier, A., Popejoy, L., Kist, S., Shumate, S., Pritchett, A., Mueller, J., & Rantz, M. (2020). Reducing avoidable hospitalizations for nursing home residents: Role of the Missouri quality initiative intervention support team. *Journal of Nursing Care Quality*, 35(1), 1–5. https://doi.org/10.1097/NCQ.0000000000000444

White, P., & Hall, M. E. (2006). Managing the literature of case management nursing. *Journal of the Medical Library Association*, 94(2), 99–106.

CHAPTER 10

Planning for Doctoral Education

Jacqueline Ferdowsali and Stephanie Stimac DeBoor

CHAPTER OBJECTIVES

Upon completion of Chapter 10, the reader will be able to:

- Differentiate between a practice- and research-focused doctorate degree in nursing.

- Describe the role(s) of the DNP and PhD in practice, the healthcare system, and education.

- Analyze the educational preparation of research-focused doctoral programs and practice-focused doctoral programs based on national competencies and accreditation standards.

- Review program evaluation and accreditation requirements for DNP programs.

OVERVIEW

For centuries, individuals sought and were conferred a doctoral degree in academics. Over that time and dependent on the specific academic focus, the aim of doctoral education has fluctuated. Specific to nursing, Carter (2013) conceptualized four periods for doctoral education transitioning from nonnursing focused degrees to ones rooted firmly in nursing. In today's modern nursing educational system, two doctoral degree concentrations have emerged, namely, research and practice. It is through education as a PhD, DNS, or DNP that a nurse can achieve the highest preparation in the profession.

Over the last decade, the number of nurses seeking to enter a doctoral program and earn a doctoral degree has increased overall. From 2018 to 2019, enrollment in DNP programs has increased from 32,678 to 36,069. While PhD enrollments (4,568 in 2019) and graduations have increased overall by 9.4% since 2009, however, since 2013, enrollments have started to decline (American Association of Colleges of Nursing [AACN], 2020a, 2020b). A reflection of the increase in DNP degrees earned rather than a decrease in popularity of doctoral education. While synergy exists between the creation of new knowledge and the translation of knowledge into practice, the PhD and DNP educational preparations have very specific and differentiated paths. The objective of this chapter is to help provide the context in which each doctoral focus within nursing is developed and actualized in the nursing profession.

Differentiating Research and Practice Doctorates in Nursing

The declaration of the title doctor translates from the Latin word of *docēre* meaning to teach (Merriam-Webster, n.d.). Historically, the passing of knowledge from teacher to student required mastery of content by the former. It is worth noting that the attainment of a doctoral degree does not imply pedagogical expertise, but it does reflect a mastery of content within the nursing profession. The conception and trajectory of the PhD and DNP are fundamentally different but ultimately require the recipient gain the knowledge, skills, and attitude to function at the highest level of nursing. The DNP's focus is on evidence translation and integration within practice whereas the PhD focuses on knowledge creation through research.

Historically, PhD-prepared faculty members were the sole tenure-track professors in institutions of higher education. The rationale for this was that research-focused institutions prefer faculty members who are prepared to develop new knowledge and theories in their respective disciplines and bring recognition to the university through their scholarly activities. Currently, some DNP-prepared faculty hold tenure-track positions in universities across the nation, yet there are still universities in the United States that limit tenure-track positions to only those PhD-prepared candidates (Auerbach et al., 2015). Many DNP graduates demonstrate extensive scholarly work in clinical practice and scholarship that contribute to the science of nursing. DNP graduates who desire to teach in schools of nursing should compare tenure-track policies in potential employing institutions to other types of positions such as clinical faculty that are not research-focused but still offer academic ranks from instructor to full professor.

Research-Focused Doctorate in Nursing

According to AACN (2020a), there are currently 135 schools in the U.S. offering a nursing-focused PhD. Research-focused doctoral programs include the DNS, DNSc, and the PhD. Each of these research-intensive doctoral degrees prepares students to pursue intellectual inquiry and conduct independent research that results in the generation of knowledge and advancement of the profession (AACN, 2010; Joseph et al., 2021, King et al., 2020; Rice, 2016). From a theoretical perspective, PhD programs are theory-based and focus on testing theory, while DNS programs are oriented more toward clinical practice research (Ponte & Nicholas, 2015). The designation as a PhD, DNSc, or DNS program often is determined by the school's specific mission and philosophy, as well as by institutional criteria for research doctoral program approval. Chapter 1 provides a historical perspective of doctoral programs specializing in education and research.

Despite recruitment efforts, the number of educated nurse researchers continues to decline, creating concern within the nursing profession (Vance et al., 2020). In October 2020, the AACN created a task force to revise the 2010 position statement on *The Research-Focused Doctoral Program in Nursing: Pathways to Excellence*. The primary goal of this group is to create a vision for research doctorates and those graduates of the programs (AACN, 2021a).

Doctor of Nursing Practice

Case Western Reserve University in 1979 introduced the concept of a practice doctoral degree in nursing. This first professional doctoral degree, called the ND, was an entry-level degree. Similar to the other early doctorate degrees in nursing, there was debate and concern about the exact title and terms to use for this new degree. Eventually a transition to the DNP degree occurred, and this is now the accepted clinical ND. There are several terms used to describe the DNP, including *practice*, *clinical*, and *professional doctorate*.

The essence of each of these terms is a clinical focus distinct from the research focus of the PhD. The AACN (2004) recommends using the terminology of practice doctorate. The AACN (2004) defines practice as

> any form of nursing intervention that influences health care outcomes for individuals or populations, including the direct care of individual patients, management of care for individuals and populations, administration of nursing and health care organizations, and the development and implementation of health policy. (p. 3)

Today, the DNP is the highest attainment within nursing practice and as reflected in the preceding definition encompasses both direct clinical care and the healthcare system structure of policies and protocols. Today DNP's hold employment in a variety of positions, from advanced practice nurses and nurse educators to health policy advocates to nurse executives, including chief nursing officers and chief executive officers of healthcare systems. Any opportunity for care enhancement through the translation of knowledge and leadership is a potential career opportunity for a DNP.

PhD Curriculum

Nurses, who are seeking to continue their education by achieving a terminal degree, must decide if their interests are practice- or research-focused. Dreifuerst et al. (2016) found that those who are exploring doctoral education take into consideration the type of program and its delivery, time to complete, faculty expertise and research interests, and the overall cost. Time and cost seem to be predominant factors for choosing a doctoral path in nursing. Many PhD programs take a minimum of 3 to 5 years to complete, whereas students achieve the DNP in 1 to 2 years depending on the curricular components and previous education.

There is a growing need to expand the number of nurse scientists. This need dictates changes in how we educate these students. The curriculum of a research-focused doctoral program is unique and based on the school's mission and philosophy as interpreted and implemented by the faculty. Usual core coursework includes the history and philosophy of nursing science, theories that guide the discipline and practice, research methods, advanced statistics, substantive nursing in a specific area of expertise, and role-related content (e.g., pedagogy). Depending on the program, required content may include mentoring, leadership, interdisciplinary research teamwork, and health policy. Unfortunately, with the decreasing numbers in PhD enrollment, there is a quest to attract nurses to these programs. Nursing leaders gathered at the University of Pennsylvania in October of 2019 to discuss the future preparation of PhD students in nursing. Much published since that meeting identifies gaps in education and future recommendations for supporting and preparing future nurse scientists. In addition, the AACN Task Force for *The Research-Focused Doctoral Program in Nursing: Pathways to Excellence* (AACN, 2021a) is tasked with multiple charges of an examination, evaluation, and revision of curricula approaches, curricular components or elements, innovation, and timeliness of degree completion.

Fairman et al. (2021) highlighted some of the challenges and changes occurring in the last decade related to a realignment and reenvisioning of the research-focused doctorate in nursing. The most notable challenges are the recruitment of high-quality students, the lack of qualified PhD faculty mentors, and funding. Faculty voice that many programs are finding ways to make PhD education more attractive, such as shortening the program of study, eliminating entrance exams (e.g., Graduate Record Examinations [GRE]), providing group mentoring, bridge programs, dissertation versus publication, and new curriculum (Fairman et al., 2021; McSweeney et al., 2020; Vance et al., 2020).

Joseph et al. (2021) identify four areas to be included in future curricula. These include the study of social determinants of health, education outside of a silo (inclusion of other disciplines within classes), innovation through strong clinical partnerships, and the ability to implement scientific research into practice. In most programs, the inclusion of these recommendations compliments the current coursework. Giordano et al. (2021) identify that while important to maintain core coursework, future scientists need to understand "precision health, omics, big data, informatics, ethics, and implementation science and health policy" (p. 231). The goal of a research-focused nursing doctorate is to prepare future nurse scientists to create new knowledge and advance the profession. In order to achieve this goal, we must evaluate current curricula and be prepared to dispose of out-of-date pedagogy.

DNP Curriculum

Frantz (2013) provides an overview of the resources needed when planning, implementing, and sustaining a DNP program:

- identified are the necessary faculty members and their qualifications;
- resources such as classrooms and simulation facilities;
- the infrastructure for delivering courses online and on-campus;
- potential collaboration between the PhD and DNP programs' course faculty and, possibly, other academic institutions;
- faculty and student practice opportunities;
- healthcare agencies' resources for clinical experiences (both advanced practice and administrative); and
- administrative and staff support specific to the DNP program.

The DNP curriculum design needs to provide students with the opportunity to immerse in clinical practice topics and develop as a nurse leader. *The Essentials: Core Competencies for Professional Nursing Education* were launched April 6, 2021 (AACN, 2021b). The new Essentials "provides a framework for preparing individuals as members of the discipline of nursing, reflecting expectations across the trajectory of nursing education and applied experience" (AACN, 2021b, p. 2).

Distinctive Considerations Within DNP Curriculum

There are currently two entry pathways for a DNP program of study, either via a baccalaureate or a master's in nursing degree. The variation in students seeking a DNP includes APRNs to nursing administrators, managers, and other nurse leaders with or without national certification. There are similarities and differences in the curriculum developed for a post-master's DNP compared to a postbaccalaureate DNP. The overall goal of either program of study is to allow students to obtain the required knowledge, skills, and attitudes within each of the DNP *Domains*.

Variations will exist related to attaining specific competencies within specialized roles, such as an APRN within the program of study. Necessary for the different roles within DNP programs is the incorporation of specialty competencies for programs that prepare DNPs for advanced practice roles such as clinical specialists, nurse practitioners, nurse midwives, nurse anesthetists, clinical nurse leaders, and others. *Domain 9: Professionalism* reflects the development of the nurse's professional identity and values of that specialization within the DNP degree. Those faculty involved with developing the curriculum will use the 10 *Domains* of the new Essentials to outline competency expectations of the program. Academic program developers' further need to examine specialty organizations for a list of competencies required for population foci of advanced nursing roles. Some of these role-specific competencies will allow the DNP student to be eligible to take a national certification exam at the end of their program of study. Exhibit 10.1 provides an example of the melding of the new Essentials and competencies of a BSN to DNP student in the role specialization of the adult-gerontology acute care nurse practitioner.

EXHIBIT 10.1: Essentials and Competencies for BSN to DNP (AGACNP Assignment).

Upon completion of this course, students will be able to:

1. Identify other healthcare professionals for collaboration to promote continuity of care for acutely ill patients and families with acute health alterations. (**Domain 6: Interprofessional Partnerships, Concept: Communication;** NONPF Competency Area: Independent Practice; NTF Criterion III.B, III.D, VI.A.4).

Assignment: Interprofessional Virtual Reality Simulation. This simulation will focus on Johanne, a 36-year-old woman, who does not fit the stereotype of someone experiencing homelessness. Not long ago, Johanne was living what would be considered a healthy life with her family. When her husband died and she lost her job, she found herself in a downward spiral, and her situation dramatically changed. Students will participate in the 1-hour simulation with an interprofessional team meeting with Johanne to identify potential referrals and resources needed. After the simulation, students will discuss as a group the following: Has working with other professions impacted your ability to address Johanne's needs? What other health professional's input may be beneficial in this case? **Competency:** Students must achieve an 83% for this 20-point assignment based on the following rubric components. **Content:** Addresses all aspects of the assignment with well-supported statements and thoughts (10 points), **Style:** Graduate-level writing with clear and well-articulated point of view (4 points), **APA Format**: Cited references and correct formatting (3 points), **Submission:** Adheres to word count, on time (3 points).

Supervised clinical experiences are an expectation of DNP education. Nationally, a minimum standard of 1,000 hours of clinical and mentored practice meets this expected requirement. When evaluating what activities will fulfill the clinical practicum requirement, a reflection on the *Domains* should precede any approval. The clinical practice requirement provides the DNP real-world experience of actualizing the DNP *Domains, Concepts, and Competencies*. Included in this consideration is any national certification or professional accreditation standards for specific roles.

Similar to PhD programs the DNP should produce a final program deliverable that allows the DNP student to demonstrate their synthesis and attainment of the DNP Essentials: *Domains, Concepts, and Competencies*. However, the focus of the DNP project is not on generating new knowledge such as the PhD student. There remains ongoing debate about the exact requirements and format of a DNP project. This ambiguity has generated frustration among nursing faculty (Dols, 2017). A struggle often exists in differentiating an MSN project from that of the DNP. The AACN Task Force report on the implementation of the DNP (AACN, 2015), the *Defining Scholarship for Academic Nursing Position Statement* (AACN, 2018b), and the DNP Toolkit (AACN, 2021c) provide current recommendations and clarifications for the DNP project.

PhD Program Evaluation

There is no professional accreditation for research-focused doctoral programs. Each institution's individual programs establishes and maintains the quality of their research-focused doctoral nursing programs. However, AACN (2010) provides quality indicators to guide the evaluation of these programs. This evaluation criterion consists of categories of faculty and administration, students, resources and infrastructure, and evaluation plan. Programs often supplement these measures with their own indicators. For example, for a state-supported program, one rubric might be the proportion of state residents in the student body and/or the number of international students enrolled. However, to date, little comparative data exist about the quality of programs other than objective measures of enrollment, race/ethnicity and gender of students, length of the program, the number of grants, and the amount of funding awarded from federal and private grants to nursing faculty.

DNP Program Evaluation and Accreditation

Program evaluation and accreditation are essential to the quality of DNP programs. Each school of nursing that has a DNP program usually has a master plan of evaluation for all programs and the DNP is included. DNP programs, in addition to the usual layers of approval within the home institution, are subject to the institution's governing board's approval, and if they are preparing entry-level advanced practice nurses, depending on state regulations, they must undergo program approval by their state board of nursing. Program evaluation provides the data for assessing the effectiveness and quality of the program. Developing evaluation plans that incorporate all the parameters of the program for assessment is important, but it is also essential that plans be in place to implement the assessment. The methods for collecting and analyzing the data, the persons responsible, and when and how the findings affect program improvements are key factors to include.

Specific to DNP program accreditation are the roles of the Accreditation Commission for Education in Nursing (ACEN, 2020) and the CCNE (2018b). The *Standards for Accreditation of Clinical Doctorate Programs* (ACEN, 2020) include six categories of standards along with details for each: Standard 1—Mission and Administrative Capacity, Standard 2—Faculty and Staff, Standard 3—Students, Standard 4—Curriculum, Standard 5—Resources, and Outcomes.

The *Standards for Accreditation of Baccalaureate and Graduate Nursing Programs* (CCNE, 2018b) identify four areas of evaluation that include Standard I—Program Quality: Mission and Governance, Standard II—Program Quality: Institutional Commitment and Resources, Standard III—Program Quality: Curriculum and Teaching-Learning Practices, and Standard IV-Program Effectiveness: Assessment and Achievement of Program Outcomes.

See Section IV of the text for more details on program evaluation and accreditation.

Challenges and Opportunities

The ever-changing landscape of doctoral education identifies the need for collaborative relationships between the research-focused and practice doctorates. There is ongoing debate concerning the role of the DNP and the differences in the PhD degree as it pertains to the profession of nursing, advanced practice, and healthcare. As the DNP is on the frontier of doctoral education in nursing, there remain challenges and opportunities for refinement. The exact structure and content of the DNP project remain a huge piece of national DNP discussions. The idea of a master's opt-out built into a DNP program structure is also something program administers will have to consider as the curriculum is developed. Additionally, national pressure to commit to the DNP as the entry level to practice degree has mounted. The Institute of Medicine (IOM) issued a recommendation in 2010, *The Future of Nursing: Leading Change, Improving Health* to double the amount of doctorally prepared nurses by 2020. In October 2004, the members of the AACN endorsed the *Position Statement on the Practice Doctorate in Nursing*. This position identified the need for an entry level to practice for APRNs to move from the master's level to the doctorate level by 2015. Furthermore, the National Organization of Nurse Practitioner Faculty

(NONPF, 2018) also issued a position statement to have the DNP degree as the entry level to practice by 2025. This shift would create questions about those advanced practice nurses currently in practice who do not have a DNP. While consensus may be to "grandparent in" those individuals for licensure to practice in the states in which they are licensed and recognized, it is anticipated that this will be a challenge for nursing to address. Despite these issues, the overall value of the DNP as a change agent addressing the most concerning quality and outcome problems within the healthcare system make these considerations worthy of continued dialogue.

SUMMARY

This chapter reviewed the growth of doctoral programs in the nation, educational preparation, curriculum, roles of both research-focused (PhD, DNS) and practice (DNP) doctorates, program evaluation, and differences between the two. Research-focused doctoral programs produce scientists. Most work in academia after graduation balances research with the other dimensions (teaching, service). The DNP prepares nurses to translate the science developed by nurse researchers into practice. Most DNP graduates work in a myriad of roles that include advanced practice, education, and leadership/management. All nursing doctorates play an important role in the changing and challenging components of healthcare within the United States. Collaboration between PhD/DNS graduates and DNP graduates contributes to the success of meeting these healthcare needs of our nation.

END-OF-CHAPTER RESOURCES

DISCUSSION QUESTIONS

1. Propose how interdisciplinary research might be supported and developed as part of a PhD/DNS program.

2. What are the strengths and limitations of having students admitted to a PhD/DNS with a baccalaureate degree in nursing, a master's degree in nursing, and a DNP degree?

3. To what extent do you believe the DNP as the terminal degree for advanced practice resulted in consensus within the nursing profession?

4. Debate research-focused degrees as contrasted to practice degrees research activities. Do they differ, or are they the same? Does this debate affect the profession of nursing discipline?

LEARNING ACTIVITIES

Student-Learning Activities

1. Compare and contrast the PhD and DNP programs. What are the similarities and differences in coursework, research training, and available faculty mentorship in your area of expertise?

2. Review the latest research and literature (the past 2 years) to identify the state of debate on the DNP and its role in research and academe.

Nurse Educator/Faculty Development Activities

1. Compare one online and one in-person PhD or DNP program. What are the strengths of each? Consider how you can make the best use of these data in your program.

2. If the student population in your program does not reflect the racial–ethnic or gender mix of the general population, what three things might you consider to rectify this disparity?

3. If your school of nursing has a DNP program, analyze its curriculum for its congruence with the AACN *Essentials* document. If your school does not have a DNP program, find a school that does and review its program of study to compare to the *Essentials*.

 A robust set of instructor resources designed to supplement this text is located at **http://connect.springerpub.com/content/book/978-0-8261-8686-7.** Qualifying instructors may request access by emailing **textbook@springerpub.com.**

REFERENCES

Accreditation Commission for Education in Nursing. (2020). *ACEN accreditation manual: Section III standards and criteria glossary.* https://www.acenursing.org/Resources-for-Nursing-Programs/sc2017-C.pdf

Auerbach, D. I., Martsolf, G., Pearson, M. L., Taylor, E. A., Zaydman, M., Muchow, A. N., Spetz, J., & Dower, C. (2015). *The DNP by 2015: A study of the institutional, political, and professional issues that facilitate or impede establishing a post-baccalaureate doctor of nursing practice program.* https://www.rand.org/content/dam/rand/pubs/research_reports/RR700/RR730/RAND_RR730.pdf

American Association of Colleges of Nursing. (2004, October). *AACN position statement on the practice doctorate in nursing.* https://www.aacnnursing.org/Portals/42/News/Position-Statements/DNP.pdf

American Association of Colleges of Nursing. (2010). *The research-focused doctoral program in nursing: Pathways to excellence.* http://www.aacnnursing.org/Portals/42/Publications/PhDPosition.pdf

American Association of Colleges of Nursing. (2015). *The doctor of nursing practice: Current issues and clarifying recommendations: Report from the task force on the implementation of the DNP.* http://www.professionalnursing.org/article/S8755-7223(15)00100-3/pdf

American Association of Colleges of Nursing. (2018a, March 26). *Defining scholarship for academic nursing task force consensus position statement.* https://www.aacnnursing.org/Portals/42/News/Position-Statements/Defining-Scholarship.pdf

American Association of Colleges of Nursing. (2018b). *Standards for accreditation of baccalaureate and graduate nursing programs.* https://www.aacnnursing.org/Portals/42/CCNE/PDF/Standards-Final-2018.pdf

American Association of Colleges of Nursing. (2020a). *PhD in nursing.* https://www.aacnnursing.org/News-Information/Research-Data-Center/PhD

American Association of Colleges of Nursing. (2020b, October). *Fact sheet: The Doctor of Nursing Practice.* https://www.aacnnursing.org/News-Information/Fact-Sheets/DNP-Fact-Sheet

American Association of Colleges of Nursing. (2021a). *Research-focused doctoral program pathways to excellence task force: Task force charge.* https://www.aacnnursing.org/pathways-taskforce

American Association of Colleges of Nursing. (2021b). *The essentials: Core competencies for professional nursing education.* https://www.aacnnursing.org/Portals/42/AcademicNursing/pdf/Essentials-2021.pdf

American Association of Colleges of Nursing. (2021c). *Doctor of nursing practice (DNP) tool kit.* https://www.aacnnursing.org/DNP/Tool-Kit

Carter, M. (2013). The evolution of doctoral education in nursing. In S. DeNisco & A. Barker (Eds.), *Advanced practice nursing: Evolving roles for the transformation of the profession* (pp. 27–35). Jones & Bartlett Learning.

Dols, J. D., Hernández, C., & Miles, H. (2017). The DNP project: Quandaries for nursing scholars. *Nursing Outlook, 65*(1), 84–93. https://doi.org/10.1016/j.outlook.2016.07.009

Dreifuerst, K. T., McNelis, A. M., Weaver, M. T., Broome, M. E., Draucker, C. B., & Fedko, A. S. (2016). Exploring the pursuit of doctoral education by nurses seeking or intending to stay in faculty roles. *Journal of Professional Nursing, 32*(3), 202–212. https://doi.org/10.1016/j.profnurs.2016.01.014

Fairman, J. A., Giordano, N. A., McCauley, K., & Villarruel, A. (2021). Invitational summit: Re-envisioning research focused PhD programs of the future. *Journal of Professional Nursing, 37,* 221–227. https://doi.org/10.1016/j.profnurs.2020.09.004

Frantz, R. A. (2013). Resource requirements for a quality doctor of nursing practice program. *Journal of Nursing Education, 52*(8), 449–452. https://doi.org/10.3928/01484834-20130713-01

Giordano, N. A., Compton, P., Joseph, P. V., Romano, C. A., Piano, M. R., & Naylor, M. D. (2021). Opportunities and challenges presented by recent pedagogical innovations in doctoral nursing education. *Journal of Professional Nursing, 37,* 228–234. https://doi.org/10.1016/j.profnurs.2020.09.003

Institute of Medicine. (2010). *The future of nursing: Leading change, advancing health.* National Academies Press.

Joseph, P. V., McCauley, L., & Richmond, T. S. (2021). PhD programs and the advancement of nursing science. *Journal of Professional Nursing, 37*(1), 195–200. https://doi.org/10.1016/j.profnurs.2020.06.011

King, T. S., Melnyk, B. M., O'Brien, T., Bowles, W., Schuber, C., Fletcher, L., & Anderson, S. M. (2020). Doctoral degree preferences for nurse educators: Findings from a national study. *Nurse Educator, 45*(3), 144–149. https://doi.org/10.1097/NNE.0000000000000730

McSweeney, J., Weglicki, L. S., Munro, C., Hickman, R., & Pickler, R. (2020). Commentary. Preparing nurse scientists. Challenges and solutions. *Nursing Research, 69*(6), 414–418. https://doi.org/10.1097/NNR.0000000000000471

Merriam-Webster. (n.d.). Doctor. In *Merriam-Webster.com dictionary.* Retrieved from https://www.merriam-webster.com/dictionary/doctor

National Organization of Nurse Practitioner Faculties. (2018, May). *The doctor of nursing practice degree: Entry to nurse practitioner practice by 2025.* https://cdn.ymaws.com/www.nonpf.org/resource/resmgr/dnp/v3_05.2018_NONPF_DNP_Stateme.pdf

Rice, D. (2016). The research doctorate in nursing: The PhD. *Oncology Nursing Forum, 43*(2), 146–148. https://doi.org/10.1188/16.ONF.146-148

Vance, D. E., Heaton, K., Antia, L., Frank, J., Moneyham, L., Harper, D., & Meneses, K. (2020). Alignment of a PhD program in nursing with the AACN report on the research-focused doctorate in nursing: A descriptive analysis. *Journal of Professional Nursing, 36*(6), 604–610. https://doi.org/10.1016/j.profnurs.2020.08.011

CHAPTER 11

A Proposed Unified Nursing Curriculum

Sarah B. Keating

Updated by Stephanie Stimac DeBoor

CHAPTER OBJECTIVES

Upon completion of Chapter 11, the reader will be able to:

- Review the issues in nursing education that led to numerous points of entry into the practice of nursing.
- Differentiate among the various levels of nursing education and their role in preparing nurses for practice in the current and future healthcare systems.
- Consider a proposed unified nursing curriculum that could streamline nursing education, verify its position as a profession, and ensure well-prepared healthcare providers (nurses) to meet the healthcare needs of the population.

OVERVIEW

As reviewed in Chapter 1, nursing education in the United States has a long history of preparing healthcare professionals through various pathways leading to professional practice and licensure (whose purpose is to ensure the safety of patients through the testing of professionals for their knowledge and competence). Diploma schools that were hospital- and training-based started in the late 19th century, while early in the 20th century, higher education, university-based programs began to appear. In the mid-20th century, additional baccalaureate programs appeared along with the recommendation from professional organizations that they serve as the entry point into the profession. However, at about the same time, associate degree, community college-based programs came on the scene that prepared nurses at the technical level in accordance with the purpose of community colleges and, at the same time, prepared them for licensure. To meet professional standards, these programs increased requirements for the associate degree to include core courses in the sciences and liberal arts. Moving on to the later 20th and early 21st centuries, nursing started to respond to the increasing complexity of the healthcare system and population healthcare needs by developing entry-level master's programs such as the clinical nurse leader (CNL) role for nonnursing college graduates and the advanced practice doctorate, previously found at the master's level.

Philosophically and realized in current nursing curricula, the profession believes in a strong foundation in liberal arts and sciences and, at the same time, prescribes the nursing major to constitute at least half of the total major. Following the usual pattern for lower and upper division majors in higher education, the usual number of units for associate degrees is 64 to 72 and bachelor's degrees range from 120 to 130 units/credits. Classically, prerequisite courses required by nursing and usually counted toward general education requirements include English composition, speech (communications), sociology, human development, psychology, anatomy, physiology, microbiology, chemistry, nutrition, and statistics. There are other courses that nursing values as foundations for practice, such as the arts, language, philosophy, genetics, economics, political science, computer science, and business. And yet, there is little or no room for these courses in the already higher unit (70 or 125) undergraduate nursing degree programs. As one begins to add up the credits, it becomes apparent that nursing as a profession and, like other professions, must be at the higher degree level. The Institute of Medicine's (2011) report validates the assumption that nursing needs to move toward the goal of requiring a higher education degree for entry into professional practice and in 2018, the National Organization of Nurse Practitioner Faculty (NONPF) committed to having the DNP be the entry level of practice for all NPs. A review of the Accreditation Commission for Education in Nursing (ACEN, 2021) and American Associate of Colleges of Nursing (AACN, 2021a) websites revealed changing numbers in levels of education. There are 31 accredited diploma programs in 2021 and 357 doctoral programs, with 106 more in the planning stages to start a DNP.

LEVELS OF NURSING EDUCATION AND THEIR ROLE IN PREPARING NURSES FOR PRACTICE

Diploma, Associate Degree, and Baccalaureate Levels

Existing levels of nursing education to prepare nurses for licensure in the United States remain at the diploma, associate degree (ADN), bachelor's (BSN), and master's levels. As noted previously, the number of diploma programs has decreased rapidly, and the number of associate degree programs has remained steady, although more programs have developed articulation agreements that provide a seamless move of the associate degree graduate into the baccalaureate nursing degree. Jeffreys (2020) describes a "proactive and holistic" approach that facilitates access for ADN graduates into the baccalaureate. This approach helps students from the onset of their education for moving into the BSN level of education prior to completion of their ADN. Coordinators provide a verbal and visual pathway that guides students through various steps in their educational transition. Bowles et al. (2020) described statewide initiatives through the Ohio Action Coalition that provide a direct progression model for students in associate degree programs the ability to move into the BSN. Through the collaboration of ADN and BSN programs, students clear academic pathways to continue their educational journey. These initiatives have contributed to increasing the number of BSNs within the state. To gain some verification of the barriers in selecting education routes between the ADN and BSN, Petges and Sabio (2020) surveyed more than 500 ADN students in Illinois. Barriers were ranked in one of three categories; situational, dispositional, or institutional. Situational barriers presented the highest concern for respondents including costs/lack of financial support or aid, job and home responsibilities, time, and childcare concerns. Dispositional barriers included no monetary benefit for getting a BSN over an ADN, fear of failing or not finishing the program, competition for admission, previous grade point average (GPA), and BSN not needed for entry-level practice. Institutional concerns were listed as the amount of time to complete, the location of the institution, courses that don't transfer, schedules being inconvenient, a lack of information, and applicants not meeting admission requirements. Despite these barriers, the respondents identified that if the entry level to practice was a BSN, two thirds stated they were likely or highly likely to enroll, whereas 32.9% said they were highly unlikely, unlikely, or unsure that they would enroll. A larger nationwide survey is recommended, as one regional area of the United States is not generalizable to all areas but does provide a view of ADN opinions regarding barriers to a higher level of education.

Issues related to undergraduate education (ADN and BSN), such as the time and money spent on undergraduate education for entry into practice, professional values, knowledge, skills, and expertise to safe practice, still raise issues related to technical versus professional practice. These issues ask nursing to consider whether it is time to move from the BSN to graduate education for entry into practice. One needs only to interview nurses who have "grown up" in nursing (CNA, LPN, ADN, BSN, etc.) to discover the excess number of credits in their degree work and realize the enormity of the problem and the injustices nurses suffered in gaining education, with little to no academic recognition of their additional work. Going one step further, nurses who hold master's and/or doctorates suffer the same overabundance of credits, completing far more than their colleagues in medicine, pharmacology, education, engineering, religion, and law.

Master's Level

According to the American Association of Colleges of Nursing (AACN, 2019), there were approximately 64 entry into practice master's-level programs in the United States. A program specifically designed by the AACN for college graduates with majors not in nursing is the clinical nurse leader (CNL) track (AACN, 2021b; Jackson & Marchi, 2020). Other entry-level master's programs offer specialties in advanced practice such as clinical nurse specialist (CNS) and NP, roles in nursing management, clinical education, and community/public health nursing. It should be noted that many advanced practice programs are converting from the master's to the DNP. For details on graduate programs, Chapter 9 provides information on master's programs, and Chapter 10 describes preparing for the DNP and PhD educational programs. Generally, except for the advanced generalist role specific to the CNL, the master's entry level of preparation trains nurses for leadership, clinical educator, and practice roles in the community.

Doctoral Levels: DNP

Yet another level of graduate nursing education is the DNP/clinical doctorate. Few, if any, entry-level doctoral programs exist, although there were several in the past. At this time, BSN graduates can continue their education and articulate directly into the DNP; however, most sit for the licensure examination, and licensure is usually required for admission into the program. It is possible that in the future, this requirement might be waived and licensure would occur after graduation from doctoral studies. However, that is very unlikely to occur anytime soon.

Since publishing the results of the *DNP by 2015* and subsequent RAND report, the AACN at its January 2020 meeting discussed next steps in assessing "the state of the DNP graduates and their contributions to advanced nursing practice" (AACN, 2020). The NONPF has strongly supported the DNP being the entry level to practice for APRNs by 2025. The AACN has issued a request for proposals to study multiple factors in relation to DNP prepared graduates to include employment, perceptions of preparation, the impact of outcomes on patients and the healthcare system, health policy, leadership, and quality. Most important, the AACN is looking for action items to support the movement of the DNP as the entry level to APRN practice.

McCauley et al. (2020) explore barriers in DNP education that contribute to the confusion as to the role of the DNP-prepared nurse. During the COVID-19 crisis, there was no question as to the value and functions of the DNP on leadership in the healthcare system, meeting the needs of individuals, improvement in healthcare outcomes, interprofessional collaboration, and evidence-based practice. The results of their study further elaborate on the barriers of adopting the DNP as the APRN entry level. One such barrier is an incurred financial burden by the student, the institution offering the DNP level of education, and those who support APRN education (tuition reimbursement). There are still questions to ask in relation to differentiating accreditation and certification for MSN versus DNP. Is there a market demand for the DNP at the student and employer levels? Finally, how do we clearly articulate the role of the DNP-prepared graduate?

Doctoral Level: PhD

Thus far, the discussion in this chapter reviewed the various levels of nursing education for entry into professional practice. It did not touch on the need for nursing scientists and educators. There is debate in the discipline about this issue as well since the questions arise as to what level should a nursing faculty member be prepared in both the sciences of nursing and education and what levels of education and research activities are expected for nursing scientists. There is an old rule of thumb in academe that the faculty members who teach should be educated to at least one degree higher than that of the students they expect to prepare. For example, faculty holding baccalaureate or master's degrees prepare students at the associate degree level, and faculty holding master's or doctoral degrees prepare students at the baccalaureate level. Obviously, doctorate programs would require the doctoral level of prepared faculty, which then raises the question, DNP or PhD or both? State boards of nursing also have regulations to the required level of education for faculty or those who teach within academe.

The question of programs to offer direct entry from the baccalaureate into the PhD level of nursing education remains an issue. Other disciplines/sciences offer these programs and produce younger graduates for the advancement of their science and professions. An interesting study by Vance et al. (2020) examined how to accelerate the process of PhD education without compromising the integrity of the educational process of the nurse scientist. This fast-tracked program of study lends itself to graduating a younger researcher who can then contribute more years of research, thus advancing the nursing profession. One must consider the faculty and institutional support system when contemplating the creation of this type of accelerated program.

Smaldone and Larson (2021) summarized the findings of the 2019 summit held at the University of Pennsylvania to discuss the education of nursing scientists. The group set out to answer two questions: What competencies should frame the educational components of the PhD? In addition, what programmatic and curricular innovations prepare and support PhD students? Their findings identified that in order to support the roles of PhD graduates, the curriculum should include content on health policy, innovation, and global relationships. Innovations included accelerated time frames and for completion and new strategies for learning. Ultimately, the competencies proposed by AACN in 2010, still remain relevant to today's education of PhD students.

Staffileno et al. (2017) conducted a qualitative study to examine the collaboration barriers between DNP- and PhD-prepared faculty. Five themes were extrapolated from the data to include a misunderstanding of the DNP in the educational role, confusion surrounding research (educational preparation), opportunities for collaboration (coteaching, research collaboration, committee work), a lack of structural support (for DNP scholarship), and personal characteristics and attitudes (qualifications, commonalities, respect). While formal education may differ between the DNP and the PhD, collaboration between the doctorally prepared nursing faculty is essential in order for knowledge generation and application to complement and advance the nursing profession. We, as a profession, must refrain from the "who's better" and "one-upmanship" trend, which has been around for years, and focus on what each level of education has to offer in the advancement of our discipline.

Often faculty who teach in the DNP program struggle with whether their students are doing research or a quality improvement (QI) project. Carter et al. (2017) identify that even the Office of Human Research Protection (OHRP), a federal agency charged with regulating research with human subjects, struggles to clearly define what is and isn't research. Oftentimes terms are used interchangeably when discussing scholarly work. Thus, the OHRP created a decision tree (www.hhs.gov/ohrp/regulations-and-policy/decision-charts/index.html) to help guide faculty, students, and other researchers.

An important point from a review of the literature and reports from practice that relates to nursing education and the faculty role is that education is also a science and consists of theories, concepts, models, and practice. Nursing academe must take this into account and ensure that nurses choosing to assume educator roles have the knowledge, expertise, and skills in both nursing and teaching. There are a few nursing programs that offer the EdD or the PhD with a major in nursing education, and there are master's degree programs that also have an education track. Nursing educators as well as their colleagues in practice must recognize the need to blend nursing and education knowledge in order to present up-to-date clinical knowledge and skills to students through effective curriculum planning and teaching and learning modalities.

PROPOSED UNIFIED NURSING CURRICULUM

Table 11.1 presents a proposed unified nursing education curriculum that addresses some of the issues raised regarding levels of nursing practice, from entry level to advanced practice and research roles, and the appropriate level of education necessary to meet the requirements of these roles. It compares a nonstop curriculum ending with a practice or research-focused doctorate to step-out options similar to today's various levels of nursing education in higher education from the ADN to the PhD. It reveals a rigorous academic program common to professional education, yet there is an efficiency of time and quality of courses that provides students with the opportunity to build on courses sequentially and integrate nursing knowledge and skills into the supporting arts and sciences. Based on the curricula in Table 11.1, the argument for "entry into practice" ends with the idea that a candidate is eligible for licensure at various points of the educational track, commencing with the completion of the associate degree (lower division) and a 3-month internship, or completion of the bachelor of science with a residency or a master's degree either as an advanced generalist (CNL) or specific functional or advanced practice nurse with prescribed residencies prior to licensure, and, finally, a doctorate that includes a clinical or research residency. Thus, students have a choice for entering practice through licensure at the associate, bachelor's, master's, or doctorate degree levels. At the same time, the curricula contain the same courses or content, thus allowing nurses to enter at the next step of their education to continue their career opportunities. If these generic curricula were adapted by schools of nursing, there would be no need for challenge examinations and repetition of courses containing the knowledge and skills already assimilated.

Schools of nursing bear the responsibility for evaluating the credentials of applicants with prior education or degrees not in nursing. There is a need for flexibility in granting credit for courses equivalent to those pre- and corequisites in nursing and nursing courses (for RNs with degrees not in nursing) to enter into the curriculum and to complete the next academic level. Examples are RNs with baccalaureates or master's

TABLE 11.1: Proposed Unified Nursing Curriculum

Career Ladder Program (with step-out options)					Nonstop Entry-Level Doctoral Program (DNP or PhD)	
Year 1						
Prerequisites		Nursing Courses			Prerequisites	
Courses	Credits	Courses	Credits		Courses	Credits
Verbal and Written Communications	6	Introduction to Nursing and Healthcare	3		Verbal and Written Communications	6
Anatomy and Physiology	6	Basic Health Assessment and Skills	3		Anatomy and Physiology	8
Microbiology	4	Nursing Process and Skills	4		Chemistry	4
Language or General Education	3	Care of the Older Adult	3		Psychology	3
Year 2						
Sociology/Anthropology	3	Parent Child Nursing	6		Human Development	3
Human Development	3	Psychiatric/Mental Health Nursing	4		Microbiology	4
General Education	3	Adult Acute Care Nursing	6		Statistics	3
Introduction to Healthcare Informatics	3	12-Week Paid Internship Prior to Licensure	Work Study/ no credit		Chemistry	4

Nutrition	3	U.S. Healthcare System and Health Professions	3
Introduction to Pharmacology	2	Nutrition	3
		Introduction to Healthcare Informatics	3

(continued)

TABLE 11.1: Proposed Unified Nursing Curriculum (*continued*)

Year 2		
Language or General Education		3
Genetics		3
Introduction to Nursing and Healthcare		3
Total Credits	16	32
Total Credits	17	

Step out for ADN : Total credits: 65

Year 4							
Cognates	Credits	Nursing Courses	Credits	Courses	Credits	Nursing Courses	Credits
General Education Electives	6	Community Health Nursing	6	Bioethics	3	Adult Acute Care Nursing	6
Bioethics	3	Nursing Leadership and Inter-professional Collaboration	3	General Education	3	Transcultural Nursing	4
Economics	3	Healthcare Delivery System	3			Community Health Nursing	6
		Nursing Informatics	3			Nursing Leadership and Interprofessional Collaboration	3

(continued)

TABLE 11.1: Proposed Unified Nursing Curriculum (*continued*)

Year 4

Cognates	Credits	Nursing Courses	Credits	Courses	Credits	Nursing Courses	Credits
		Capstone Practicum	3			Nursing Informatics	3

Year 4

Cognates	Credits	Nursing Courses	Credits	Courses	Credits	Nursing Courses	Credits
		12-Week Paid Residency Prior to Licensure	Work Study/ no credit			Critical Care Nursing	4
Total credits	12		18		6		26

Step out for BSN: Total credits: 65 (lower division) + 60 (upper division) = 125

Year 5							
Nursing Cognates	Credits	Nursing Courses	Credits	Nursing Cognates	Credits	Nursing Courses	Credits
Nursing Theory	3	Functional Role Theory I, for example, Advanced Practice, Clinical Nurse Leader, Clinical Specialty, Education, Management	2	Nursing Theory	3	Capstone Practicum (upper division)	3
Analysis of Healthcare Organizations	3	Functional Role Practicum I	4	Analysis of Healthcare Organizations	3	Functional Role Theory I, e.g., Advanced Practice, Clinical Nurse Leader, Clinical Specialty, Education, Management	2
Nursing Research Evidence-Based Practice	3			Nursing Research Evidence-Based Practice	3	Functional Role Practicum I	4
Advanced Nursing Informatics	3			Advanced Nursing Informatics	3		

(continued)

TABLE 11.1: Proposed Unified Nursing Curriculum (*continued*)

			Year 5				
Nursing Cognates	Credits	Nursing Courses	Credits	Nursing Cognates	Credits	Nursing Courses	Credits
Advanced Pathophysiology[a]	3			Advanced Pathophysiology[a]	3		
Total Credits	15/12		6	Total Credits	15		9

[a]*This course is not required for nonadvanced practice MSN roles.*

				Year 6			
Cognates	Credits	Nursing Courses	Credits	Nursing Cognates	Credits	Nursing Courses	Credits
Advanced Health Assessment[a]	3	Functional Role Theory II, e.g., Advanced Practice, Clinical Nurse Leader, Clinical Specialty, Education, Management, etc.	2	Advanced Health Assessment[a]	3	Functional Role Theory II, e.g., Advanced Practice, Clinical Nurse Leader, Clinical Specialty, Education, Management, etc.	2
Advanced Pharmacology[a]	3	Functional Role Practicum II	4	Advanced Pharmacology[a]	3	Functional Role Practicum II	4
Population Health	3	Master's Project or Thesis[b]	3–6	Population Health	3	Nursing History and Philosophy	3
		For entry-level master's: 12 Week Paid Residency Prior to Licensure	Work Study/ no credit	Healthcare Economics	3		
Total Credits[a]	9/3		6/9-12[b]	Total Credits	12		9

[a]These three courses are not required for nonadvanced practice roles.
[b]Required of nonadvanced practice master's degree candidates.

Step out for master's degree with 30-42 credits

(continued)

TABLE 11.1: Proposed Unified Nursing Curriculum (*continued*)

Year 7							
DNP				Research-Focused Degree (PhD or DNS)			
Cognates	Credits	Nursing Courses	Credits	Cognates	Credits	Nursing Courses	Credits
Healthcare Economics	3	Translational Science	3	Quantitative Research	3	Nursing Science, Analysis of Theories	3
		Foundations for the DNP in Practice and Leadership	3	Qualitative Research	3	Seminar: Dissertation I	3
		Advanced Communications and Interprofessional Healthcare	3	Mixed Methods	3	Advanced Communications and Interprofessional Healthcare	3
		Advanced Nursing Informatics	3			Quality Nursing Care and Outcomes Management	3

DNP Project I, II	6				12
Quality Nursing Care and Outcomes Management	3		9
Total	3	21

(continued)

TABLE 11.1: Proposed Unified Nursing Curriculum (*continued*)

Year 8 DNP and PhD/DNS							
DNP				Research-Focused PhD or DNS			
Nursing Courses	Credits	Cognates	Credits	Cognates	Credits	Nursing Courses	Credits
Role-Specific Evidence-Based Practice Residency	6	Electives (education courses for faculty roles or cognates to support research)	6	Electives (education courses for faculty roles or cognates to support research)	6	Nursing Science Theory Development	3
DNP Project III	3		6			Advanced Practice and Leadership Role Development	3
Advanced Practice and Leadership Role Development	3					Seminar Dissertation II	3

For entry-level DNP: 12 Week Paid Residency Prior to Licensure	Work Study/ no credit	For entry-level PhD: 12 Week Paid Residency Prior to Licensure	Work Study/ no credit	
Total	12	6	6	9

Postmaster's DNP: Total 36 credits

Nonstop DNP: Total 195 credits

Nonstop PhD: Total 207

(Created by S. Keating, 2018)

in other disciplines and nonnurses with baccalaureates or higher degrees who matriculate directly into master's programs rather than repeating the baccalaureate. Of course, RNs need upper division–level nursing courses or their equivalent and nonnurses need nursing courses equivalent to the baccalaureate but offered at the graduate level prior to entering master's- or doctorate-level nursing courses.

The advantages of the entry-level doctorate program are numerous. It would facilitate high school graduates' entry into a nursing program with graduation 8 years away, thus producing expert clinicians, researchers, and educators who are relatively young in age. The 8-year total curriculum plan provides the time for in-depth education and the production of quality graduates prepared for practice, teaching, and research roles. If the profession embraces this transformation of nursing education, then it must come to grips with the reality that there are roles for personnel such as the licensed practical/vocational nurses. It is logical that these programs fall into the community college genre, thus raising the specter of the "Civil War" in nursing yet again. This author leaves that debate to the nursing educators reading this text and the profession over the next few decades.

SUMMARY

This chapter summarized the current state of nursing education with its many points of entry into professional practice and the educational programs that produce the nursing workforce. While the world order, the national society, and the healthcare system change rapidly, it is difficult to predict the future. There are prevailing trends that should have an impact on the development and evaluation of nursing curricula over the next decade. If nursing chooses not to respond to these changes, the profession will continue to be splintered with less opportunity for it to help in shaping public policy toward optimal healthcare for the populace. Nursing educators have a responsibility to work with their colleagues in practice and research to develop curricula that prepare nurses for the future, who are competent and caring, excellent clinicians and practitioners, leaders and change agents, and scholars and researchers. A nursing education system for the future will have the following characteristics:

- Clearly defined levels of education and differentiated practice in the healthcare system based on education and experience
- Entry into practice for staff nurse positions following a 3-month residency in a selected arena of practice
- Quality institutions of higher education that specialize in the preparation of staff nurses for entry into evidence-based practice in a timely fashion
- Quality higher education institutions that focus on the faculty role of excellence in teaching, community service, research, and the translation and application of knowledge from nursing science and related disciplines
- Quality institutions of higher education that specialize in the preparation of nurses to provide evidence-based advanced practice nursing and interprofessional services for individuals, families, communities, and aggregates
- Students, graduates, and faculty who are active participants and generators of new knowledge in nursing and related disciplines' research
- Quality institutions of higher education that specialize in the preparation of nurse leaders who will influence healthcare policy and change the healthcare system for the benefit of the populations they serve
- Academic and health science centers that specialize in nursing research and the advancement of nursing science through translational science and evidence-based practice; testing of theories; the development of new theories, concepts, and models; and educational innovations on the national and international levels

END-OF-CHAPTER RESOURCES

DISCUSSION QUESTIONS

1. Given the recent pandemic and rapid changes that occurred in both healthcare and education, what changes do you foresee for nursing education within the next 3 to 5 years?

2. It is often said that "what's old is new again." Do you see any strategies for changing nursing education based on what worked in the past and how can they apply to needed changes in nursing education today? What are the lessons from the past that prohibited nursing from moving its educational agenda forward? How can today's nursing educators use these lessons to bring about change?

LEARNING ACTIVITIES

Student-Learning Activities

1. Synthesize the information in this text into a "Dream School of Nursing." Develop a curriculum that prepares nurses for practice 10 years from now. Remember to keep in mind that practice and the setting in which it is delivered will be different. Martha Rogers long ago envisioned "nursing in space," so let your imagination run wild!

Faculty Development Activities

1. Hold a faculty meeting focused on brainstorming and let creative thoughts flow freely. List the characteristics of the ideal nurse prepared to practice 5 to 10 years hence. Examine the new AACN Essentials and decide how a curriculum can be developed that provides the kind of education necessary to prepare the future nurse. Focus on creativity and newer theories of learning. Compare these ideas to your existing curriculum. How can it be transformed into the one you envision and still meet accreditation and professional standards and criteria?

A robust set of instructor resources designed to supplement this text is located at **http://connect.springerpub.com/content/book/978-0-8261-8686-7.** Qualifying instructors may request access by emailing **textbook@springerpub.com.**

REFERENCES

Accreditation Commission for Education in Nursing. (2021). *Accredited programs*. http://www.acenursing.com/accreditedprograms/programsearch.htm

American Association of Colleges of Nursing. (2019). *Accelerated baccalaureate and master's degrees in nursing*. https://www.aacnnursing.org/Portals/42/News/Factsheets/Accelerate-Programs-Fact-Sheet.pdf

American Association of Colleges of Nursing. (2020). *AACN seeks proposals to assess the current state of graduates from DNP programs*. https://www.aacnnursing.org/News-Information/News/View/ArticleId/24706/RFP-DNP

American Association of Colleges of Nursing. (2021a). *DNP fact sheet: Current DNP program statistics*. https://www.aacnnursing.org/News-Information/Fact-Sheets/DNP-Fact-Sheet

American Association of Colleges of Nursing. (2021b). *CNL frequently asked questions*. https://www.aacnnursing.org/CNL/About/FAQs

Bowles, W. S., Sharpnack, P., Drennan, C., Sexton, M., Bowler, C, Mitchell, K., & Mahowald, J. (2020). Beyond articulation agreements: Expanding the pipeline for baccalaureate nursing in Ohio. *Nursing Education, 41*(5), 274–279. https://doi.org/10.1097/01.NEP.0000000000000713

Carter, E. J., Mastro, K., Vose, C., Rivera, R., & Larson, E. L. (2017). Clarifying the conundrum: Evidence-based practice, quality improvement, or research? The clinical scholarship continuum. *JONA, 47*(5), 266–270. https://doi.org/10.1097/NNA.0000000000000477

Institute of Medicine. (2011). *The future of nursing: Leading change, advancing health*. National Academies Press.

Jackson, M., & Marchi, N. (2020). Graduate-entry education for nonnurses: Preparation, pathways, and progress. *Nursing Education Perspectives, 41*(1), 30–32. https://doi.org/10.1097/01.NEP.0000000000000510

Jeffreys, M. (2020). ADN-to-BSN articulation, academic progression, and transition: A proactive, holistic approach. *Nurse Educator, 45*(3), 155–159. https://doi.org/10.1097/NNE.0000000000000708

McCauley, L. A., Broome, M. E., Frazier, L., Hayes, R., Kurth, A., Musil, D. M., Norman, L. D., Rideout, K. H., & Villarruel, A. M. (2020). Doctor of nursing practice (DNP) degree in the United States: Reflecting, readjusting, and getting back on track. *Nursing Outlook, 68*(4), 494–503. https://doi.org/10.1016/j.outlook.2020.03.008

National Organization of Nurse Practitioner Faculty. (2018). *The doctor of nursing practice degree: Entry to nurse practitioner practice by 2025*. https://cdn.ymaws.com/www.nonpf.org/resource/resmgr/dnp/v3_05.2018_NONPF_DNP_Stateme.pdf

Petges, N., & Sabio, C. (2020). Examining the barriers to BSN prelicensure education among ADN students: A quantitative follow-up. *Teaching and Learning in Nursing, 15*(4), 262–267. https://doi.org/10.1016/j.teln.2020.06.011

Smaldone, A., & Larson, E. L. (2021). What PhD competencies should guide the preparation of nurse scientist? *Journal of Professional Nursing, 37*(1), 201–203. https://doi.org/10.1016/j.profnurs.2020.06.010

Staffileno, B. A., Pencak Murphy, M., & Carlson, E. (2017). Determinants for effective collaboration among DNP- and PhD-prepared faculty. *Nursing Outlook, 65*, 94–102. https://doi.org/10.1016/j.outlook.2016.08.003

Vance, D. E., Heaton, K., Antia, L., Frank, J., Monyham, L., Harper, D., & Meneses, K. (2020). Alignment of a PhD program in nursing with the AACN report on the research-based doctorate in nursing: A descriptive analysis. *Journal of Professional Nursing, 36*(6), 604–610. https://doi.org/10.1016/j.profnurs.2020.08.011

CHAPTER 12

Staff Development: The Specialty of Nursing Professional Development

Rochelle Walsh

CHAPTER OBJECTIVES

At the end of this chapter the reader will:

- Identify the qualifications and responsibilities of those who work in the nursing professional development communities.
- Identify learning theories used for curriculum development outside of academia.
- Describe the components of a needs assessment in curriculum development.
- Discuss the impact of internal and external forces when developing curriculum.

OVERVIEW

Much like the education colleagues of academe, the educator serving in the role of staff development or nursing professional development (NPD) is responsible for curriculum development in healthcare settings. This chapter applies previous information on the development and evaluation of a curriculum. It examines the role of educators in staff/NPD. This chapter provides the readers with the modern history of staff development, qualification of roles and responsibilities of those within NPD, and learning theories used for curriculum design and evaluation.

NURSING PROFESSIONAL DEVELOPMENT

Beginnings

As nurses, we are lifelong learners. To stay current with changes in evidence-based practice, nurses must participate in continuing education and staff development activities. Those who provide this extended learning are often referred to as clinical educators, nurse educators, staff development specialists, or nursing professional development specialists (NPDS). The latter is the terminology used within this chapter.

The modern history of staff development can be traced to the founding of the Council on Continuing Education by the American Nurses Association (ANA) in 1971 (Brunt & Morris, 2020). In 1974, Helen Tobin, a pioneer of staff development, published *The Process of Staff Development: Components for Change.* This, along with continuing contributions to the profession, launched staff development into a well-respected discipline of professional nursing (Puetz, 2009).

Qualifications and Responsibilities of Those Within Staff Development

The NPD community comprises practitioners who have an extensive range of educational backgrounds. Specialty certification often differentiates between one who is a generalist and one who is a specialist. A generalist is defined as a practitioner that does not have a certification, whether they hold a baccalaureate degree or a graduate degree. A practitioner who holds a graduate degree and an NPD certification classifies as a specialist (Harper & Maloney, 2017; Maloney & Woolford, 2019). Outside the NPD role, the focus of their profession delineates between the generalist and the specialist. A generalist, by definition, has a variety of roles, duties, and abilities. In contrast, a specialist is a nurse educator with a specific concentration in one or more areas in which there is a perceived competency (Merriam-Webster, n.d.). Other specialties, such as clinical nurse specialists and clinical nurse leaders, serve in the NPD roles. Determining this variability depends on the organization, the needs of the organization, and the organization's definition of nursing practice.

A staff development specialist, often referred to as a nurse educator, clinical nurse educator, or NPDS, is one who teaches outside of the academic system. A clinical nurse educator within a professional development department whether it be in the traditional hospital, home care, ambulatory care, long-term care, or subacute care setting, wears many hats in their role. Their role includes conventional and continuing education (ANA, 2017) but may also involve nontraditional methods and types of teaching. Simulation, grand rounds, journal clubs, online learning management systems, and the creation of educational games are a few examples teaching and learning strategies. In the completion of the previously listed duties, the educator utilizes criteria as outlined by the ANA in the Scope and Practice for Nursing Professional Development, the Association for Nursing Professional Development, *NPD Scope and Standards of Practice* (2016), and the human resource guidelines of accreditation agencies that certify hospitals (i.e., The Joint Commission). These organizations provide guidance for the educator's involvement in policy creation and revisions, regulatory and accreditation requirements, and ongoing compliance/competence monitoring of current and new staff.

Learning Theories in Nursing Professional Development

The learning theories that relate specifically to NPD are primarily those that concern adult learning and adult education. Philosophical perspectives from behaviorism, constructivism, and adult learning theory guide the delivery of instruction.

Behaviorism learning theory is associated with the process of changing behavior through positive reinforcement. This behavioral change correlates to the development of responses to stimuli (Braungart & Braungart, 2011), which serve as a motivator for the learner. Both positive and negative reinforcements affect learning depending on the delivery. Industry, business, and the military often use this type of education. A demonstration of this theory in NPD is with new graduate nurses (NGNs) in a skills lab learning how to set up an arterial pressure line. The procedure utilizes hands-on approach with the educator's instructional guidance, support, and encouragement to the point that the student can implement the skill and at which time the student no longer needs to have close instruction but has an available resource (Aliakbari et al., 2015).

Constructivism is a cognitive learning theory based that on the idea that the learner builds on an understanding of previous knowledge. The process of forming this learning can be through personal reflection or facilitated through the educator, instructor, or coach. Significant in nursing is the potential for adding new information to the foundation (Candela, 2020). It relies on the participant to depend on intrinsic motivation versus rewards generated from the instructor in the form of praise, grades, and reinforcement. The nursing staff (NGN or RN), takes an active role in their learning. Outside of academe, the NPD educator is no longer the "sage on the stage" who stands before a gathering and expounds the information. They are instead responsible for giving resources that guide the nursing staff in the process of incorporating the new information with older beliefs and experiences. The NPD educator may provide various reading materials and questions to monitor the nursing staff's understanding of the issue. An example of evaluating their understanding would be the use of a "what if" situation, in which they explain the answer in their own words (GSI Teaching and Resource Center, 2020), such as What if your patients' blood pressure (B/P) started to drop? What if you found your patient crying after receiving a terminal diagnosis? As stated, this process of question allows the NPD educator to assess the nurse's knowledge, understanding, and plan for intervention.

A significant theory that describes adult learning is Knowles's (1973) Theory of Andragogy, which discusses the desire to be involved with learning (self-directed) and relevance to the learner's needs (immediate application). Knowles recognized that there are distinct differences in adult learning from those of a child. The premise is that successful adult learning occurs when there is an engaged learner, attracted to the material, has established a need for the information, and has some control of the process (Warren, 2016). Motivation for the adult learner comes from the need to know. For a nurse in the workforce, it helps to gear it toward the new, safe, and evidence-based information that they need to care for their patients (Candela, 2020). Instead of "teaching," the NPD educator acts as a facilitator to assist staff nurses in content acquisition.

There is no "right" theoretical approach, just as there is no "right" learning style for all situations or students. Nurse educators will likely need to merge the method and style to meet the learning requirements at that given time. The NPDS must know about learning theories and learning styles to meet the needs of their population and provide regard for the individual's learning styles and needs.

Needs Assessment

The development of curriculum in the staff development arena is much the same as in the academic setting. It starts with a needs assessment. A needs assessment is the "process by which a discrepancy between what is desired and what exists is identified" (American Nurses Credentialing Center [ANCC], 2015, p. 46). In the NPD role, the material found in a needs assessment comes from various participants (the nurses, administration, accrediting bodies, and other disciplines). In addition to regulatory bodies, including The Joint Commission and Occupational Safety and Health Administration (OSHA), the NPDS looks for commonalities in issues that have led to the filing of an occurrence report for an adverse event. Physicians and staff, along with customer comments and complaints, may also affect the choice of topics. Another source of material in a needs assessment is the determinants of certifications, Magnet®, Nursing Excellence, American Heart Association's Get with the Guidelines-Stroke, and Heart Failure, to name a few.

The NPDS goes through what is very similar to the nursing process (Table 12.1). The first step is the assessment, or, in this case, the needs assessment. This will identify any gaps in practice, knowledge, and desired performance. Depending on the situation, a needs assessment may be informal as an individual providing an opinion or focused as a SWOT analysis. The latter focuses on the **S**trengths, **W**eaknesses, **O**pportunities, and **T**hreats within an organization, empowering health professionals to contribute to the

TABLE 12.1: A Comparative View

Nursing Process	Staff Development
Assessment	Needs Assessment
Diagnosis	Analyze data to determine needs and validate if environmental, process, or learning
Planning	Plan intervention
Intervention	Create learning plan (multidimensional)
Evaluation	Evaluate results of plan

analysis. It is a simple instrument used when assessing needs for change or professional development programs. Bos et al. (2016) state that the completion of a needs assessment identifies current knowledge deficits, unknown learning needs, validates previous learning needs, prioritizes the learning needs, and identifies performance standards that meet the organization's standards, mission, vision, and goals. In addition, a needs assessment provides validation of previous educational programs and learning. Often, the requirements of the individual, organizational, and community at large provide division of learning needs. The needs of the individual may be associated with a specific learning deficit. Whereas determining the organizational needs usually is associated with accreditation standards outside the agency. The community level includes the need for information that affects health, as exemplified by the COVID-19 global pandemic. Both nurses within the organization and the surrounding community needed information regarding disease preparedness, safety measures, disease processes, and ultimately vaccines.

It is essential to use several methods to identify the data needed to understand the issue at hand. With that in mind, the NPDS needs to focus on all the issues when conducting the needs assessment. A mixed-methods needs assessment allows for the collection multidimensional data pertaining to a specific problem or issue (Campos Zamora, 2020). Collecting qualitative and quantitative data provides strong evidence for appropriate actions associated with the issue, whatever the cause of the practice gap (Diagnosis). It is crucial to collect as much data as possible based on the time allotted and available resources. Some organizations may use the "rapid improvement" or "Kaizen event" (Martin & Osterling, 2007), which is a small group working intensely over 3 to 7 days on an identified issue and developing a solution for improvement (Planning and Intervention). Without a varied source of data, it is possible that all interests are not assessed and that may lead to gaps that could be overlooked.

Agencies should be aware that not all data help design a response to a problem. Data bombardment is a situation described by Bleich (2016). In data bombardment, healthcare agencies are the recipients of data that they subscribe to for benchmarking purposes. Collected information comes from social media, emails, telephone calls, and websites. Furthermore, filtering through this extensive amount of data creates reviewer saturation and becomes a barrier to the creation of a working needs assessment.

Data collection methods from questionnaires, interviews with leaders and stakeholders, focus groups, direct observation, and quantitative sources such as internal reports, chart audits, and benchmark records provide rich sources of information. The easiest method and most used are questionnaires. A simple questionnaire provides a way to reach multiple people and retrieve large amounts of information, providing one has a high enough return rate for analysis. Experience dictates that the less complicated the questionnaire, the more likely the participation.

Used interchangeably are the terms needs assessment and learning needs assessment. The two, although very similar, are not the same. Not everything is about education/or learning. Sometimes the issue is performance. Once the needs assessment is completed, the NPDS determines if the problem is associated with learning or nonlearning needs, such as performance issues. It is imperative for an ongoing needs assessment to flush out any potential deficits before the development of an adverse event based on a performance issue.

External Frame Factors

External factors, forces outside of the parent institution, play a large role in determining curriculum development for nursing staff/professionals within a healthcare agency. For example, the health needs of the population served; competitive agencies; development of new programs; regulatory, governmental, and accreditation bodies; organizations engaged in the oversight of care; and the nursing profession are key external factors for consideration.

The changing healthcare of the population as a determinant of educational needs is evident in today's society. As COVID-19 has raged through our country, NPDS has created and implemented programs to help healthcare providers learn about the disease process. They have created education for personnel to understand treatment options and protecting themselves from this deadly disease. While COVID-19 is today's health crisis, the NPDS examines continuous data to identify future health issues. The focus surrounds major causes of morbidity and mortality within the community, state, and country that influence services provided by the healthcare institution.

External factors in healthcare include organizations involved in the oversight of care such as Medicare, Medicaid, and private insurance; regulatory practices; and accreditation bodies (e.g., The Joint Commission), that affect educational needs. While the NPDS cannot be an expert on all, having stakeholders within the organization who are familiar with these requirements aid and guide the NPD experts to understand where gaps may arise.

The nursing profession itself presents as an external force. NGNs educated from different colleges and universities, updates in skills and evidence-based practice related to new published literature, and nursing's accrediting/regulatory bodies present challenges for the NPDS regarding curriculum development and evaluation. Additionally, the NPDS considers issues challenging the learners themselves, such as nurses' increasing age, burnout, stress, and violence (within and outside of the workplace). Knowledge of these factors allows for the efficacy of the NPDS in providing support and promotion of self-care along with education and resources to combat the stressors of the workplace.

Internal Factors

The internal factors that influence curriculum development in a healthcare organization are those that affect the content, workflow, and delivery of education. Resource availability has an effect on the delivery of information. These internal factors include the organizational and administrative structures, physical structure and resources, governance, staff (professional and nonprofessional) population served, internal approval (advisory board), and financial stability (DeBoor, 2022). Curricular creation and revision are dependent on resource availability, such as equipment such as simulation mannequins for skill training, human resources with the expertise to teach, and the financial prowess to ensure both. Educational programs for both patients and staff development depend on the costs and benefits of the programs.

The nursing staff also influences professional development curriculum and education. The best question for the NPDS to ask is , "Do they have the knowledge, skills, attitudes, and judgment (ANA, 2017) to provide safe, competent care?" For instance, NGNs come from schools of nursing with generalist education and training. Their formal education may not have prepared them to care for patients in complex environments like the ICU or specialty care such as oncology. The NPDS takes over where formal education has ended to close the knowledge deficit by offering protected time during orientation for additional didactic and hands-on skill experiences. This fosters confidence in new nurses toward managing common clinical scenarios in these complex specialty areas. In addition, many NPD departments are responsible for yearly competency programs for currently employed nurses, nursing apprenticeships, residencies, and transition-to-practice programs that socialize the new nurse into their role.

Readiness to Learn

Many researchers over the years have explored readiness to learn. Lictenthal (as cited by Kitchie et al., 2011), explains this as an individual's capacity to take in new information. Physical, emotional, experiential, and knowledge aspects of the learner can affect how much learning occurs. Bartosiewicz et al. (2019), examined two aspects of readiness" a willingness to apply learning to the workplace and readiness to use the information in life experiences. Is this something the individual needs to know today to perform their job? Both explanations are reasonable but rely on the point at which a learner is ready to learn. The learner must be a willing participant and join in the process for it to be effective. Without that willing participation, the information, no matter how important deemed, does not yield application of said knowledge to the situation, the workplace, or the life experience.

Institutional Economics and Resources for Nursing Professional Development

While there are many factors that determine the financial stability of a healthcare organization, the economics of healthcare are partially dependent on the productivity of their employees. A memory from one of the first classes in nursing school is learning that people go to the hospital for nursing care. In many healthcare institutions across the United States, nurses represent the highest percentage of the workforce within the institution. Thus, the recruitment and retention of a nurse lend to the financial security of the organization. Conversely, a high turnover rate in nursing contributes to a financial strain on the organization. Nurses possess what is termed in some economic theoretic perspectives as part of the institution's human capital. (Rondeau et al., 2009). Human capital refers to the knowledge, skills, abilities, and judgment that an individual possesses that supports the daily activities within an agency setting and contributes to the overall productivity and financial stability. NPDS contributes to the organization's productivity, financial stability, and nursing human capital through programs that enhance quality patient care outcomes and lead to increase recruitment and retention rates.

Economic and budgetary limitations influence the NPDS's role. A large NPD department provides a variety of internal and external (community) programs, which generate additional income (e.g., basic life support [BLS], advanced cardiac life support [ACLS], pediatric advanced life support [PALS], advanced trauma life support). Unfortunately, often these revenue-generating streams only cover the cost of hosting these programs, and the bulk of funding comes through general operational funds. This being the case, NPD departments must constantly validate their role in increasing the agency's human capital. The implementation of a continuous assessment and improvement plan to identify educational needs and prevention of an adverse event is one way to provide value-added evidence and validation of the NPDS role.

A request for education typically addresses a practice gap and an internal or external source initiates that said request. An identified problem determined to be an educational issue results in recruiting the NPDS to join or lead the team in assessing the issue. The NPDS and team must always consider financial resources and risk when tasked with a new educational concern. One way to do this is to perform a quick performance analysis before the needs assessment is completed (Rossett, 2009). This allows for an examination of a system or application to be in relation to performance and provides a starting point by asking questions" What is the current process? What is not working in the current process? What are the perceived barriers or challenges identified? Is it a training or a performance issue? Do we need to change the process? Is there going to be a need for new policies? What precisely is it going to take to reach the goal? After the performance analysis and appropriate needs assessment, a plan is determined. The scope of the problem and benefit realized from the new plan determines the overall costs. Does the issue affect the organization at the micro-level (orientation to a new piece of equipment in the ICU) or macro-level (reduction of readmission rates for congestive heart failure patients)? One important measure to evaluate is the return on investment (ROI). This compares the financial gains against the investment costs on the issue. Opperman et al. (2016a) explain that the NPDS will accomplish this measure by applying an evaluation model that "builds a compelling chain of evidence for the value relation between the learning activity and the organization's bottom line" (p. 123). The stakeholders will use the ROI calculations to determine if the educational program's impact has met the criteria for achieving the performance metrics (Opperman et al., 2016b).

COMPONENTS OF NURSING PROFESSIONAL CURRICULUM DEVELOPMENT

Mission, Philosophy, and Goals of the Nursing Professional Development Department

An NPD department is an extension of the agency that employs NPDSs. As an extension of an agency, the department will create its own mission, vision, philosophy, and goals statement that describes the department's role within the parent institution. These independent statements often mirror or parallel those of the parent organization. The content of those noted statement differences in mission and vision usually relate to the scope of services provided and the overall program goals of the population served. For example, the institution's mission is "to deliver compassionate quality care to patients, which optimizes the healthcare outcomes of the community" whereas the NPD mission is to "provide educational opportunities for the health system's nurses that contribute to quality patient care." Both are providing optimization of healthcare outcomes, but the focus varies based on the populations served. The core values expressed in the mission and vision should be descriptive of the agency's activities. These would include the clinicians' values and theories on which they base their education pursuits that produce evidence of leadership, practice excellence, and a sense of inquiry (Association of Nursing Professional Development [ANPD], 2016a, 2016b).

NPD goals are in league with the parent organization. Determining a goal provides the basis for formulating specific outcomes, again, much like the nursing process. In practice, the levels of function of an NPD department and the NPDS may range from minimal responsibilities of teaching American Heart Association, Basic and Advanced Life Support courses to those that oversee and are responsible for the development of orientation, preceptorship of NGNs, continuing education programs, preparation for accreditation, and competency management. These functions, in turn, support the overall goals of education through the NPD department.

Organizing Framework

The organizing framework for an NPD program mirrors that of the overall organizational framework. The ANA's *Scope and Standards* and revised 2016 NPD Standards of Professional Performance provide structure and standards of practice that mimic the nursing process. This list includes identifying and assessing practice gaps, identifying learning needs, outcome identification, planning, implementation, and evaluation. Two modifications from the previous standards included, first, the assessment process related to practice gaps and, second, expanding the role of implementation to include the leadership of collaborative interprofessional resources to provide education. Both are easily doable within the role of an NPDS.

Program Objectives

For any educational opportunity, the NPDS identifies objectives or learning outcomes as part of the planning phase. Objectives for NPD are much like those written in academic settings and use action verbs; they are specific, measurable, achievable, relevant, and time-oriented. For example, "By the end of the Basic EKG class, the new graduate nurse will be able to apply the five steps in rhythm identification to normal and abnormal heart rhythms." Learning objectives serve as an evaluation tool and measure of the educational activity or program success (Bowers & Honyak, 2017).

Implementation Plan

The implementation of a plan for an educational activity or program depends on the objectives, the scope of the task, and the specific learning domain (cognitive, affective, psychomotor). The NPDS uses different teaching and communication methods for different learner needs and the required task. For example, in the case of policy changes, are the policy changes unit-specific or systemwide? Is it a minor change or a total revision? Does the policy change affect any stakeholders outside of the organization? The answer to those questions dictates the plan and implementation. If a new policy involves a system change in practice and skills, a formal class provides an opportunity to deliver a consistent message and evaluate individuals' understanding and or competency of a new skill. For a simple policy change, a flyer, a staff email, or an announcement during "change of shift huddle" is appropriate. The plan and implementation depend on the type of request and the associated impact on internal and external stakeholders. Regardless of the teaching and learning activities are simple or complex, an evaluation follows all educational activities.

Evaluation of Staff Education Programs

Program evaluation falls within the scope, standards, and responsibility of the NPD. This standard requires the NPD to use reliable and valid instruments in the evaluation process. Not all instruments function equally for evaluating all activities. Based on the needs assessment, the identified practice gap dictates the instrument for evaluation. The NPDS may consider a pretest to identify a knowledge gap, followed by a posttest to assess the efficacy of the intervention. Whereas a return demonstration is better suited in evaluating employees for a skill deficit (Schumacher et al., 2018). It is essential that the evaluation tool identified is evidence-based, focused on the stated outcomes of the program, and reviewed by content experts and stakeholders. Finally, the use of formative and summative assessments provides valuable information in identifying knowledge deficits.

A formative assessment often used to guide "instruction" and provide feedback to the learner happens during the learning session and allows the NPDS the opportunity to identify deficits in the moment. It also gives learners the opportunity to self-assess during the activity. A formative evaluation offers facilitation, active encouragement, discussion, and clarification throughout the learning process. For example, the NPDS completes rounds on a unit in which two NGNs are being oriented and conducts a quick 5-minute "interview" assessment. They might say, "Tell me about your patient," or "What is the plan of care for your patient today?" How the new graduate answers the question gives insight into their understanding of the disease process and interventions ordered for the patient. It allows for open dialogue and the opportunity to suggest further learning.

A summative evaluation is the most common method of evaluating an individuals' learning, whether knowledge or skill acquisition. This finding informs if the participant achieved the outcome outlined by presenters. For instance, giving an EKG exam after a 16-hour Basic EKG class. Can the participants identify common and lethal arrhythmias after participating in the class? Summative assessments usually have an associated grade or required level of achievement. The NPDS institutes a remediation plan if the learner falls below the set objective. Both formative and summative evaluations have a purpose in nursing professional/staff development. They can guide changes to the program or future classes and provide information that allows the NPDS to synthesize the education program's impact on the participants.

CURRICULUM DEVELOPMENT APPLIED TO NURSING PROFESSIONAL DEVELOPMENT

Orientation, Employee Training Programs, and New Graduate Programs

One of the main functions of a professional NPDS is to manage an orientation program or orient the new and newly hired nurses to the area they are to practice. The agency's goal is that each nurse following orientation will be able to provide safe, patient-centered, high-quality care (Monforto et al., 2020). Depending on the agency's setup, this may include front-loading with OSHA requirements, including fire and safety mandates, providing access to policies, computer access and training, and skills training prior to the start of the unit orientation process.

Orientation to individual units depends on the specialty of the unit, the skills required to do the job, the experience level of the nurse (new graduate or license RN with previous employment history), and the time allotted. The NPDS individualizes much of orientation toward the learner's needs, but the length of orientation is unit-specific. Usually 6 weeks of orientation for a general medical–surgical area, 6 to 8 weeks for a specialty area (orthopedics, oncology), and 12 or more weeks for a critical care area (cardiac, trauma, postanesthesia, or OR). In the needs assessment, the NPDS evaluates the individual's education level, previous experiences, and current competencies.

A graduate nurse is likely to enter into a nursing residency program, often developed, implemented, and managed by the NPDS. These programs support the new nurse for the first 6 to 12 months of employment. Residency programs have been so successful in creating a positive impact in the onboarding of new nurses that the American Academy of Nursing issued a directive that all employers should provide a transition to practice or nurse residency program for all newly graduated nurses (Goode et al., 2018). The ANA asserts that each nurse needs to demonstrate the necessary knowledge, skills, attitudes, and judgment to determine competency. They further outline the basis of that competency on the measure of fundamental performance, and it can be measured (ANA, 2017). Nurse residency programs are a great example in which an NPDS can clearly evaluate the competencies of the NGN and create a plan of remediation as needed. An NPDS lead residency program makes a difference for the agency in terms of preparing nurses to have increased decision-making skills, expanding the use of evidence-based knowledge in everyday practice, and overall retention. The latter providing further evidence of the benefit of an NPD department and NPDSs within the organization. Like all educational activities or programs, implementing a transition to practice or nurse residency begins with a needs assessment. One must consider yearly hiring practices of how often and how many. Is a residency program a cost-efficient venture for the organization?

Budget Planning for Nursing Professional Development

NPD departments and the educational programs created, require a portion of the institution's overall financial resources. It is the NPD's role to show that the benefit to the agency outweighs the costs. Therefore, budget planning is essential. Yearly, the NPD department, like all other departments of the institution provides its planned budget. The department administrator will meet with all NPDSs of the institution and determine the anticipated program needs for the next year. There are many components to factor into the yearly budget. What are ongoing program needs (residency, BLS, ACLS, etc.) for the upcoming year? Are there any accreditation programs up for review requiring additional education? The pandemic taught us to plan for contingency funds. Contingency planned finances use a calculation based on a percentage of the entire project. In the business world, those calculations range from 15% to 40% of the entire project budget. This would be highly unlikely for an NPD department or any department within a healthcare organization. This type of department may be lucky to factor any percentage of the total operating budget, but considering this information is important for the upcoming year's budgetary needs.

The question arises, Does a review of each teaching and learning activity need a financial assessment? The answer is no. It is reasonable to complete an economic assessment on 5% to 10% of the programs (DeSilets, 2010). A focus would be on those larger programs that match your agency's mission and philosophy, including issues with safety issues, hospital-associated errors, and high-risk activities.

Maintaining Quality Programs and Future Planning

Need for Program Development

An NPDS's essential role is to maintain the competency and performance of the healthcare professionals who work within the agency, organization, or health system. They work with nurses and interprofessional colleagues that include physicians, social work, respiratory therapists, pharmacists, and unlicensed personnel to maintain a high level of performance. As a group, their charge is to advocate for patient safety and quality of care for patients. Through the assessment process, they determine gaps in practice. Using their knowledge of education through the curriculum process, they lead the healthcare team through process change and better outcomes influencing the community at large.

Approval Process

While similarities exist in much of curriculum development and evaluation between academe and NPD, there are differences within the approval processes. A consistent formal approval process exists on the academic side (Chapter 2), but the same is not necessarily true for NPD.

The approval process for an NPD is dependent on what the the institution needs. For example, the orthopedic unit receives a new piece of equipment for the rehabilitation of a total knee patient. The educator assigned to that unit or for the institution would meet with the orthopedic unit leadership team and vendor to discuss educational needs for the staff and create a plan for that individual unit. For this example, no formal procedure for approving the educational plan is required. In some cases, the vendor completes the education with the NPDS providing organization and oversight of the staff.

The following is an illustration of the approval process for a larger educational project. One common problem for hospitals is throughput, patients staying in the ED because of a lack of inpatient beds. This project examines the cost of a program to educate medical–surgical nurses on cardiac rhythms to facilitate the rollout of remote cardiac monitoring to alleviate the crush of noncardiac admissions to the telemetry units. Currently, nurses on the medical and surgical units are not familiar with cardiac rhythms, and there are misgivings from the nursing staff on their ability to care for the patients who could be having arrhythmias.

The Problem: Although the hospital has 116 telemetry beds, admission to the telemetry units of patients without documented heart disease hamper throughput for those beds. Nurses on the medical and surgical units are unfamiliar with cardiac monitoring and care of patients with arrhythmias.

Stakeholders: Leadership, NPDSs, nursing and ancillary staff, physicians and NPs from the ED, telemetry, medical, and surgical units. If there is a shared governance system within the organization, consider the leadership team of nursing's shared governance committee as well.

Stakeholders' Meeting: Discussion of the problem, potential solutions, and appointment of a small group to create a cost analysis and business plan. The use of an improvement process (rapid workflow analysis, rapid improvement process, Plan–Do–Check–Act cycle, Lewin's Change Theory) guides the educational plan. Include an evaluation of barriers or challenges with accreditation or regulatory agencies in designing and implementing this educational plan.

Cost Analysis: The most basic of economic evaluations for educational programs helps identify the cost per participant (the program's total cost divided by the number of participants; Opperman et al., 2016a). A cost–benefit ratio uses the value of the program's impact divided by the total cost of the program. Opperman identifies that a cost analysis helps determine how to keep costs down but does not figure in the benefit achieved by the implementation of the training program. It is important to include current literature and practices similar to the educational program planned as justification for costs. For example, decreased ED throughput results in an increase in medicine errors (Kustad et al., 2010). It is estimated that 400,000 medication errors cost up to $3.5 billion (Patient Safety, 2016), the average cost of each error then costing up to $8,750. Therefore, improved throughput leads to a decrease in ED medication errors show the benefit in the cost of the program. Other outcomes for consideration include patient satisfaction, job stress, productivity, and patient volumes.

Development of a Business Plan: Statement of purpose, benefits, challenges and risks of project/program, number of participants, cost per participant (including overtime costs), operating procedures, new portable telemetry packs, cardiac monitors and installation costs, incidentals (office supplies, copying, ancillary staff, include all costs no matter how large or small). This is a 2-hour course and because each nurse works at a 0.9 FTE (full-time equivalent; 36 hours per week); overtime is avoided for this activity as employees attend on an off-shift session. Additional cost factors include replacement costs, if the nurse(s) attend the class during their shift and education for new hires, new nurses, and yearly competency updates.

Approval Process: Return to stakeholders for business plan and cost analysis presentations. There may be additional meetings required based on the overall costs of the project/program that include members of senior leadership (Chief Nursing Officer [CNO], Chief Operating Officer [COO], CFO) for final approval before implementation.

Implementation of Educational Program: When instituted, the plan includes a mandated class developed by the two NPDSs, for all RNs on included remote monitoring units. Content includes common heart rhythms, processes for initiation and discontinuation of monitor, and plans to initiate for emergencies.

Evaluation of Learners and Educational Program: The NPDS utilizes summative assessments for learners that include a posttest with a required level of achievement. The NPDS institutes a remediation plan if the learner falls below the set objective. The program evaluation consists of student evaluations and data collected from set benchmarks (e.g., throughput, decreased medication errors, employee satisfaction) to ensure program quality.

SUMMARY

This chapter provided readers with the modern history of NPD, qualification of roles and responsibilities of those within NPD, and learning theories used for curriculum design, and evaluation. Similar to their academic colleagues, the educator serving in the role of staff development or NPDS is responsible for curriculum development and evaluation in healthcare settings. This chapter described the impact of internal and external forces when developing curriculum and the components of a needs assessment in curriculum development.

END-OF-CHAPTER RESOURCES

DISCUSSION QUESTIONS

- How do healthcare issues such as the pandemic impact staff development?

- Describe the barriers accreditation or regulatory agencies impose on curricular development or redesign within the institution.

- Discuss the financial impact of the NPDS at the micro- and macro-levels of an institution.

- Discuss the role of the NPDS in the development and maintenance of a new graduate residency program. Include your thoughts regarding the length of the program, the number of new graduates accepted, and the evaluation of participants.

LEARNING ACTIVITIES

Student-Learning Activities

1. Imagine yourself in the role of a new NPDS. List the topics that you believe you need to know in order to be most effective in this role. Prioritize the list and explain the rationale for the order of priority.

2. Choose a current issue or new evidence-based practice in healthcare and develop a housewide or individual unit educational plan for the nursing staff.

A robust set of instructor resources designed to supplement this text is located at **http://connect.springerpub.com/content/book/978-0-8261-8686-7.** Qualifying instructors may request access by emailing **textbook@springerpub.com.**

REFERENCES

American Nurses Association. (2017). *ANA recognition of nursing specialty, approval of a specialty nursing scope of practice statement acknowledgment of specialty nursing standards of practice, and affirmation of focused practice competencies.* https://www.nursingworld.org/~4989de/globalassets/practiceandpolicy/scope-of-practice/3sc-booklet-final-2017-08-17.pdf

American Nurses Credentialing Center. (2015). *2015 ANCC primary accreditation provider application manual.*

Association of Nursing Professional Development. (2016a). *ANPD vision, mission, and core values.* https://www.anpd.org/page/about

Association of Nursing Professional Development. (2016b). *The nursing professional development: Scope and standards of practice* (3rd ed.).

Aliakbari, F., Parvin, N., Heidari, M., & Haghani, F. (2015). Learning theories application in nursing education. *Journal of Education and Health Promotion, 4,* 2. https://doi.org/10.4103/2277-9531.151867

Bartosiewicz, A., Łuszczki, E., Różański, A., & Nagórska, M. (2019). Analysis of determinants of readiness for professional development among polish nurses. *International Journal of Environmental Research and Public Health, 16*(10), 1800. https://doi.org/10.3390/ijerph16101800

Bleich, M. R. (2016). Helping leaders learn. *The Journal of Continuing Education in Nursing, 47*(12), 531–533. https://doi.org/10.3928/00220124-20161115-03

Bos, B. S., Wangern, T. M., Elbing, J., Carl, E., Rowekamp, D. J., Kruggesl, H. A-L., Conlon, P. M., Scroggins, L. M., Schad, S. P., Neumann, J. A., Barth, M. M., Grubbs, P. L., & Sievers, B. A. (2016). Pressure ulcer prevention: Where practice and education meet. *Journal for Nurses in Professional Development, 32*(2), 94–98. https://doi.org/10.1097/NND.00000000000000228

Bowers, R., & Honyak, K. (2017). Establishing measurable outcomes for educational activities and departments. In P. Dickerson (Ed.), *Core curriculum for nursing professional development* (4th ed., pp. 184–196). Association for Nursing Professional Development.

Braungart, M. M., & Braungart, R. G. (2011). Applying learning theories to healthcare. In S. B. Bastable, P. Gramet, K. Jacobs, & D. Sopczyk (Eds.), *Health professional as educator: Principles of teaching and learning* (2nd ed., pp. 51–89). Jones and Bartlett Learning.

Brunt, B. A., & Morris, M. M. (2020, September 25). Nursing professional development. In StatPearls [Internet]. StatPearls Publishing. https://www.ncbi.nlm.nih.gov/books/NBK531482/

Campos Zamora, M. (2020). *Interprofessional continuing professional development in rural hospitals: A mixed methods educational needs assessment.* Master's thesis, Harvard Medical School.

Candela, L. (2020). Theoretical foundations of teaching and learning. In D. Billings & J. Halstead (Eds.), *Teaching in nursing: A guide for faculty* (5th ed., pp. 247–270). Elsevier.

DeBoor, S. S. (2022). Curriculum development in nursing. In M. Oermann, J. De Gagne, & B. Phillips (Eds.), *Teaching in nursing and role of the educator: The complete guide to best practice in teaching, evaluation, and curriculum development,* (3rd ed., pp. 321–344). Springer Publishing Company.

DeSilets, L. (2010). Calculating the financial return on educational programs. *The Journal of Continuing Education in Nursing, 41*(4), 149–150. https://doi.org/10.3928/00220124-20100326-08

Goode, C., Glassman, K. S., Ponte, P. R., Krugman, M., & Peterman, T. (2018). Requiring a nurse residency for newly licensed registered nurses. *Nursing Outlook, 66,* 329–332. https://doi.org/10.1016/j.outlook.2018.04.004

GSI Teaching and Resource Center. (2020). *Constructivism.* https://gsi.berkeley.edu/

Harper, M. G., & Maloney, P. (2016). *Nursing professional development: Scope and standards of practice* (3rd ed.). Association for Nursing Professional Development.

Harper, M., & Maloney, P. (2017). The updated nursing professional development scope and standards of practice. *The Journal of Continuing Education in Nursing*, *48*(1), 5–7. https://doi.org/10.3928/00220124-2070110-02

Kitchie, S. (2011). Determinants of learning. In S. Bastable, P. Gramet, K. Jacobs, & D. Sopczyk (Eds.), *Health professional as educator: Principles of teaching and learning* (pp. 103–150). Jones and Bartlett Learning.

Knowles, M. S. (1973). *The adult learner: A neglected species*. Gulf Publishing .

Kustad, E. B., Sikka, R., Sweis, R. T., Kelley, K. M., & Rzechula, K. H. (2010). ED overcrowding is associated with an increased frequency of medication errors. *The American Journal of Emergency Medicine*, *28*(3), 304–309. https://doi.org/10.1016/j.ajem.2008.12.014

Maloney, P., & Woolforder, L. (2019). Ninety years and counting: The past, present and future of nursing professional development specialty. *Journal for Nurses in Professional Development*, *35*(2), 56–65. https://doi.org/10.1097/NND.0000000000000532

Martin, K., & Osterling, M. (2007). *The Kaizen event planner: Achieving rapid improvement in office, service, and technical environments*. Productivity Press.

Monforto, K., Perkel, M., Rust, D., Wildes, R., King, K., & Lebet, R. (2020). Outcome-focused critical care orientation program: From unit based to centralized. *Critical Care Nurse*, *40*(4), 54–64. https://doi.org/10.4037/ccn2020585

Merriam-Webster. (n.d.). Generalist. In *Merriam-Webster dictionary*. Retrieved from https://www.merriam-webster.com/dictionary

Opperman, C., Liebig, D., Bowling, J., Johnson, C. S., & Harper, M. (2016a). Measuring return on investment for professional development activities: A review of the evidence. *Journal for Nurses in Professional Development*, *32*(3), 122–129. https://doi.org/1.1097/NND.0000000000000262

Opperman, C., Liebig, D., Bowling, J., Johnson, C. S., & Harper, M. (2016b). Measuring return on investment for professional development activities: Implications for practice. *Journal for Nurses in Professional Development*, *32*(4), 176–184. https://doi.org/1.1097/NND.0000000000000274

Patient Safety. (2016). *Final report national quality forum (3-15-2017)*. http://www.qualityforum.org/Publications/2017/03/Patient_Safety_Final_Report.aspx

Puetz, B. E. (2009). Editorial. *Journal for Nurses in Staff Development*, *25*(3), 105–106. https://www.nursingcenter.com/pdfjournal?AID=865251&an=00124645-200905000-00001&Journal_ID=54029&Issue_ID=865250

Rondeau, K. V., Williams, E. S., & Wagar, T. H. (2009). Developing human capital: What is the impact on nurse turnover? *Journal of Nursing Management*, *17*(6), 739–748. https://doi:10.1111/j.1365-2834.2009.00988

Rossett, A. (2009). *First things fast: A handbook for performance analysis* (2nd ed.). Pfeiffer.

Schumacher, C., Shinners, J., & Graebe, J. (2018). Evaluating the effectiveness of educational activities: Part one. *The Journal of Continuing Education in Nursing*, *49*(6), 245–247. https://doi.org/10.3928/00220124-20180517-02

Tobin, H. (1974). *The process of staff development: Components for change*. Mosby.

Warren, H. (2016). Middle-range theories: Frameworks for examining a nonsurgical cosmetic problem. *Plastic Surgical Nursing*, *36*(1), 9–11. https://doi.org/10.1097/PSN.0000000000000124

CHAPTER 13

Distance Education, Online Learning, Informatics, and Technology

Stephanie Stimac DeBoor

CHAPTER OBJECTIVES

Upon completion of Chapter 13, the reader will be able to:

- Review the various types of distance education programs utilized in the delivery of nursing education programs.
- Analyze the application of technology and informatics and their effectiveness in the implementation of the nursing curriculum.
- Review the literature related to the efficacy of distance education programs.
- Examine the issues facing nursing educators that relate to the application of informatics and technology in nursing education.

OVERVIEW

This chapter discusses the effects of informatics and technology on curriculum development and evaluation. Provided is a review of distance education formats, including land-based satellite campuses of home institutions, blended (hybrid), web-based with immersion, and online platforms. In addition, other technological approaches, such as smart classrooms, patient simulations, electronic medical record systems, and information systems applied to education and healthcare, are analyzed. Finally, a brief review of the research findings on the efficacy of these programs, student satisfaction, and issues related to distance education and technology is given.

DISTANCE EDUCATION PROGRAMS

Distance education is defined as any learning experience that takes place at a distance away from the parent educational institution's home campus. In the true fashion of distance education, it can be as close as a few blocks away in an urban center to as far away as another nation. Curriculum is typically implemented through a planned strategy for the delivery of courses or classes that can include off-site satellite classes managed by the home faculty or credentialed off-site faculty, broadcast of classes through videoconferencing and teleconferencing to off-campus sites, web conferencing, web-based instruction, and faculty-supervised clinical experiences including preceptorships and internships. During the pandemic with "shelter in place" orders, many of us became quick studies of how to accomplish distance or online education. Most recently utilized for the purpose of distance education were Big Blue Button (2021), Zoom (2021), Microsoft® Teams (2021), and GoToMeeting (2021), to mention a few. Distance education offers continuing education programs, degree programs, single academic courses, or a mixture of on-campus and off-campus course offerings. In the early 1700s, we find tracings of distance education through correspondence study (Bower & Hardy, 2004). The instructor would mail the students their lessons, and once completed, the students would, in turn, return the assignments via mail. While a good way to include those who did not otherwise have access to a home campus, lost mail and time delays proved to be limitations of the postal system. Technology continued to advance with satellite communication in the 1960s, advancing to fiberoptic systems of the 1980s. Today, the internet and a few keystrokes from any computer allow students to connect to faculty from all over the world. While online education became a trend in universities across the United States to increase enrollment in RN-to-BSN and graduate nursing programs, it became the norm in March 2020 as a way to continue to provide education to all programs and levels of nursing during the COVID-19 pandemic.

The following discussion reviews planning considerations for distance education. Also discussed are types of distance education, including satellite campus programs; web, video-, and teleconferencing; and online, web-based programs.

Needs Assessment and Compatibility With the Components of the Curriculum

When planning for any type of educational program delivered off the main campus, nursing educators must have supporting data from an assessment of the external and internal frame factors that document the need for a program. It should include the projected success of the program based on a business case, cost analysis, assured applicant pool, and a business plan. Once the needs assessment is completed and a time frame is in place, planners review all of the components of the curriculum to ensure congruence with the originating educational program. For details on conducting a needs assessment, budgeting, and the components of the curriculum, see Section II, Chapters 3 and 4. In addition, developing an evaluation plan ensures the quality of the program and compliance with accreditation standards.

External Frame Factors

Whether considering distance education for individual students from multiple locations or a group of students within one geographical location, utilizing the components of assessment from the internal and external frame factors, a needs assessment reveals the feasibility for developing a distance education program. If the program plans an off-campus but on-land satellite, the external frame factors include an assessment of the community where the program is to take place with such factors as community location and receptivity to distance education. Also included are the population's characteristics and its sophistication in technology, the delivery of education far from the home campus, and the ability to create an academic setting away from the home campus. The most up-to-date technology and information technology (IT) system support teams are necessities if delivering the program in a completely online format. Additional external frame factors include an assessment of support and area competition from vendors of distance education programs and other nursing education programs that serve the region. The healthcare system and health needs of the populace have an influence on the program as to how graduates of the program can serve them. Assessments of collaborative relationships that will supply the program with available practicum locations in the off-site healthcare agencies are critical to the success of the program within that community area.

A demonstrated need for a distance education program includes support from members of the nursing profession; national, regional, and state regulating bodies; and accreditation agencies' approvals. One must consider the most recent updated regulations and requirements of the U.S. Department of Education (USDE, 2020) and the National Council for State Authorization Reciprocity Agreements (NC-SARA, 2021), especially for those who will sit for licensure and national certifications. Usually, the sponsoring program must notify all accrediting and approval agencies of its plans to offer the distance education program, with each of these agencies requiring specific descriptions of the program, including the potential student body, faculty, curriculum plan, academic and capital infrastructure support systems, timelines, plans for evaluation, and, most important, financial feasibility with a business plan.

Internal Frame Factors

Much like the external frame factors, a review of the internal frame factors provides additional information in the planning for a distance education program. Of prime concern is the support of the parent academic institution and its experience with distance education programs. If it has a history of managing these types of programs, it is more likely to be supportive of the nursing program. A check of the mission and purpose, philosophy, and goals of the parent institution and the nursing program is in order to ensure the distance education program's congruence with those of the parent. The internal economic situation and its influence on distance education programs are critical to the financial feasibility of the program. Once again, the most up-to-date technology and IT system support teams are necessities for the delivery of a completely online program. An assessment of faculty familiarity and comfort with the use of current technology, along with support from instructional designers and programmers, will be required to support an effective distance education program.

Cost Issues

If the recommendations from the need's assessment demonstrate that the distance education program is viable, the school of nursing administration prepares a project proposal, or business plan to present to the parent institution. The purpose of a project proposal is to persuade key administrators and stakeholders that establishing a distance education program meets the mission of the institution, has a substantial potential student body, and adapts the existing accredited program to an online or satellite format without compromising its quality. The project proposal describes the program in detail and demonstrates that it is economically feasible. If prior distance education programs demonstrated success in bringing revenues to the program or are, at the least, self-sufficient, it is more likely to receive support for new programs. After the presentation to and approval by the administration, the developers create a detailed business plan from the proposal.

The first and foremost cost issue to address in the business plan is the economic feasibility of the distance education program based on an analysis of expected start-up costs, administrative costs, required number of faculty and staff, capital expenses (on-site facilities, technology support systems), and academic support (recruitment, admission, records, library access, student support systems). Many times, the needs assessment becomes a write-off at the expense of the nursing program with financing secured contingency funds or program development funds generated from grant overhead costs. The plan should include possible initial grant support for start-up funds and plans for eventual self-sufficiency.

Student enrollment is often limited due to the physical constraints of the classroom. Distance learning reduces or eliminates this issue as students can access their course from anywhere that has an internet connection. Increasing the number of students provides added tuition dollars, but one must consider if those additional funds in tuition offset the costs for other needed resources required for distance learning. The capital required from the parent institution is listed and includes clinical-experience facilities; technological support systems for videoconferencing, teleconferencing, and/or web-based instruction; administrative, faculty, and staff expenses; and academic support systems, such as library, academic, and student services. Included in the assessment is a list of potential administrators, staff, faculty, and the proposed program's student body characteristics.

The administration's role and costs include supervisory or management functions to implement the program such as budget and personnel management, liaison activities with regional stakeholders, public relations, coordination, marketing plans, and preparation of reports to seek approval and accreditation of the distance education program from relevant agencies. Some of the staff and/or faculty cost considerations are the required full- and part-time equivalents, benefits, travel, and other expenses, supplies, and equipment.

Curriculum and Evaluation Plans

In addition to the economic feasibility for the program, an analysis of the curriculum is in order to ensure that the proposed distant program is congruent with the mission, goals, organizational framework, and student-learning outcomes of the parent program. Although the format and delivery of the curriculum may differ from the original, it must meet the same goals and objectives of the program. Administrators and faculty must make decisions regarding the format and have a rationale for why they chose those formats. Developing an online program requires consideration of faculty pedagogy. This transformation may be difficult for some faculty members who always taught as the "sage on the stage."

Consideration of how the new program fits into the master plan of evaluation of the parent program ensures its quality. Additionally, an evaluation plan provides monitoring the program as it is implemented for corrections along the way (formative evaluation) and to have summative evaluation plans in place that measure the success of the program in terms of student-learning outcomes and success, satisfaction of the stakeholders, and its continued congruence with the components of the parent program's curriculum. See Table 13.1 for guidelines for the development of distance education programs.

TYPES OF DISTANCE EDUCATION PROGRAMS

The following is a description of the major types of distance education programs and those that fall under the formats of synchronous (live, real time, simultaneous) or asynchronous (occurring at various times) delivery. Online courses are those in "which at least 80% of the course content is delivered online. Face-to-face instruction includes courses in which 0% to 29% of the content provides online delivery; this category includes both traditional and web-facilitated courses. Blended, (sometimes called hybrid) instruction has 30% to 80% of the course content delivered online" (Allen & Seaman, 2016, p. 7). Universities utilize learning management systems (LMSs) to deliver web-based, online educational courses. Listed are some of the pros and cons for each type of distance education options.

TABLE 13.1: Guidelines for the Development of a Distance Education Program

Guideline Topic	Questions for Data Collection and Analysis	Desired Outcome
Needs Assessment: External Frame Factors	To what extent are the distant sites supportive of the program and sophisticated in the use of technology? To what extent has the healthcare system demonstrated support for the program and the nursing profession? To what extent is the healthcare system open to student clinical experiences and what resources do they have available for the experiences? To what extent is the program competitive with other educational programs?	The distant site or sites are receptive to distance education programs, sophisticated or open to the technology of distance education, and has a healthcare system supportive of the program, the nursing profession, and student clinical experiences, if indicated. The program is competitive with other programs.
External Frame Factors	Did program approval and accreditation bodies receive notification of the program? Do they approve, or is there an indication that they will approve the program in the future?	Notification of relevant program approval and accrediting agencies and receipt approve the program or there are indications for approval in the future.
Needs Assessment: Internal Frame Factors	To what extent does the distance education program's mission, philosophy, organizing framework, goals, and objectives reflect those of the parent institution? To what extent does the parent institution have experience in the selected modality or modalities of distance education and/or have the resources to support it? Are there plans in place that indicate adequate resources for the program including infrastructure, human resources, and academic program support?	The mission, purpose, philosophy, organizing framework, goals, and objectives of the distance education program are congruent with the parent institution. The parent institution has experience with and/or the resources to support the program. Plans are in place and resources are adequate for academic infrastructure, human resources, and academic program support.
Economic Feasibility	To what extent will the parent institution support a needs assessment for the distance education program? If there are no funds from the institution, are there other possible resources? Are there start-up funds available from the institution, or are there other sources such as funds from partner healthcare or educational institutions?	There is support from the parent institution or other sources for a needs assessment. There are start-up funds from the parent institution or other sources.

(continued)

TABLE 13.1: Guidelines for the Development of a Distance Education Program (*continued*)

Guideline Topic	Questions for Data Collection and Analysis	Desired Outcome
	Does the business case justify the need for the program including its congruence with the mission of the institution, a demonstrated need for the program in the community, an adequate potential student body, and assurance of the maintenance of its quality?	The business case is persuasive and includes justification for the development of the program, i.e., meets mission, meets a need, has an adequate potential student body, and maintains quality.
	Has the business plan accounted for personnel costs (staff, technicians, faculty); administrative costs; facilities (if indicated); academic support systems, e.g., library, enrollment services, financial aid; and the required technology system(s)?	The business plan includes funds for the required personnel, administrative costs, facilities (if indicated), academic support systems, and the required technology system.
	To what extent are there plans for self-sufficiency? Are there projections for the size of the student body and other resources necessary to maintain the program?	There are financial plans in place for self-sufficiency and maintenance of the program.
Congruence With the Components of the Curriculum	To what extent does the curriculum plan for the distance education program reflect that of the parent institution, e.g., course descriptions, credits, objectives, and content?	The distance education program's curriculum plan is congruent with that of the parent institution.
Delivery Model Options	To what extent were modalities reviewed that included, off-site, on-land satellite campuses, videoconferencing and/or teleconferencing, and online or web-based methods reviewed?	Review of all modalities for the delivery method, leading to a rationale for the selected model or combination of several.
Delivery Model Options: Selection and Its Rationale	To what extent does the selected model fit the learning needs of the students?	The selected model fits the learning needs of the students.
	To what extent are there faculty members who can utilize the model(s)? If not, are there faculty development plans and technical support in place?	The selected model is within the scope of the faculty's expertise or there are faculty development plans in place.
	To what extent is the selected model "user-friendly" for students and faculty?	The selected model is "user-friendly" for students and faculty.
Delivery Model: Implementation Plan	To what extent is the selected model(s) congruent with the curriculum plan?	The selected model is congruent with the curriculum plan.
	Does the selected model fit the implementation plan of the curriculum, i.e., is it possible to deliver theory, lab, and clinical experiences?	Implementation of the curriculum plan occurs through the utilization of the selected model(s).

(*continued*)

TABLE 13.1: Guidelines for the Development of a Distance Education Program (*continued*)

Guideline Topic	Questions for Data Collection and Analysis	Desired Outcome
Delivery Model: Evaluation	Is there an evaluation plan in place, and to what extent is it congruent with the master plan of the parent institution? Does the evaluation plan include both formative and summative evaluation measures? To what extent does the evaluation plan include strategies and personnel for follow-up and revisions based on the data analyses and recommendations from the evaluation plan? Is the selected delivery model(s) relevant to current education practices? To what extent is the selected model adaptable to future changes in the profession and education and healthcare systems?	There is an evaluation plan in place and it is congruent with the master plan of evaluation for the parent institution. The evaluation plan includes both formative and summative measures. The evaluation plan has mechanisms in place to revise the program according to data analyses and recommendations from evaluation activities. The selected delivery model is relevant to current education practices and adaptable to future changes in the education, profession, and healthcare systems.

Source: DeBoor, S. (2018). Distance education, online learning, informatics, and technology. In S. Keating & S. DeBoor (Eds.), *Curriculum development and evaluation in nursing education* (4th ed., pp. 185–202). Springer Publishing Company.

Satellite Campuses

For the purposes of this discussion, *satellite campuses* are defined as those programs that offer the curriculum in whole or in part on off-campus sites from the parent institution. While they can incorporate technology methods such as videoconferencing and web-based instruction, the majority of the teaching and learning takes place in classrooms and involves in-person (synchronous) interactions between the faculty and students. For nursing, clinical experiences may occur in healthcare facilities in the community in which the satellite campus is located. Faculty members who teach in the parent institution serve as on-site faculty or act as consultants to off-site faculty who teach the same curriculum. For home campus faculty who teach on the satellite campus; travel costs and the related travel time are included in the costs for implementing the program and weighed against the cost of the salary and benefits for hiring on-site faculty. With the emergence of virtual learning environments (VLE) such as Zoom, and other similar LMSs, there is less use of satellite campuses for nursing education.

Online/Web-Based Programs

Online and web-based instruction had its beginnings through faculty and student use of communication tools such as electronic mailing lists, email, and access to resources and references on the internet. In the 1990s and early 21st century, the use of web-based instruction through LMSs became more prevalent. LMSs software serve for the development of online/web-based instruction, which the institution has a contract, or some institutions develop their own. The Babson Survey Research Group (2018) reported on the state of online learning in institutions of higher education, identifying that the growth of online enrollments is outpacing overall enrollments. This report identified 6.3 million students enrolled in distance education during the fall of 2016. In 2020, COVID-19 reshaped the teaching and learning of higher education and resulted in the highest transition to online learning in history. As control over the pandemic emerges, universities debate whether to return to campus for face-to-face instruction, remain online, or continue in a blended format.

Web-Based With Immersion

This form of distance education has students complete the majority of studies entirely online through asynchronous discussion boards and written assignments. Students are required to come to the home campus for one or more days, once or twice per semester for immersion. Some programs bring students for a week-long immersion one time per year. During on-campus meetings, students participate in skill labs, clinical assessments with standardized patients (SPs), and lectures from clinical experts to enhance their learning. Immersion days allow students to interact and collaborate with faculty and other peers of the cohort. Faculty has an opportunity to assess students' knowledge, skills, and expertise within their specialty of study and provide remediation as needed. Students enjoy speaking with faculty and getting immediate feedback as opposed to the delayed response of online communication. The downside to this format is that students must incur the expense of traveling to the home campus in addition to the standard university tuition and fees they pay each semester.

Blended or Hybrid Distance Education

Hybrid courses utilize blended synchronous and asynchronous formats for educational delivery. Students have both online and required times to meet face to face either on campus or within an online "virtual" classroom. The "virtual" classroom is a web-conferencing platform through which faculty and students can meet live. Big Blue Button (2021), Blackboard Collaborate (2021), and Zoom (2021) are examples of this technology. This type of distance education allows for more flexibility for those who do not have easy access to a home campus. Students can log in at any time to lessons from anywhere as long as they have access to a computer and the internet. Echoed for this format are those similarly expressed pros and cons of the web-based with immersion format, in particular travel expenses for campus meetings.

Development of Online Programs

Web-based teaching and learning require a VLE or an LMS, computer access to the web by faculty and students, IT support by way of instructional support staff, and training sessions for faculty and students who are not familiar with the system. Some institutions of higher learning use experienced IT staff and faculty who mount and manage courses for teachers whose only responsibility is for the actual teaching of the course. This method provides technical support for teaching faculty; however, it may remove some of the academic freedom from the teacher of record. For example, the teacher does not have the ability to change course assignments or formats without going through the support staff to make the changes. It can also prove to be expensive since the institution is paying for several staff members when only one may be required.

Quality Matters (QM, 2021) provides best practices for developing online courses. It is an overview of and part of providing quality in distance education and online programs. This includes standards and rubrics for online courses, support from online experts, and focus on course design and evaluation.

One must consider that there are differences in traditional classroom and online education; thus, faculty need to adopt a pedagogical shift in teaching strategies. As mentioned earlier, it is essential to have a supportive IT infrastructure within the institution to assist faculty with successful adaptation to technological innovation in nursing education. It often takes time to convert a traditional course or a new course to a web-based course and, as with all courses, requires updating and revisions each subsequent time taught. Many of us learned to accomplish this task in a few short days as COVID-19 closed campuses and halted traditional face-to-face education. Multiple learning activities are available through the internet such as synchronous real-time chat rooms and live classrooms where students and faculty meet at a prearranged time and discuss topics or review questions about course assignments. Asynchronous entries (occurring at various times and labeled as "threaded discussions") about selected topics provide the students and faculty with opportunities to discuss topics and present their ideas and views. The assignments related to these usually require reading assignments and/or a review of the literature so that the discussions are scholarly submissions on the subject at hand. Faculty can post a lecture through an essay or PowerPoint presentation that includes voice-over recording, notes, illustrations, references to uniform resource locators (URLs), videotapes, movies, and other audiovisual media and pose thought questions for discussions related to the "lecture." Group work assignments are possible using chat rooms, live classrooms, threaded discussions, and email communications. Although of all online assignments, group work seems to be the least liked and produces more stress when all members do not participate and contribute to the final product.

Many LMSs have programs that allow faculty to develop surveys and examinations that are secure and provide statistical analyses of the results. A few examples of web-based educational and live-time platforms are Blackboard Collaborate (2021). Canvas (2021), Moodle (2020), and Pearson Education Inc. (2021). There are online exam proctoring services available to protect the integrity of the program. Examity (2021), Honorlock (2021), Proctorio (2020), and ProctorU (2021) are some examples of these proctoring services. Make sure to consider the costs of these programs when developing the needs assessment and eventual program budgetary plan.

Learning Theories for Online Formats

Distance education programs employ *andragogy* (adult learning) strategies for the delivery of courses and classes through off-campus satellite sites, videoconferencing, online, telecommunications, and web-based technology. The majority of teaching and learning strategies offered in these formats are learner-centered and facilitate active student participation in the process rather than the traditional pedagogical methods for presenting information to the student. See Chapter 6 for learning theories that apply to online educational formats and for ideas for research on the use of learning theories for online instruction.

Cheng (2021) identifies that constructivism theories of learning lend themselves to the *Own It, Learning It, Share It* (OLSit) framework, which promotes student engagement and autonomy. This framework easily transferred to an online learning environment where students must be more self-directed than compared to traditional face-to-face education. The framework applies well to electronic learning since it focuses on the ability of the learner to develop autonomy, strategies for goal setting, scaffolding, and monitoring achievements. The OLSit framework also benefits faculty to assist students owning the educational process for their learning, autonomy, and to be outcome-focused.

Research Findings on the Efficacy of Online Formats

As online teaching and learning continue to become the norm of delivery, it is important to examine the effectiveness of this educational modality. One need only type in "the effectiveness of online learning in higher education" to view thousands of results, many during the 2020–2021 timeframe and relating to the COVID-19 transition. Articles worldwide describe the successes of online learning through multiple formats (asynchronous, virtual synchronous, hyflex, blend-flex, and podcasting). Most of the literature depicts positive outcomes for students and overall a positive transition to online teaching, but there are identified struggles that occurred during the abrupt change in teaching format.

Over the last 10 years, the literature has shown that in order for online education to be effective, there needs to be an organized plan for implementation. Crotwell Pullis and Hekel (2021) provided an example of how they adapted assignments in a community health course for nursing students to an online format. It was important to these authors that they preserved the integrity of the activity while converting it to an online format. They identified that online teaching and learning is a flexible and effective format, as long as faculty present clear instructions and expectations for the course. Multigenerational students, but mostly Millennials or Generation Z, who are adept with the use of technology, identified that even with the stressors faced during the pandemic, they enjoyed the course. Faculty identified the highest course evaluation scores ever received. Overall, a face-to-face course can be converted to an online format, and through the use of technology, students remain engaged.

Advantages and Disadvantages of Web-Based Education

In 2019, the USDE provided a guide for faculty regarding how to use technology to support student learning in colleges and university settings. They made five recommendations that focus on interventions and pedagogical strategies for incorporating technology regardless of online, blended, or face-to-face delivery.

Advantages of web-based education include flexible times for students and faculty, multiple learning and teaching strategies, active participation on the part of all students, personal/individual communications between students and faculty, moderate maintenance times for managing and updating the course once it is mounted, and relative assurance of curriculum integrity. For the home institution, the advantage of web-based education includes the ability to enroll more students without creating a need for on-campus space.

There are reported disadvantages of online learning. One is the need for technological support: the large amount of faculty time consumed in mounting the course and the need for faculty and student development in the use of technology. Additionally, there are the initial and ongoing costs related to contracts for LMSs and computers. Finally, the lack of face-to-face encounters between faculty and students, the possible loss of core nursing tenets and communications, and a minimal sense of belonging to the home campus raise concerns.

Regmi and Jones (2020) conducted a systematic review to examine the "enablers and barriers" of online learning for those in the health sciences. Results indicated that there were equal or better results in the social construction of knowledge acquisition and the transfer of that knowledge into practice for those who participated in online learning. Of the barriers identified were a lack of student motivation and self-discipline to participate, being resource-intensive, IT skills and support and that it may not fit or be adaptable to all disciplines (nursing was not included as one of the disciplines).

Jowsey et al. (2020) conducted a literature review of the effectiveness of online learning within a blended format. They identified four key themes in relation to student's experiences: active learning, technological barriers, support, and communication. Active learning in this format is dependent on the student's participation. Students enjoyed the social aspect when face-to-face but did not feel as connected with their peers when completing their work online. Conversely, some students enjoyed the flexibility of the program format and the ability to learn when they wanted. In relation to technology, not all students or faculty were comfortable with all the technology platforms. Students expected the faculty to be experts with this technology and have the ability to quickly problem-solve when things went wrong. As with any type of online learning, the ability of the faculty and students to engage is dependent on a stable internet connection. It was determined that in a blended format, students felt supported when able to interact with peers and faculty and receive timely feedback. This support resulted in positive communications. Communication was deemed more effective by students when done face-to-face and least effective when limited to online. These authors highlight the positive aspects of a blended format as well as the identified challenges through a review of the literature. It is important for faculty who are developing or revising a course and entertaining the idea of presenting the content through a blended format to consider the findings of this review.

Langegård et al. (2021) examined the lived experiences of transitioned nursing students from face-to-face learning to distance learning during the pandemic. Many students reported that there was a reduction in their ability to socialize with other classmates. This rapid transition did not allow faculty to prepare for the use of web-based platforms and tools, leading to less positive faculty and student experiences. While some students enjoyed the opportunity to learn online, they noted that it increased their accountability for learning and adaption to the associated change in content format.

CLINICAL COURSES AND DISTANCE EDUCATION

Faculty develop clinical courses, including skills laboratory content, according to the implementation plan of the curriculum. Assignments of students to clinical laboratories for the acquisition of assessment and clinical skills, as well as to healthcare agencies for supervised clinical experiences, provide hands-on learning. The latter are under the supervision of faculty who either directly supervise a group of students in the clinical setting or coordinate student preceptorships for those assigned to qualified staff nurse preceptors.

With careful planning, it is possible to provide clinical experiences for students enrolled in online courses through videoconferencing or teleconferencing and web-based instruction, keeping in mind that course objectives must remain the same to ensure the integrity of the curriculum. Delivered through the selected distance education technology, faculty responsible for clinical courses can design the course so that the didactic and discussion components of the course align. Assignments, logs, or journals describing the clinical experiences, examinations, and pre- and postconferences can also take place via technology and can be *asynchronous* (occurring at various times) or *synchronous* (simultaneous). The actual clinical experiences occur through faculty-coordinated preceptorships, through local faculty hired by the institution for clinical supervision of students, or by faculty traveling to the clinical site to supervise a group of students.

Whether a local or distance site of the nursing program, if faculty members serve as coordinators for clinical experiences with preceptors and students, they must secure affiliation agreements between the educational program and the healthcare agency and preceptor. The following are additional considerations for choosing preceptors. Has the program created standards for the qualifications of the preceptors? How will preceptors be oriented? Does the preceptor's national certification and current role match the specific population foci of the students they are precepting? Finally, the faculty role includes providing guidance throughout the experience for the preceptors and students; developing a communications network for all participants; supervising preceptors and students; assigning grades with input from the preceptors; and evaluating and revising the program based on feedback.

If the pandemic taught us nothing else, we learned that it is possible to provide relevant clinical experiences for students through distance education modalities. For example, the National Council of State Boards of Nursing (NCSBN®; 2021a) provides guidelines for regulatory bodies of nursing to use for assessment of readiness in prelicensure nursing programs. During the pandemic, many nursing programs were forced to use simulation, virtual patients (e.g., IHuman, vSim, Shadow Health), and telehealth to deliver clinical experiences for undergraduate and graduate students. State boards of nursing increased the allotted simulation time for prelicensure students to compensate for the loss of clinical sites. As states lifted shelter-in-place orders, small groups or clinical groups (6–10 students) participated in on-campus simulations. Simulated clinical experiences in a laboratory setting can take place with the use of task trainers, high- and low-fidelity mannequins accompanied by case scenarios to prepare for hands-on clinical experiences in "real-life" practicum settings. While we do not know the complete impact on students graduating from a nursing program during the pandemic, there has been a decrease in the percentage of NCLEX® pass rates. The NCSBN in early 2021, posted results for all quarters of 2020 and there is a notable decline in NCLEX pass rates between the first and last quarters of 2020 (NCSBN, 2021b). There is a need for more research in this area and how educators plan, develop, and evaluate future curricula to support learning during any future global health crisis.

THE GROWTH OF INFORMATICS AND TECHNOLOGY

Technology in the Classroom

While the pandemic took us off campus and into the complete world of online teaching and learning, as of this writing, the plan for the fall of 2021 is the return of on-campus students. With that return, classroom technology will also return with the possibility of a very different look from prior to the pandemic.

The utilization of technology in the classroom and through distance education guides the implementation of the curriculum by determining the format for delivery of its courses. Technology applied to the classroom and distance education programs has grown exponentially over the past few decades. It moved from teacher-centered lectures accompanied by movies and slide shows in the classroom to the use of online PowerPoint presentations with voice-over features (e.g., Camtasia, Kaltura, and Zoom), YouTube videos, MP3, and flash drives containing course materials for faculty and students' personal computers. Online technology is available through eLearning software that provides the educator with the ability to broadcast lectures or brief discussions complemented by movies, slides, website access, and so on. The development of these multimedia teaching/learning aids promotes active student participation in the learning process and facilitates the change from teacher-focused strategies to student-centered learning processes.

Most faculty are adept at utilizing technology within the smart classroom. Smart classrooms are technology-enhanced classrooms that provide opportunities for teaching and learning through the integration of technology, such as computers, specialized software, audience response technology, networking, and audio/visual capabilities. As previously mentioned, video-capture software, such as Camtasia, SnagIt, and Adobe Presenter, allows faculty members to record their lecture videos and broadcast them on the web or save them to a video file. Students can be present for the live classroom lecture, view on a website in real time outside of the classroom, or watch at a later time. The recorded feature allows students to review the information for clarity or study purposes at their convenience.

Engaging students inside or outside of the classroom is important in the promotion of the learning process. Current technology has provided ways to promote student engagement. For example, Kahoot and Poll Everywhere are exemplars of open-source, cloud-based, or commercial audience response system (ARS) applications quickly replacing classroom response systems such as handheld "clickers." These ARSs allow students to respond to questions using a range of personal computing devices such as smartphones, tablets, and laptops. This provides students with immediate distributions of their and peers' answers. This technology provides a venue for students who would normally remain silent to now join in and be part of the group. In addition, an ARS encourages engagement, participation, and provides instant feedback, which Millennial and Generation Z learners' desire.

Another example of promoting student engagement through active learning is the use of a digital teaching application such as Nearpod. This interactive application allows the faculty to create gaming, simulations, polls, and drawings; providing students real-time results of their learning. Garrison et al. (2021) found that using this type of technology is as effective as traditional teaching in increasing students' knowledge attainment.

Electronic library resources provide faculty, researchers, and students with internet access to journals, electronic versions of textbooks, and reference databases. The most frequently used databases in nursing are Cumulative Index to Nursing and Allied Health Literature (CINAHL), Cochrane Database of Systematic Reviews, Health Sciences, Medline, Nursing and Allied Health, Ovid Nursing Journals Full Text, and PubMed. Social sciences and the sciences databases such as Behavioral Sciences and ScienceDirect are frequently used, as well as Educational Resources Information Center (ERIC) for references on education.

The "cloud" internet databases store files and other data in remote computer servers in order to synchronize and download them onto other electronic devices. They provide a virtual place for faculty, researchers, and students to store and exchange files and databases and submit and grade written assignments such as papers, journals, and logs. These services can be free or, if there is a large amount of data to store, a fee may be charged. Examples of some of these virtual files internet services are Apple's iCloud, DropBox, Google Drive, and Microsoft One Drive.

APPLICATION OF TECHNOLOGY TO EDUCATION

Simulated Clinical Experiences

The NCSBN (2021b) identified that up to 50% of high-quality simulation may be substituted for prelicensure nursing clinical hours. The application of technology to the implementation of the curriculum occurs both on-campus and through distance education delivery systems. An example is the use of realistic interactive patient simulations in the laboratory setting for students to practice skills in a safe environment prior to providing nursing care in the clinical setting. Patient simulators come with ready-made case scenarios or faculty members can develop their own scenarios that can be programmed into the simulators. Many schools of nursing located on multidisciplinary health sciences campuses pool resources with other disciplines that result in shared state-of-the-art facilities to practice skills and foster interprofessional educational opportunities.

Newer models of mannequins available for all levels of nursing skills labs consist of low-fidelity or high-fidelity models. Examples of low-fidelity models are partial models such as an arm for practicing insertion of an arterial line or a pelvis for physical examination. Whole-body mannequins can be low fidelity for practicing such skills as bathing, turning, and positioning. High-fidelity mannequins are programmed to exhibit symptoms of bleeding, irregular pulses and respirations, emotions such as cries of pain and tears, and so forth. They are programmed according to preset scenarios and can be controlled by faculty from a control room adjacent to the simulated patient room. There is not one pedagogy specific to simulation, but when developing scenarios, one must consider whether the purpose of the simulation is for high- or low-stakes testing and learning. A key component of all simulations is debriefing. Verkuyl et al. (2020) discuss the importance of group and self-debriefings as a way to enhance the effectiveness of student learning. A self-debriefing takes place prior to the group meeting so that the student has an opportunity to process their individual involvement during the simulation experience. The goal of combining these two debriefings is thought to enhance individual learning and reflection. It is important for faculty to be present as a resource and facilitator for both processes.

Virtual patient simulations (VPS), virtual reality (VR), and augmented reality (AR) are evolving technologies used to support students who have limited access to clinical experiences. Students don VR goggles and physically take part in a virtual world where they have the opportunity to practice skills without the need for real patients or equipment other than the goggles. There are multiple applications that can be purchased to enhance these learning opportunities (e.g., UbiSim). AR is a cross of virtual and physical reality blended. Products such as 3D4 Medical, Human Anatomy Atlas, and Visible Body represent this blended technology. Virtual simulation, such as *IHuman, Shadow Health Digital Clinical Experience, vSim® for Nursing,* and Zygote Body are three-dimensional worlds of healthcare that are entered through the users' laptops or personal computers. Students interact with their patients (an avatar) and receive feedback on their interactions and interventions with the virtual patient. These situations allow students to make clinical decisions in a situation that does not place the patient at risk. These technologies continue to transform education and improve learning outcomes.

Other hands-on simulated experiences include products like SynDaver (an anatomically correct synthetic model of a human often used for anatomy lab) or human patient simulation with SPs. SPs are real people who have been educated with a scenario to present with specific health problems. Students interview and examine the patients for diagnosing health problems, and although real patients cannot simulate actual symptoms, they can provide realistic opportunities for history taking and communication skills. SPs are briefed ahead of time on what role they will be playing. During the simulation, the SP provides the student with additional information to assist in student learning. Technology can be integrated during the encounter to provide the student with altered heart tones, lung sounds, and the like to enhance the student experience. At the end of the simulation, SPs can provide feedback related to communication, interactions, and overall performance of the student. Oftentimes, the use of SPs is in connection with an inter- or intra-professional education activity that allows for enhancing communication between professions and learning more about each other roles within healthcare. In some institutions, the nursing school partners with a drama school to fill the role of SPs. This is a cost-saving venture, and students from both departments benefit from this partnership.

Research Findings on the Efficacy of Case Scenario Simulations

There is much published on the use of simulation to enhance knowledge, clinical reasoning, self-efficacy, confidence, and reduce stress in nursing students. The success of these identified outcomes is specifically connected to high- or low-stakes testing in simulation and the debriefing that follows. Simulation is thought to be an opportunity for students to experience hands-on scenarios similar to what will be encountered in clinical settings. Some view simulation as a "test run," in which learning occurs when mistakes are made. That learning is then transferred into the clinical arena. More often, simulation is being used in high-stakes testing, in which students are unable to progress unless they successfully meet the requirements of the simulation exercise (e.g., medication preparation and administration).

While during the moment of testing, the student's anxiety may rise, following successful completion of the task results in bolstering the student's confidence moving forward.

Bryant et al. (2019) present best practices in simulation education along with the latest trends and research that are linked to safe patient outcomes. For developers of simulation, in order to optimize student-learning outcomes, one must consider the International Nursing Association for Clinical Simulation and Learning (INACSL, 2016) standards of best practice for simulation. These standards provide criteria with required elements for producing purposeful and systematic planning for effective simulation outcomes.

Electronic Medical Records and Information Systems

As electronic patient records and information systems are prevalent throughout the healthcare system, there is a necessity for schools of nursing to provide the theoretical and technical knowledge related to these systems for nursing students. Programs of nursing can purchase simulated electronic medication administration record technology to enhance student learning. Booth et al. (2018) identify the lack of experience nursing students have with this platform and stress the importance of educational preparation and students' exposure to this technology before entering the clinical setting. The authors created a "gamified" approach to medication administration with multiple points of feedback throughout the scenario. Given the seriousness of medication administration, the more practice nursing students have to perform this task the more proficient they become, thus increasing patient safety by reducing medication errors. Everett-Thomas et al. (2021) identified the use of electronic health records within a simulation as a way to assess both critical thinking and documentation of nursing students. They also identified that the more practice students have with documentation, the more proficient they become at the skill. This, in turn, enhances the readiness of the student for actual clinical experiences.

TRENDS, ISSUES, AND CHALLENGES FOR THE FUTURE

To remain competitive and current in the higher education market, nursing programs need to determine how they will expand their programs to meet the needs of students who may live and work some distance away from the home campus. Distance learning through technology offers the best opportunity for working nurses to continue their education and, as described earlier in the chapter, has been successful. Through consortia of varying levels of education, regional collaboratives, and the healthcare industry, these programs can be cost-effective and reach many more nurses than ever imagined.

The pandemic brought about an increase in the market for LMSs. Many vendors provided cost-effective opportunities to continue quality educational programs through web-based technology. Proven to be an effective modality for engaging students in transformative learning experiences, universities now consider continuing these options even with the return to face-to-face education. However, they require the technology, staffing, and faculty development programs to realize their full potential.

No matter the modality, the program must be within the context of the program's mission, philosophy, organizational framework, and goals and objectives. As with all curriculum development projects, faculty must examine the purpose of the distance education program in light of these components. Teaching strategies implemented during the pandemic must be evaluated to ensure they are compatible with the mission. If not, they must be revised or discontinued. For those programs that are compatible, the usual formative evaluation strategies must take place to ensure that the planning and implementation phases of the program are congruent with the overall curriculum plan. An evaluation plan to measure outcomes must be in place to maintain quality, meet program approval and accreditation standards, and ensure a quality program for its stakeholders such as students, consumers, and faculty.

The majority of distance education programs have copyright and intellectual property policies in place that are congruent with the parent institution. For new programs, along with faculty development and implementation support, it is advised that these policies be developed early in the process. The ideal policy is one that gives the individual faculty member the rights to the course syllabus and learning activities; however, the course description and objectives remain the property of the institution.

Privacy issues are addressed through the maintenance of the same policies of the parent institution. For web-based courses, owing to identification theft and computer hackers, many institutions issue identification numbers for students, staff, and faculty rather than using their Social Security Numbers. Most LMSs have built-in privacy safety and security mechanisms that allow only students and faculty access to courses through personal identification numbers and passwords, and to protect debit and credit card information when paying tuition and fees. In using platforms to meet with students or to discuss patient information during seminar time, one must consider both Family Education and Privacy Rights Act and Health Insurance Portability and Privacy Act rules for online platforms. Not all platforms are compliant for both, without spending additional dollars for those upgraded services.

As distance education programs increase in the future, new issues and challenges face faculty and institutions of higher learning. Less attention will be needed on the actual technology of the delivery systems, and more attention will be necessary on the quality of the programs as they match the mission and purposes of the educational programs. Outcomes from distance education programs will be measured by increased opportunities for nurses to continue their education and the continued partnerships between education and service that result in a nursing workforce ready to meet the challenges of an ever-changing healthcare system and the health promotion and disease prevention needs of the populace.

SUMMARY

This chapter reviewed the various types of distance education programs and their relationship to curriculum development and evaluation. The influence of informatics and technology on nursing education was discussed. Some of the issues facing these types of programs were reviewed including cost-effectiveness, faculty workload, the application of teaching and learning principles, and student-learning outcomes.

END-OF-CHAPTER RESOURCES

DISCUSSION QUESTIONS

1. To what extent does technology continue to support distance education programs? What impact did the global pandemic have on established distance programs? To what extent do you see the abrupt shift to online learning during the pandemic have on education in the next 5 years?

2. Of the multiple technology-supported distance education programs, which do you believe

   - is most cost-effective?
   - meets desired outcomes?

- reaches the highest number of students?
- fosters faculty development?
- Explain your rationale.

3. Understanding there was a decrease in NCLEX pass rates during the pandemic, discuss the pros and cons for the delivery of clinical courses through simulation and distance education strategies.

LEARNING ACTIVITIES

Student-Learning Activities

1. Search the current literature (past 5 years) for at least three research articles about distance education programs, web-based education, or the application of informatics and technology in nursing education.

   a. Analyze them for a description of the outcomes for specific distance education modalities.

   b. Compare the modalities according to the outcomes that relate to teaching and learning effectiveness and student and faculty satisfaction.

Faculty Development Activities

1. Select one course that you teach and adapt it to either synchronous virtual or asynchronous web-based technology. Explain your rationale for selecting one or the other as it applies to the course.

2. If you teach a course or courses online, evaluate them for their student-learning outcomes and other measures of its effectiveness. Compare it to the program mission and program goals/objectives. Develop a plan for revising the course based on your evaluation.

3. If you teach simulation, evaluate it using the INACSL standards of best practice. Develop a plan for revising the course based on your evaluation.

A robust set of instructor resources designed to supplement this text is located at **http://connect.springerpub.com/content/book/978-0-8261-8686-7.** Qualifying instructors may request access by emailing **textbook@springerpub.com.**

REFERENCES

Allen, I. E., & Seaman, J. (2016). *Online report card: Ten years of tracking online education in the United States*. http://onlinelearningsurvey.com/reports/onlinereportcard.pdf

Babson Survey Research Group. (2018). *Grade increase. Tracking distance education in the United States*. https://bayviewanalytics.com/reports/gradeincrease.pdf

Big Blue Button. (2021). *Teaching platform*. https://bigbluebutton.org/

Blackboard Collaborate. (2021). *Virtual classroom tool designed for education*. https://www.blackboard.com/teaching-learning/collaboration-web-conferencing/blackboard-collaborate

Booth, R. G., Sinclair, B., McMurry, J., Strudwick, G., Watson, G., Ladak, H., Zwarenstein, M., McBride, S., Chan, R., & Brennan, L. (2018). Evaluating a serious gaming electronic medication administration record system among nursing students: Protocol for a pragmatic randomized controlled trial. *JMR Research Protocols*, 7(5), e138. https://doi.org/10.2196/resprot.9601

Bower, B. L., & Hardy, K. P. (2004). From correspondence to cyberspace: Changes and challenges in distance education. *New Directions for Community Colleges*, 128, 5–12.

Bryant, K., Aebersold, M. L., Jeffries, P. R., & Kardong-Edgren, S. (2020, April). Innovations in simulation: Nursing leaders' exchange of best practices. *Clinical Simulation in Nursing, 41*(C), 33–40. https://doi.org/10.1016/j.ecns.2019.09.002

Canvas. (2021). *Higher ed Canvas LMS*. https://www.instructure.com/product/higher-education/canvas-lms

Cheng, Z. (2021). Leveraging theories in instructional design: A reflective response to OLSit framework. *Educational Technology and Research Development, 69*, 109–112. https://doi.org/10.1007/s11423-020-09932-9

Crotwell Pullis, B., & Hekel, B. D. (2021). Adapting a community health nursing course to an online format. *Public Health Nursing, 38*(3), 439–444. https://doi.org/10.1111/phn.12868

DeBoor, S. (2018). Distance education, online learning, informatics, and technology. In S. Keating & S. DeBoor (Eds.), *Curriculum development and evaluation in nursing education* (4th ed., pp. 185–202). Springer Publishing Company.

Everett-Thomas, R., Joseph, L., & Trujillo, G. (2021). Using virtual simulation and electronic health records to assess student nurses' documentation and critical thinking skills. *Nursing Education Today, 99*, 104770. https://doi.org/10.1016/j.nedt.2021.104770

Examity. (2021). *Better test integrity*. http://examity.com

Garrison, E., Colin, S., Lemberger, O., & Lugod, M. (2021). Interactive learning for nurses through gamification. *JONA, 51*(2), 95–100. https://doi.org/10.1097/NNA.0000000000000976

GoToMeeting, by Log Me In. (2021). *HD video conferencing. On any device*. https://www.gotomeeting.com/video-conferencing

Honorlock. (2021). *About us*. https://honorlock.com/about-us/

International Nursing Association for Clinical Simulation and Learning Standards Committee. (2016, December). INACSL standards of best practice: Simulation[SM] simulation design. *Clinical Simulation in Nursing, 12*(S), S5–S12. http://doi.org/10.1016/j.ecns.2016.09.005

Jowsey, T., Foster, G., Cooper-Ioelu, P., & Jacobs, S. (2020). Blended learning via distance in pre-registration nursing education: A scoping review. *Nurse Education in Practice, 44*, 102775. https://doi.org/10.1016/j.nepr.2020.102775

Langegård, U., Kiani, K., Nielsen, S. J., & Svensson, p-A. (2021). Nursing students' experiences of a pedagogical transition from campus learning to distance learning using digital tools. *BMC Nursing, 20*(23), 1–10. https://doi.org/10.1186/s12912–021–00542-1

Microsoft® Teams. (2021). *Video conferencing*. https://www.microsoft.com/en-us/microsoft-teams/video-conferencing

Moodle. (2020). *About Moodle*. http://moodle.org/about

National Council of State Authorization and Reciprocity. (2021). *What is SARA?* https://nc-sara.org/

National Council of State Boards of Nursing. (2021a). *National simulation guidelines for prelicensure nursing programs*. https://www.ncsbn.org/9535.htm

National Council of State Boards of Nursing. (2021b). *2020 number of candidates taking NCLEX examination and percent passing, type of candidate*. https://www.ncsbn.org/Table_of_Pass_Rates_2020_Q4.pdf

Pearson Education Inc. (2021). *Products & services for institutions*. http://www.ecollege.com/index.php

Proctorio. (2020). *Not just proctoring. A comprehensive learning integrity program*. https://proctorio.com/

ProctorU. (2021). *Exam security done right*. https://www.proctoru.com

Quality Matters. (2021). *Helping you deliver on your online promise*. https://www.qualitymatters.org/

Regmi, K., & Jones, L. (2020). A systematic review of the factors—enablers and barriers—affecting e-learning in health sciences education. *BMC Medical Education, 20*(91), 1–18. https://doi.org/10.1186/s12909-020-02007-6

U.S. Department of Education. (2019). *Using technology support postsecondary student learning: A practice guide for college and university administrators, advisors, and faculty.* https://files.eric.ed.gov/fulltext/ED594748.pdf

U.S. Department of Education. (2020, August 24). *Secretary DeVos issues new distance learning regulations to spur high-quality distance and competency-based programs, better serve diverse population of higher education students [Press release].* https://www.ed.gov/news/press-releases/secretary-devos-issues-new-distance-learning-regulations-spur-high-quality-distance-and-competency-based-programs-better-serve-diverse-population-higher-education-students

Verkuyl, M., St-Amant, O., Hughes, M., Lapum, J. L., & McCulloch, T. (2020). Combining self-debriefing and group debriefing in simulation. *Clinical Simulation in Nursing, 39,* 41–44. https://doi.org/10.1016/j.ecns.2019.11.001

Zoom. (2021). *Video conferencing and web conferencing service.* https://www.zoom.us

SECTION IV

PROGRAM EVALUATION AND ACCREDITATION

Stephanie Stimac DeBoor

OVERVIEW

This section examines the theories, concepts, and models used to evaluate and approve nursing education programs. Although evaluation appears as the last step, it occurs throughout the processes of curriculum development and its implementation. Evaluation activities are part of the program approval through state regulatory and accreditation processes. These processes serve, in part, as proof of the program's credibility for consumers and document the institution's ability to meet professional and educational standards. Feedback from evaluation activities provides the reason for programmatic changes, whether minor or major, that must occur to maintain an up-to-date and high-quality curriculum.

Changes that occurred during the COVID-19 global pandemic created change in the delivery of curriculum, as well as evaluation criteria for online delivery. Current economic and educational systems in the United States continue to recover from the effects of the pandemic. Educational programs place an emphasis on outcomes and benchmarking those outcomes to assess whether the program remains relevant. Part of this continual evaluation of program quality provides information that allows for the correction of errors and improvement of the overall program. In addition to measuring outcomes, it is necessary to assess the processes that bring about the final product, such as, instructional strategies that enable learners to become actively involved and self-directing to acquire new knowledge, behaviors, attitudes, and skills. Assessment of the technology used, for example, web-based platforms, smart classrooms, simulated clinical situations, and so forth are part of the evaluation. Additional outcome measures include graduates' performance and satisfaction, the quality of the program as compared to professional standards, and the program's competitors provide a summative evaluation on how well the program meets its mission and goals.

To ensure quality, the parent institution should hold regional accreditation that demonstrates achievement in standards for higher education. This accreditation achievement is important to the nursing program's quality as well. There are many levels of program approval and accreditation that nursing programs undergo. For example, the parent institution approves and periodically evaluates the nursing program, and the state board of nursing, a regulating agency, must approve the program initially and at periodic intervals. Although the state board assesses quality, its primary charge is to view the program's performance in light of consumer protection. It also determines the program's eligibility for graduates to sit for RN licensure and, in many states, approves nursing programs for advanced practice.

While accreditation is voluntary, it provides credibility to a nursing program on the regional, national, and professional levels. Its purpose is to ensure quality as measured by higher education and nursing accrediting agencies' standards and criteria set by professional peers. An accredited program provides advantages, including its reputation for quality, eligibility for grants and other external funding and for its graduates' eligibility for licensure, certification, admission into higher degree programs, and scholarships.

THE ROLE OF FACULTY, STUDENTS, CONSUMERS, AND ADMINISTRATORS IN EVALUATION

Multiple stakeholders play a role in ongoing educational program evaluation. As is true for curriculum development, the faculty is key to the assessment of program processes, outcomes, along with the collection and analysis of the data. Students are as important for their part of the evaluation process, providing measures of their performance on tests, clinical skills, satisfaction with the program, assessment of teaching effectiveness, and the quality of the courses in which they participate. Evaluation of the program must also come from the major consumers of the program, which include alumni, employers of the graduates, and the recipients of the graduates' nursing care. Graduates' performance on licensure and certification exams, job skills, professional achievements, and recommendations of the program to other potential students can be used further identify a program's success. Employers of the graduates and the population receiving their services provide valuable feedback and serve as an indicator of the program's match to the current community healthcare needs and the system's demand for employment of its graduates.

The role of administrators, chief nursing officers, or deans in program evaluation is to provide the leadership and financial resources necessary for the process and, if warranted, consultation services (internal or external expertise). Administrators must ensure that there is adequate support staff for the ongoing collection and analyses of data along with the final dissemination of findings in a timely manner.

THE MASTER PLAN OF EVALUATION AND PROGRAM REVIEW

Chapter 14 reviews definitions, concepts, and theories related to evaluation, quality assurance, and accreditation applicable to nursing education. It describes the system of program approval and periodic review within the parent institution. Traditionally, reviews of established programs occur every 5 years within the institution to ensure quality and, in some instances, justify the continuation of the program when enrollments decline or economic times require the downsizing of academic programs.

With an emphasis on outcomes, evaluation is essential for measuring success, establishing benchmarks, and continually improving the quality of the program. Because programs need to meet academic and accreditation standards, professional discipline expectations, and consumer demand, most institutions have a master plan of evaluation. An evaluation model, theory, or criteria set by accrediting bodies serve as a guide for the master plan. Often integrated with the school's strategic plan, the master plan provides the procedures for collecting information to prepare required reports such as program approval or review, accreditation, and to demonstrate the worth of the program to the parent institution and the community. Institutions use the evaluation results for continual program quality improvement, demonstration of excellence, and marketing programs to the public.

PREPARING FOR AN ACCREDITATION VISIT

Chapter 15 follows through on the concepts from Chapter 14 by providing a case study of the process for preparing for accreditation in nursing education. Due to the global pandemic, accreditation site visits became virtual visits. This chapter provides educators with guidelines for preparing for accreditation, whether conducted on-site or virtual. It includes timelines; preparing the report, roles, and responsibilities of faculty; submission of the report; and preparation for the visit.

CHAPTER 14

Program Evaluation and Accreditation

Susan M. Ervin

CHAPTER OBJECTIVES

Upon completion of Chapter 14, the reader will be able to:

- Analyze common definitions, concepts, and theories of quality assurance and program evaluation.

- Analyze several models of evaluation for their utility in nursing education.

- Analyze the various forms of accreditation and typical accreditation processes that are used to indicate a program meets specific standards and criteria.

- Compare research to program evaluation processes.

- Justify the rationale for strategic planning and developing a master plan of evaluation for educational programs.

- Compare the roles of administrators and faculty in program evaluation and accreditation.

OVERVIEW

This chapter reviews definitions, concepts, and theories related to evaluation, quality assurance, and accreditation as they apply to nursing education. Conceptual models of evaluation; utilization of standards, criteria, and benchmarks for evaluation and accreditation; comparison of evaluation research to program evaluation; and types of program evaluation and their purposes are included. The chapter continues with a discussion of strategic planning, the development of master plans of evaluation, and the roles of nursing faculty and administrators in these activities. As discussed in the section overview, educational evaluation occurs while assessing the program for its quality, currency, relevance, compliance with regulatory agency requirements and accreditation standards, projections into the future, and the need for possible revisions. Although the administration usually assumes the leadership for strategic planning, faculty become part of the process, especially in relation to responding to information provided by curricular evaluation and the future plans for the institution. A master plan of evaluation provides the information necessary for curriculum evaluation and revision, if indicated, and for program or institutional strategic planning.

COMMON DEFINITIONS, CONCEPTS, AND THEORIES RELATED TO EVALUATION, QUALITY ASSURANCE, AND ACCREDITATION

While many of the terms, concepts, and theories of educational evaluation originated from business models, they have been adapted to education, especially in light of the emphasis on outcomes. For the purpose of this text, definitions of commonly used terms in evaluation are provided as they apply to nursing education. *Evaluation* is a process of gathering information about an entity to determine its worth. The end product of an evaluation is a judgment of the entity's worth. In comparison, *assessment* is a process that gathers information resulting in a conclusion such as a nursing diagnosis or problem identification. It does not end with a judgment but rather with a conclusion.

Quality is a term that takes on many meanings depending on the context in which it is used. Schindler et al. (2015) conceptualized quality as "purposeful, transformative, exceptional, and accountable" (p. 8). *Quality assurance* in nursing education is the process of collecting data on how well the institution or program meets its defined standards, criteria, goals, or mission. *Total quality management* (TQM) and *continuous quality improvement* (CQI) are processes or systems that involve all the program stakeholders in the assessment of the quality and effectiveness of the program according to criteria or standards. These processes identify gaps or errors and correct problems to ensure that the program maintains its purpose and quality. Stakeholders continuously ask the following questions: How are we doing? Are we measuring the right data to meet our goals? What barriers or challenges are we encountering? What are the processes or systems that inhibit or enhance our progress? What can we do to improve? One indicator of a nursing program's quality is first-time pass rates for the NCLEX® or national certification for APRN students. State regulatory and accrediting bodies use a school of nursing's pass rates to evaluate program quality.

Educational programs use formative and summative evaluation methods for assessment of performance. Scriven (1996) developed the classic and still used definitions for formative and summative evaluation. *Formative evaluation* is described as "intended—by the evaluator—as a basis for improvement" (p. 4). For example, in nursing, the faculty compares students' progress in meeting course outcomes and whether students have succeeded in the processes that occurred. Based on the findings, faculty may take corrective measures so students can meet outcomes, or possibly, they may change the outcomes. Scriven describes *summative evaluation* as a holistic approach to the assessment of a program and it uses results from the formative evaluation. For example, faculty evaluates the development of critical thinking and clinical decision-making skills in graduates as an outcome of the educational program. In this instance, these skills would need to be measured both before and after the program to determine proficiency in the skills. Both formative and summative types of evaluation "involve efforts to determine merit or worth" (Scriven, 1996, p. 6). Scriven points out that summative evaluation can serve as formative evaluation. For example, if a nursing program finds that graduates' clinical decision-making skills are inadequate (summative evaluation), it can use that information to analyze the program for the strategies (formative evaluation) that were utilized to promote these skills and make improvements as necessary.

Additional definitions commonly used in evaluation are *goal-based evaluation* and *goal-free evaluation*. Scriven (1974) described goal-based program evaluation as that which focuses only on the examination of program goals and intended outcomes. An alternative method, goal-free evaluation, could be used to examine not only the intended effects, but also unintended effects, side effects, or secondary effects. An unintended effect in nursing might be an increase in the applicant pool owing to the community's interactions with students in a program-sponsored, nurse-managed clinic. While this was not a stated goal of the program, it was a positive unintended outcome.

CONCEPTUAL MODELS OF EVALUATION

Conceptual Models

Historically, nursing education programs used many of the models of evaluation developed in healthcare and education. Examples were Donabedian's (1996) Structure, Process, and Outcome model for healthcare evaluation and Stufflebeam et al.'s (1971) Context, Input, Process, and Product (CIPP) educational model. Some of these models continue to serve nursing well, but as nursing develops the uniqueness of the discipline, it is using its own models for evaluation.

Hodges et al. (2020) describe the application of the CIPP model in higher education to evaluate "emergency remote teaching" (ERT) that many faculty had to employ during the pandemic. They identify that it would be difficult to evaluate ERT against typical online learning but provide criterion examples that would be useful for evaluation. They point out the need to include internal and external metrics for a more complete evaluation. Lippe and Carter (2018) found the CIPP model useful in the evaluation of end-of-life care in a prelicensure nursing program. They identified strengths, curricular redundancies, and missing content. These examples provide practical application and a guide for using the CIPP model for the evaluation of higher education programs.

A model for evaluating the quality of nursing doctoral education (QNDE) developed by Kim et al. (2014) surveyed faculty and students in doctoral programs across the United States. The QNDE questionnaire for the survey consisted of four domains of measurement: the program, faculty, resources, and evaluation. Results from the survey revealed that the overall quality of the schools assessed was good, but there was room for improvement. It is a model of evaluation that could be applied to other nursing programs at the graduate level. In 2020, Kim et al. further evaluated the content and construct validity and reliability of a revised version of the QNDE. The results of this study continue to support that the revised QNDE is a credible instrument for evaluating the quality of a nursing research-focused, doctoral program.

Benchmarking

Programs can set benchmarks to measure their own success and standards of excellence or compare themselves to similar institutions. Benchmarks can be used in competition with other programs for recruiting students or seeking financial support or they can be used to motivate the members of the institution to strive toward excellence. Another function of benchmarking is the ability to collaborate with other institutions to share strengths with each other and to continually improve programs.

Accrediting bodies such as the Commission on Collegiate Nursing Education (CCNE) also use benchmarks to evaluate nursing programs. Benchmarks used by CCNE include the financial health of the institution, completion rates, NCLEX and certification pass rates, and student and employer satisfaction with the program (CCNE, 2018). Other benchmarks that institutions may use include applicant pools, admission and retention rates, commitment to diversity, and student, faculty, staff, and administrator satisfaction rates.

An Evaluation Processes Model

Earlier was a discussion on quality improvement. A routine evaluation process of the nursing program is critical for measuring the quality of the program. Similar to the Centers for Disease Control and Prevention (2017) framework for program evaluation, Adams and Neville (2020) provide an updated version called the "Easy Evaluation." This updated approach, developed from multiple evaluation models, provides six phases to guide the evaluation process. While it focuses on the processes of evaluation, it includes a framework for assigning value or worth to the findings from the process. The major phases of the process include logic model; evaluation priorities and questions; evaluation criteria and performance standards; collect, analyze and interpret data; draw evaluative conclusions; and share lessons learned (Adams & Neville, 2020, p. 3). For nursing programs, there are many standards and include accreditation standards or criteria and professional and educational essentials or standards.

Formative Evaluation for Nursing Education

Formative and/or process evaluation strategies include course evaluations, student achievement measures, teaching effectiveness surveys, staff, student, administration, and faculty satisfaction measures. Stakeholder evaluation includes impressions of student and faculty performance by clinical agencies' personnel, assessment of student services, and other support systems. Students' critical thinking development and other standardized tests such as gains in knowledge and skills, NCLEX readiness, Barkley Predictor, retention/ attrition rates, and cost-effectiveness of the program provide further formative evaluation. Antecedent or input evaluation items include the admission (grade point averages), ATI Test of Essential Academic Skills (TEAS: www.atitesting.com/educator/solutions/ teas) Health Education Systems Incorporated (HESI, evolve.elsevier.com/education/ training/hesi-exam-testing/), and Graduate Record Examination (GRE; www.ets.org/ gre/revised_general/about) scores for applicants and accepted students. Other input evaluation includes retention and/or attrition rates; scholarship, fellowship, and loan availability; and endowments and grants for program development and support.

Nursing education's need to improve the evaluation measures in formative education proves to be a challenge in clinical learning experiences. During the pandemic, this became even more of a challenge because of removing students from clinical sites and faculty trying to find ways to provide relevant clinical experiences. The use of Zoom to hold seminars and discuss case studies and oral and written concept mapping proved useful in evaluating students' clinical reasoning outside of the formal clinical site. Virtual clinical utilizing products such as vSim and IHuman provided a chance for faculty to evaluate student's clinical reasoning and critical thinking as a group and independently. Konrad et al. (2021) identified that evaluating students in the clinical setting often focuses on the tasks they do rather than the reasoning behind the task itself. Thus, faculty must employ multiple teaching strategies inside and outside clinical facilities to facilitate an effective evaluation of learning objectives.

SUMMATIVE EVALUATION USING STANDARDS, ESSENTIALS, AND CRITERIA

Summative evaluation differs from formative evaluation in that its purpose is to assess and judge the outcomes of the educational program, while formative evaluation assesses the processes used to achieve the outcome. The "product" of the educational program can be measured according to the overall goal and outcomes of the program/curriculum and other standards and criteria of regulating bodies such as boards of nursing, professional standards such as nursing organizations' code of ethics and practice standards, essentials or competencies defined by professional and educational organizations, and, last but not least, accreditation standards and criteria.

Measures to determine outcomes of the program include success rates of the graduates including their pass rates on licensure and certification exams, graduates' satisfaction with the program, and employers' satisfaction with program graduates' performance. Additional outcome measures include graduation rates, accreditation and program approval status, stakeholders' perceptions of the graduates, ratings of the program by external evaluators or agencies, faculty and student research productivity, community service, and public opinion surveys. Many of these outcome measures can be used to serve as benchmarks for setting achievement levels, for example, setting the pass rates on NCLEX 2% to 3% higher than the national average or local and state competition as a measure of quality.

TYPES OF PROGRAM EVALUATION

Program Approval by Regulatory Agencies

Each state, according to its constitution, regulates higher education and approves programs. They usually require that the institutions meet regional accreditation standards and for professional programs, professional accreditation standards. For information on individual states, the U.S. Department of Education (USDE) database of accredited postsecondary institutions provides information for the various state, territory, and commonwealth departments of education and their higher education agencies at https://ope.ed.gov/dapip/#/home.

Presently, for nursing, there is no national licensure for practice as a nurse or as an advanced practice nurse. Thus, licensure to practice as a nurse usually falls onto the state in which the nurse practices. Each state has a Nurse Practice Act (NPA) that delineates the role of the nurse through defined regulations. The state board of nursing acts to enforce the regulations in the interest of patient safety and public protection. The membership of the National Council of State Boards of Nursing (NCSBN), (2021a) consists of all 50 state boards as well as those in Washington, D.C., and the four U.S. territories. In addition to the definition of *nursing practice*, the advanced practice role is defined using the consensus standards as a model. In 2021, all state boards have definitions of advanced practice and use parts of the consensus model. As of this writing, 24 states allow full practice authority. For an updated list of the states utilizing major components of the Consensus Model, go to www.ncsbn.org/5397.htm.

In 2017, the institution of the Nurse Licensure Compact (NLC) took affect, and currently, 33 states participate in the NLC. This allows the nurse reciprocity, or mutual recognition, of nurse licensure among member states (NCSBN, 2021b). Adoption of the APRN Compact occurred in 2020 and proposed to allow an APRN the same privilege, reciprocity. At present, only two states, Delaware and North Dakota have pending APRN Compact legislation. Once seven states have enacted legislation, the APRN Compact will be implemented (NCSBN, 2020). With the advent of the COVID-19 pandemic in early 2020, governors in some states temporarily waived licensing requirements to increase the number of frontline caregivers. The waiver applied to nurses (and other providers) who held a valid license in another state; the waiver temporarily allowed them to practice in states where they were not licensed (Nevada State Board of Nursing, 2020). The advent of the NLC and the pandemic affected state boards of nursing, NPAs, and the scope of practice across the United States.

Program Approval by Accreditation

A major factor that affects curriculum development and evaluation in nursing education is the imperative that a nursing program meet state board of nursing regulations and accreditation standards set by a national accreditation agency. In addition, in the case of certain specialties, specialty accreditation organizations such as those for nurse midwives and nurse anesthetists accredit programs with those specialties. While not necessarily part of accreditation agencies' standards, professional organizations set forth some standards and criteria for program evaluation. The organizations include the American Association of Colleges of Nursing (AACN), the National Task Force (NTF) on Quality Nurse Practitioner Education, the National League for Nursing (NLN), and the Consensus Model for APRNs: Licensure, Accreditation, Certification, and Education (LACE) that can, in turn, be part of accreditation expectations. While accreditation in the United States is voluntary, failure to be approved or accredited can lead to the closure of the institution by the state regulatory agency, ineligibility for program development funds, or disqualification of the program's students for Title IV financial aid support, traineeships, and scholarships. If students attempt to transfer credits or have degrees from nonaccredited schools, it is likely that the credits and degrees will not be recognized when applying to other institutions of higher education that are accredited.

Accreditation agencies set the standards or criteria by which to evaluate the quality of educational programs. The Council for Higher Education Accreditation (CHEA) is an organization of institutions in higher education whose purpose and mission is to ensure academic quality through accreditation. An overview of its membership and role in advocacy for quality higher education in the United States may be found on its homepage at www.chea.org/. In addition to its role in quality assurance in the United States, CHEA has an international quality group to address quality issues in higher education in other nations. Information about this group may be found at www.chea.org/about-ciqg. CHEA recognizes accrediting agencies and serves as a representative for higher education concerned with national accreditation issues as well as in the world community. A list of its recognized accrediting bodies may be found on its website (www.chea.org/chea-recognized-accrediting-organizations). An example of the issues in which CHEA becomes involved is its advocacy role in ensuring the maintenance of quality education and accreditation status even during the pandemic (CHEA, 2020).

The USDE is the official governmental agency that recognizes accrediting agencies in the United States. On the institutional level, colleges and universities are usually accredited by a regional accrediting agency, including the Middle States Commission on Higher Education; the New England Association of Schools and Colleges, Commission on Institutions of Higher Education; the North Central Association of Colleges and Schools, The Higher Learning Commission; the Northwest Commission on Colleges and Universities; the Southern Association of Colleges and Schools, Commission on Colleges; the Western Association of Schools and Colleges, Accrediting Commission for Community and Junior Colleges; and the Western Association of Schools and Colleges, Senior Colleges and University Commission. A list of these agencies and details about them can be found on the USDE website (www2.ed.gov/admins/finaid/accred/accreditation_pg6.html#RegionalInstitutional). These regional agencies have the infrastructure and paid staff to support their mission, which is to ensure the quality of higher education institutions. The agencies are staffed by experts in the field including not only those in education but also staff experts in distance learning systems, educational technology, and informatics. Volunteer directors or commissioners who are experts in higher education such as presidents, provosts, administrators, deans, and faculty set the standards and policies of the accreditation agencies. Additional volunteers are selected and trained according to their expertise in higher education to act as visitors to institutions undergoing accreditation. The USDE recognizes accrediting agencies to ensure educational quality, including the regional agencies as well as specialized accreditors.

The majority of nursing programs are housed in multipurpose colleges or universities that are regionally accredited. Since PhD and DNS programs are not accredited by a specialized accrediting agency for nursing, it is important that they are regionally accredited to ensure they meet the standards of quality in higher education doctoral programs. (As an aside, the AACN, 2021, provides information regarding curricula, admission requirements, selection of a research-focused degree in nursing.) In order to determine if an institution meets regional accreditation standards, it prepares a self-study report that responds to each of the accreditation standards and involves the stakeholders in its preparation including administrators, faculty, staff, and students. After receiving the report, a team of volunteer peer evaluators from the accrediting agency visits the institution to conduct a comprehensive on-site evaluation. The evaluators meet with institution and nursing administrators, nursing faculty, students, staff, and the community of interest; visit didactic and clinical settings; and access school resources that support the self-study report (CCNE, 2019, 2021). The team prepares a report on its findings that is presented to the board or commission of the accrediting agency that reviews the findings and determines if the institution meets the standards and should receive either first-time accreditation, continuing accreditation, or submit a progress report if indicated. There are two major accrediting bodies in nursing recognized by the USDE, Accreditation Commission for Education in Nursing (ACEN), and the CCNE. A third accrediting body, the National League for Nursing, Commission for Nursing Education Accreditation (NLN CNEA) earned designation as an accrediting body from the USDE in May 2021.

The COVID-19 pandemic drastically changed the accreditation process for schools of nursing. ACEN and CCNE moved from on-site to virtual visits beginning in the fall of 2020. Nursing programs still submitted a self-study and planned for evaluators to meet with faculty, students, and other constituents. All meetings and observations were to be virtual, however. Schools utilized a virtual, rather than an on-site, resource room to upload videos of students in clinical and simulation. The actual simulation experience was videotaped along with pre- and postbriefings. Utilizing platforms such as Zoom allowed the evaluators to meet with constituents and provided evaluators the opportunity to observe students in didactic and laboratory settings. Development of narrated videos or PowerPoints of the campus, and physical facilities and resources afforded evaluators access to physical resources of the school and parent institution. Within 24 months of the virtual visit, each school will have an on-site follow-up visit, which is a requirement of the USDE (CCNE, 2020). See Chapter 15 for more information on preparation for, and a case study of, a virtual accreditation visit.

Program accreditation, like institutional accreditation, is voluntary, but for students and graduates of nursing programs, coming from an accredited program is essential for scholarships, traineeships, financial aid support, career opportunities, and future continuing education plans that involve a higher degree. Each of the nursing accrediting agencies (ACEN and CCNE) are similar to the regional accreditors as they have an infrastructure and staff but depend on volunteer experts from the profession to set standards, make site visits, and participate in recommendations and policymaking.

As mentioned earlier, there are specialized accreditors for nursing programs with specialty tracks in their graduate programs. Nursing specialty accrediting agencies recognized by the USDE include the American Association of Nurse Anesthetists and the American College of Nurse-Midwives (USDE, 2021). The Consensus Model for APRNs: LACE was developed in 2008 by representatives from professional nursing organizations, nursing educators, certification agencies, and state boards of nursing. The model identified four areas of advanced practice: nurse anesthetists, clinical specialists, nurse midwives, and nurse practitioners. It also recognizes certified nurse practitioners who practice in both acute care and primary care settings and are educated and certified for both roles. Advanced practice nurses are required to have licensure by the state board of nursing where they practice, a national certification recognized by the National Council of State Boards of Nursing, and an education from an accredited institution recognized by the USDE and in accordance with the standards delineated in the Consensus Model. A detailed description of the Consensus Model: LACE may be found at the NCSBN: www.ncsbn.org/Consensus_Model_for_APRN_Regulation_July_2008.pdf.

Program Approval in Academe

Within academe are two types of program evaluation that differ from regulatory and accreditation processes: *program approval* and *program review*. Before a new program is initiated, its parent institution must approve it. The faculty develop the curriculum for a new program based on a needs assessment that provides the rationale for the program, how it meets the mission of the institution, and identifies the key stakeholders. In addition to the curriculum plan, a budget projecting the start-up and maintenance costs and income for the next 5 to 10 years accompanies the proposal as justification.

In academe, the processes of approval are as follows: The first step is for the faculty within the originating department/school's curriculum committee to approve the proposal. The next step depends on the hierarchal structure of the institution. The following levels of approval are based on a moderate- to large-scale institution, and it is understood that smaller institutions may not have as many approval rungs. After faculty approval, the proposal may go to a curriculum or program-approval committee within its college or division if not an independent school. Preliminary approval may have to be granted by administrators before it enters other formal approval levels in order to determine its economic feasibility and its fit with the mission and/or strategic plan. After approval at the program's local level by committees and faculty as a whole, it proceeds to the next level, which is usually a program or curriculum committee at the division or college level. With its approval, it goes to the overall university or college graduate or undergraduate committee for its review and approval. Next, it may go to a subcommittee of the faculty senate that reviews program proposals. On its approval, the senate reviews it for its role in the university and quality and, if approved, sends it to the chief executive for academic affairs such as a vice president or provost. Upon that person's approval, the president of the institution approves the program. The governing board such as a board of trustees or regents is the final rung of approval, and it may have a subcommittee that reviews it with recommendations prior to its going to the full board. These levels of approval are for academic approval only. For professional programs, such as nursing, accreditation, and state regulatory bodies complete these approvals to ensure the academic entities that the program is qualified for professional approval and accreditation. If a school of nursing is adding an additional specialty to an established program, a substantive report goes to the accrediting body to show the new program meets the accreditation standards.

Program Review

Program review in academe occurs on average every 5 years within the parent institution. The purpose of a program review is to ensure the quality and sustainability of the program and to demonstrate to the institution's constituency its place in the academic community. Faculty prepares an overview of the program especially related to its mission, student-learning outcomes, enrollments, the quality of the faculty, and enrollment and graduation projections. When economic times are tough, such as during the "Great

Recession" and currently the COVID-19 pandemic, these reviews help demonstrate the relationship of the program to the mission of the institution, its contributions to the community, and the quality of the program. Nursing often finds itself having to justify its program owing to the relatively small faculty-to-student ratios required for clinical supervision. Nursing programs provide data as evidence to support the program, its cost-effectiveness, its place in meeting the mission of the institution (serving the public), and its contributions of student enrollments to the core general education, prerequisite requirements, program development funds, and research and scholarship production.

The requirements and processes for program approval and review use the same data sets as many of the other assessment and evaluation activities related to professional accreditation and standards of excellence. Thus, it is not unusual for a parent institution to request copies of the most recent self-studies and accreditation reports that either substitute for program review criteria or supplement the requirements. Program approval and review should be integrated into the school's strategic plan so that data sets gathered from the master plan can serve all assessment and evaluation activities.

Research and Program Evaluation

Research in evaluation differs from the evaluation process. It begins with a description of a problem and a research question related to program evaluation theories, concepts, and processes for the purpose of comparing them, testing them, and perhaps developing a new theory, concept, or model of evaluation. As is common in most research, the purpose for investigation and a research question/inquiry is stated. There is a literature review, and based on the review, a theoretical/conceptual framework is postulated followed by descriptions of the methodology, data collection and analysis, findings, and recommendations. Research in evaluation is usually viewed as applied research and differs from basic research as it is searching for practical solutions to problems. Looking to contribute to the discipline of educational theory and conceptual bases, it has a broader focus than program evaluation.

The evaluation process starts with an identification of the program or entity, the purpose of the evaluation, and the stakeholders within the program. It requires many of the same steps of research including a review of the literature, identification of a theory or model of evaluation to guide the process, collection and analysis of credible data related to the program, synthesizing the analysis to come to a conclusion, and a judgment with recommendations for further assessment and strategies for improvement. It differs from program evaluation research as it focuses on one program, and its purpose is to evaluate or judge the program in terms of the program's quality and ability to meet its purpose and goals.

Strategic Planning

Strategic planning for an institution provides the guidelines for carrying out the mission of the institution and, at the same time, is used to evaluate how well the institution is meeting its mission and goals. The mission statement provides a means for formulating the strategic plan. When initiating the planning, it is important to question how the institution will continue to meet its mission. A strategic plan incorporates the institution's vision statement and core values that look to the future and where it plans to be 3 to 5 years hence. From that vision, goals are set that guide the processes necessary to reach the vision. Strategic planning takes a hierarchical approach. In academe, the parent institution's top administrators (president, vice presidents, provosts, deans, etc.) initiate the plan. Key stakeholders in the institution participate in the planning process to ensure that the plan and its action plans are relevant and realistic in terms of meeting the goals within the period specified. A yearly examination of progress identifies if the plan and actions are meeting the vision. If a shortfall occurs, the team remediates the plan as necessary after careful examination of what created the setbacks or plan to fail.

Each program within the institution may choose to develop its own strategic plan. It should be congruent with the parent institution but unique to the program's mission and goals. The chief nursing officer of the nursing program and administrative team act as the initiators of a strategic plan and involve faculty, staff, and students in the planning process. It is useful to consult with community stakeholders, graduates, and consumers of the program as well for their perspectives on how well the program meets its mission, goals, and what they foresee for the future. In addition, consulting with other disciplines assists the planners in identifying the role of nursing in both higher education and healthcare systems.

Like the parent institution, it is wise for nursing programs to review, at least annually, progress toward the goals and adjust or develop new goals as needed. To avoid the pitfall of excessive planning processes that result in implementation failure, the use of a master evaluation plan provides the structure, details, and timelines for assessing and evaluating the progress toward reaching the vision and short and long-term goals.

MASTER PLAN OF EVALUATION

Rationale for a Master Plan of Evaluation

When developing a master plan of evaluation, one must consider the integration of accreditation or program approval standards. These standards or criteria are the baseline requirements of the profession to ensure that programs are of sufficient quality to meet the expectations of the discipline. They demonstrate to the public that external reviewing bodies recognize a program for the quality of its graduates and that it meets educational and professional standards. Graduation from an accredited program is usually a requirement of admission for a continued degree or educational work. Many funding agencies for programs require accreditation as it indicates that the program is of high enough quality to assume the responsibility for the administration of grants and completion of projects. Most accrediting agencies require that a program have a master plan of evaluation or evidence of institutional policies with their regular review and reports on compliance or revisions if indicated (ACEN, 2020; CCNE, 2018). A master plan helps identify the components of the program that need to be evaluated, who will do the data collection and when, what methods of analysis of the data will be employed, and the plans for responding to the findings for quality improvement. Having a master plan of evaluation in place greatly facilitates these processes when submitting accreditation self-study reports, program approval reports, or proposals for funding.

With an emphasis on outcomes, the evaluation process is essential for measuring success, establishing benchmarks, and continually improving the quality of the program. A master plan of evaluation is used to provide data for faculty's decision-making as part of an internal review and for meeting external review standards. It is important to have a master plan that continually monitors the program so that adjustments can be made as the program is implemented as it is part of the total quality improvement process. It is equally important to measure outcomes in terms of meeting the vision, strategic plans, goals, and objectives of the program, with certain benchmarks that help pinpoint the quality of the program.

Components of a Master Plan of Evaluation

The master plan must specify what is being evaluated and an organizing framework is useful so that as nearly as possible, no crucial variable is omitted for review. Additionally, it is important to identify the persons who will

1. collect the data,
2. analyze the findings,
3. prepare reports,
4. disseminate the reports to key people, and
5. set the timelines for previous steps.

Finally, there must be a feedback loop in place for recommendations and decision-making. Reports from the evaluation should include the following:

1. Identification of existing and or anticipated barriers/challenges
2. New and previously missed needs
3. Accomplishments and rationale for the success
4. Recommendations for improvement, discontinuance of a program, or proposals for new programs
5. Action plans for changes that include the people responsible and timelines
6. A summary of the evaluation and findings on the program's success or progress toward meeting its goals

Table 14.1 provides guidelines for developing a master plan of evaluation and the major components to be assessed for evaluation. In addition to including the curriculum and its components, it incorporates external and internal frame factors (Johnson, 1977), the infrastructure, the core curriculum, students, alumni, and human resources. As indicated in the table, these are only the major components. It is possible that as educational evaluation evolves, other components will emerge. The elements within each component are not listed. Each institution must determine which elements fall under the major components.

ROLES OF ADMINISTRATORS AND FACULTY IN PROGRAM EVALUATION AND ACCREDITATION

Administrators in academe provide the vision and leadership for the educational program. However, it is imperative that the administration and the major stakeholders of the institution be in agreement about its mission, vision, purpose, and goals. Stakeholders include the governing board, the chief executive officer, the administrators of the infrastructure and the academic programs, the faculty, students, alumni, and consumers served by the institution. These stakeholders make up the "personality" and body of the institution that marks it as unique in its contributions to society, and they, too, must be in agreement with the vision and purpose of the institution to maintain a strong educational program. The administration periodically reviews the mission and vision of the institution to match them to current needs and provides the leadership for revising them according to need. Additionally, the administration monitors assessment and evaluation activities to ensure program quality and provides adequate resources in a timely manner for accreditation and program evaluation activities.

All faculty members participate in the evaluation of the curriculum and the program through their input into specific areas and needs for assessment, the collection of data, data analyses, and the formulation of recommendations for decision-making regarding the program. In many schools of nursing, there are evaluation committees that lead the

TABLE 14.1: Major Components and Guidelines for Developing a Master Plan of Evaluation

Component	Action Plans							Follow-Up Plans
	Responsible Party	When and How Often	Instruments and Tools for Data Collection	Data Findings and Analysis	Criteria, Outcomes, or Benchmarks	Reports and Recommendations	Maintain and Monitor or Improve	By Whom, How, and When
Program Mission/Vision/Goals/Organizational Framework								
Program								
Strategic Plan								

External Frame Factors							
Internal Frame Factors							
Infrastructure Systems: Buildings							

(continued)

TABLE 14.1: Major Components and Guidelines for Developing a Master Plan of Evaluation (*continued*)

Component		Action Plans						Follow-Up Plans
	Responsible Party	When and How Often	Instruments and Tools for Data Collection	Data Findings and Analysis	Criteria, Outcomes, or Benchmarks	Reports and Recommendations	Maintain and Monitor or Improve	By Whom, How, and When
Facilities								
Support Systems								
Student Services								

Financial								
Administration								
Technology/Informatics								

(continued)

TABLE 14.1: Major Components and Guidelines for Developing a Master Plan of Evaluation (*continued*)

Component	Action Plans							Follow-Up Plans
	Responsible Party	When and How Often	Instruments and Tools for Data Collection	Data Findings and Analysis	Criteria, Outcomes, or Benchmarks	Reports and Recommendations	Maintain and Monitor or Improve	By Whom, How, and When
Library								
Baccalaureate[a] Curriculum: Congruency With Mission/Vision/ Philosophy/Organizational Framework								
Overall Purpose/Goal								

End-of-Program (student-learning outcomes) and Level Objectives							
Prerequisites							
General Education							

(continued)

TABLE 14.1: Major Components and Guidelines for Developing a Master Plan of Evaluation (*continued*)

| Component | | Action Plans | | | | | | Follow-Up Plans |
	Responsible Party	When and How Often	Instruments and Tools for Data Collection	Data Findings and Analysis	Criteria, Outcomes, or Benchmarks	Reports and Recommendations	Maintain and Monitor or Improve	By Whom, How, and When
Electives								
Baccalaureate Nursing Major Courses Course Objectives and Content								
Learning Activities								

Teaching Effectiveness							
Graduate[a] Curriculum: Congruency With Mission/ Vision/Philosophy/ Organizational Framework							
Overall Purpose/Goal							

(continued)

TABLE 14.1: Major Components and Guidelines for Developing a Master Plan of Evaluation (*continued*)

Component		Action Plans						Follow-Up Plans
	Responsible Party	When and How Often	Instruments and Tools for Data Collection	Data Findings and Analysis	Criteria, Outcomes, or Benchmarks	Reports and Recommendations	Maintain and Monitor or Improve	By Whom, How, and When
End-of-Program (student-learning outcomes) and Level Objectives								
Prerequisites								
Cognates								

Electives							
Core Nursing Courses Course Objectives and Content							
Specialty/Functional Courses Course Objectives and Content							

(continued)

TABLE 14.1: Major Components and Guidelines for Developing a Master Plan of Evaluation (*continued*)

Component		Action Plans						Follow-Up Plans
	Responsible Party	When and How Often	Instruments and Tools for Data Collection	Data Findings and Analysis	Criteria, Outcomes, or Benchmarks	Reports and Recommendations	Maintain and Monitor or Improve	By Whom, How, and When
Learning Activities								
Teaching Effectiveness								

[a]The same components for the baccalaureate and graduate curricula apply to associate degree, master's, and doctorate programs.

process or, in other cases, curriculum committees may be charged with the evaluation of the curriculum and program. As part of the parent institution, nursing representatives provide input into university/college-wide evaluation activities. As a professional program, nursing faculty has valuable input into evaluation processes owing to the necessity for meeting professional accreditation and organizations' standards and criteria.

SUMMARY

This chapter reviewed classic definitions, concepts, and models of evaluation with definitions of commonly used terms. The rationale for strategic planning and a master plan of evaluation was presented. Types of tools and instruments for data collection for evaluation of educational programs and the roles of administrators and faculty were reviewed.

END-OF-CHAPTER RESOURCES

DISCUSSION QUESTIONS

1. Explain the differences between conceptual models of evaluation and the use of benchmarks. Give examples of their application to the evaluation of an educational program.

2. To what extent do you believe faculty should be involved in a strategic planning process? Explain why.

3. Describe how a master plan of evaluation contributes to the external review of a nursing program.

LEARNING ACTIVITIES

Student-Learning Activity

1. Using Table 14.1, develop a master plan of evaluation for the case study of a fictional school of nursing outreach program found in the Appendix.

2. Nurse Educator/Faculty Development Activity

3. Using Table 14.1, find your school of nursing's evaluation plan and assess it for any missing components or action plans.

 SPRINGER PUBLISHING CONNECT™ A robust set of instructor resources designed to supplement this text is located at **http://connect.springerpub.com/content/book/978-0-8261-8686-7.** Qualifying instructors may request access by emailing **textbook@springerpub.com.**

REFERENCES

Accreditation Commission for Education in Nursing. (2020). ACEN accreditation manual 2017 standards and criteria (Rev. ed.) https://www.acenursing.org/acen-accreditation-manual/

Adams, J., & Neville S. (2020). Program evaluation for health professionals: What it is, what it isn't and how to do it. *International Journal of Qualitative Methods, 19*, 1–11. https://doi .org/10.1177/1609406920964345

American Association of Colleges of Nursing. (2021). *PhD education.* https://www.aacnnursing .org/Nursing-Education-Programs/PhD-Education

Centers for Disease Control and Prevention. (2017). *A framework for program evaluation*. https://www.cdc.gov/eval/framework/index.htm

Commission on Collegiate Nursing Education. (2018). *Standards for accreditation of baccalaureate and graduate nursing programs*. https://www.aacnnursing.org/Portals/42/CCNE/PDF/Standards-Final-2018.pdf

Commission on Collegiate Nursing Education. (2019). *General advice for hosting a CCNE on-site evaluation*. https://www.aacnnursing.org/Portals/42/CCNE/PDF/advice.pdf

Commission on Collegiate Nursing Education. (2020). *Frequently asked questions—Virtual evaluations: Nursing education programs*. https://www.aacnnursing.org/Portals/42/CCNE/News/Virtual-Evaluation-FAQs-for-Education-CCNE.pdf

Commission on Collegiate Nursing Education. (2021). *CCNE accreditation process*. https://www.aacnnursing.org/CCNE-Accreditation/What-We-Do/CCNE-Accreditation-Process

Donabedian, A. (1996). Quality management in nursing and health care. In J. A. Schemele (Ed.), *Models of quality assurance* (pp. 88–103). Delmar.

Hodges, C., Moore, S., Lockee, B., Trust, T., & Bond, M. A. (2020, March 27). The difference between emergency remote teaching and online learning. *EDUCAUSE Review*. http://www.cetla.howard.edu/workshops/docs/The%20Difference%20Between%20Emergency%20Remote%20Teaching%20and%20Online%20Learning%20_%20EDUCAUSE%20(2).pdf

Johnson, M. (1977). *Intentionality in education: A conceptual model of curricular and instructional planning and evaluation*. Center for Curriculum Research and Services.

Kim, M. J., Hugh, M., Park, C. G., Shake, K., Park, S. H., Galvin, K., & Burke, L. (2020). Global assessment instrument for quality of nursing doctoral education with a research focus: Validity and reliability study, *Nurse Education Today*, *91*, 2–9.

Kim, M., Park, C., Park, S., & Ketefian, S. (2014). Quality of nursing doctoral education and scholarly performance in U.S. schools of nursing: Strategic areas for improvement. *Journal of Professional Nursing*, *30*(1), 10–18.

Konrad, S., Fitzgerald, A., & Deckers, C. (2021). Nursing fundamentals-supporting clinical competency online during the COVID-19 pandemic. *Teaching and Learning in Nursing*, *16*(1), 53–56. https://doi.org/10.1016/j.teln.2020.07.005

Lippe, M., & Carter, P. (2018). Using the CIPP model to assess nursing education program quality and merit. *Teaching and Learning in Nursing*, *13*, 9–13.

National Council of State Boards of Nursing. (2020). *APRN compact*. https://www.ncsbn.org/aprn-compact.htm

National Council of State Boards of Nursing. (2021a). *Membership*. https://www.ncsbn.org/membership.htm

National Council of State Boards of Nursing. (2021b). *Nurse licensure compact* (NLC). https://www.ncsbn.org/nurse-licensure-compact.htm

Nevada State Board of Nursing. (2020). *COVID-19 resources and information*. http://nevadanursingboard.org/covid-19-resource-and-information/

Schindler, L., Puls-Elvidge, S., Welzant, H., & Crawford, L. (2015). Definitions of quality in higher education: A synthesis of the literature. *Higher Learning Research Communications*, *5*(3), 3–13.

Scriven, M. (1974). Evaluation perspectives and procedures. In W. J. Popham (Ed.), *Evaluation in education: Current applications* (pp.). McCutchan.

Scriven, M. (1996). Types of evaluation and types of evaluator. *Evaluation Practice*, *17*(2), 151–161. https://journals.sagepub.com/doi/pdf/10.1177/109821409601700207

Stufflebeam, D. L., Foley, W., Gephart, W., Guba, E., Hammond, R., Merriman, H., & Provus, M. (1971). *Educational evaluation and decision making*. Peacock.

U.S. Department of Education. (2021). *Accreditation in the United States*. https://www2.ed.gov/admins/finaid/accred/accreditation_pg6.html

CHAPTER 15

Planning for the Accreditation Visit

Susan M. Ervin

CHAPTER OBJECTIVES

Upon completion of Chapter 15, the reader will be able to:

- Discuss the benefits of accreditation in nursing education.
- Prepare for an accreditation evaluation visit, including developing a timeline, writing the self-study, and preparing a resource room.
- Differentiate between onsite and virtual accreditation evaluation visits.
- Discuss preparation of faculty, students, and programs' communities of interest for the accreditation evaluation visit.
- Relate the role of continuous quality improvement to accreditation.

OVERVIEW

The primary purpose of accreditation for nursing education programs is to protect the interests of the public. Accreditation demonstrates program quality, provides eligibility for receipt of federal funding, increases marketability, and facilitates academic progression for graduates (Halstead, 2017). Nursing education programs directly affect public health and safety; thus, they must demonstrate rigorous standards in the preparation of graduates.

This chapter reviews nursing education programs' preparation for accreditation. In addition, there is a discussion of the description and comparison of regulatory bodies and accreditation at the institutional and program level. Although addressed in Chapter 14, "Program Evaluation and Accreditation," presented here is a review of bodies that accredit nursing programs and a discussion of the benefits of accreditation to nursing education. COVID-19 affected the accreditation process, including site visits by evaluators. Provided in this chapter is a case study of a nursing program preparing to host a site visit during the pandemic and the process of holding a virtual visit.

ACCREDITATION

Accreditation is a voluntary, nongovernmental peer-review process undertaken by higher education institutions (universities and community colleges) and programs (e.g., academic nursing programs) within those institutions. It focuses on the quality of universities and community colleges and the ability of institutional educational programs to meet their mission, goals, and outcomes (Beasley et al., 2019; Commission on Collegiate Nursing Education [CCNE], 2018).

The U.S. Department of Education (USDE) is the official government body that recognizes accrediting bodies in the United States at the institutional and program levels. Institutional accreditation focuses on the entire university or community college. In the United States, regional accrediting bodies recognized by the USDE usually accredit colleges and universities. These include the Middle States Commission on Higher Education; the New England Association of Schools and Colleges, Commission on Institutions of Higher Education; the North Central Association of Colleges and Schools, The Higher Learning Commission; the Northwest Commission on Colleges and Universities; the Southern Association of Colleges and Schools, Commission on Colleges; the Western Association of Schools and Colleges, Accrediting Commission for Community and Junior Colleges; and the Western Association of Schools and Colleges, Senior Colleges and University Commission. These regional bodies have the infrastructure and paid staff to support their missions to ensure higher education institutions' quality.

Nursing educational programs within institutions receive accreditation by one of two bodies recognized by the USDE: the Accreditation Commission for Education in Nursing (ACEN) and the CCNE. The Council for Higher Education Accreditation (CHEA; www.chea.org/), an organization of institutions in higher education whose purpose and mission is to ensure academic quality, recognizes both of these accrediting bodies. A third accrediting body, the National League for Nursing Commission for Nursing Education Accreditation (NLN CNEA), received recognition from the USDE in May 2021; however, the discussion in this chapter focuses on the ACEN and the CCNE.

Both the ACEN and CCNE have established standards and criteria that nursing programs must meet to obtain accreditation. The ACEN (2020) provides accreditation for all levels of nursing education, from practical nursing to clinical doctorate programs within the United States, U.S. territories, and internationally in countries such as Jordan, Saudi Arabia, and Turkey. The ACEN also serves as a Title IV-HEA Gatekeeper for some practical nursing programs and hospital-based programs eligible to participate in financial aid from the USDE. This ensures that these programs comply with the Higher Education Reauthorization Act, Title IV, which addresses federal student aid programs for higher education (www.acennursing.org). CCNE provides accreditation for baccalaureate, master's, doctor of nursing practice (DNP), and post-graduate APRN programs in the United States. Both accrediting bodies support and encourage continuous quality improvement (CQI) that contributes to the continued growth and improvement of nursing education programs (ACEN, 2020; CCNE, 2018). Typically, nursing education programs seek accreditation from either the ACEN or the CCNE, although a few attain accreditation by both bodies (Spector et al., 2018).

As discussed in Chapter 14, "Program Evaluation and Accreditation," there are specialized accreditors for nursing programs with specialty tracks in their graduate programs. Nursing specialty accrediting bodies recognized by the USDE include the American Association of Nurse Anesthetists and the American College of Nursing Midwives (USDE, 2021). The Consensus Model for APRNs Licensure, Accreditation, Certification & Education (LACE)—was developed in 2008 by representatives from professional nursing organizations, nursing educators, certification bodies, and state boards of nursing and identified four areas of advanced practice. These include nurse anesthetists, clinical specialists, nurse midwives, and nurse practitioners. It also recognizes certified nurse practitioners who practice in acute care and primary care settings and are educated and certified for both roles. Advanced practice nurses must be licensed by the state board of nursing where they practice, certified by a certification program recognized by the National Council of State Boards of Nursing (NCSBN), and educated in an accredited institution recognized by the USDE and according to the standards delineated in the Consensus Model. A detailed description of the Consensus Model: LACE may be found at the NCSBN (www.ncsbn.org/Consensus_Model_for_APRN_Regulation_July_2008.pdf).

The Accreditation Process

Nursing education programs that seek accreditation submit an application and a self-study document that defines how the program meets the accrediting body's standards. The accreditation process enables the nursing program to engage in an in-depth self-analysis and evaluation; it results in a self-study document that articulates its compliance with the accrediting body's standards. A scheduled accreditation evaluation visit (also called a site visit) usually occurs approximately six weeks after the self-study is submitted to the accrediting body (the ACEN or the CCNE). Evaluators who participate in these visits have in-depth knowledge of accrediting body standards and are experts in nursing education and practice (Beasley et al., 2019). The purpose of the evaluation visit is to validate the information in the self-study, assess compliance with accreditation standards, and review processes programs have in place for continuous quality improvement (CQI; ACEN, 2020; CCNE, 2019). After the self-study is submitted, but prior to the evaluation visit, the program notifies its community of interest (e.g., students, faculty, alumni, clinical bodies) that an accreditation visit is scheduled and the opportunity exists to provide comments directly to the accrediting body about the quality of the nursing program.

In preparation for the site visit, the nursing program establishes a resource room in which materials such as those referenced in the self-study, the program's systematic plan for evaluation, course syllabi, faculty vitae and achievements, and student work samples are available for review by the evaluators. During the site visit, evaluators review documentation in the resource room. They also visit classroom, lab, and clinical sites and meet with administrators, faculty, students, and other program constituents to ask questions and explore constituent experiences with the nursing program. The evaluators provide informal feedback at the conclusion of the visit. A formal report is provided to the chief nurse administrator of the program 2 to 3 weeks following the site visit, and there is a period (at least 15 days) in which they can respond to the report. The chief nurse administrator, in their response, may offer corrections of errors and comments that agree or disagree with the evaluators' findings or provide additional documentation that supports program compliance with accreditation standards (CCNE, 2019).

An accrediting body review committee (CCNE) or panel (ACEN) receives the self-study document, evaluation team report, and response to the team report. The committee or panel reviews all materials and develops a proposed accreditation action forwarded to the ACEN or CCNE board of commissioners. The action usually includes accreditation status and length, identification of any program areas of concern, and a schedule for submission of progress reports (ACEN, 2020; CCNE, 2019). The board of commissioners notifies the program of the final accreditation decision approximately 6 months following the site visit. The board of commissioners may grant the program accreditation. Programs receive accreditation for 5 years if applying for initial accreditation and 10 years for those that applied for reaccreditation. The board of commissioners may make other decisions as well. They may deny accreditation to programs that fail to meet accreditation standards, or they may continue accreditation with conditions or warnings if a program partially meets standards (ACEN, 2020). Accreditation may also be withdrawn if the program does not meet standards, the parent institution loses accreditation, or programs close (CCNE, 2019).

The COVID-19 pandemic drastically changed the accreditation process for programs of nursing. The ACEN and the CCNE moved from on-site to virtual accreditation evaluation visits beginning in the fall of 2020. Programs still submitted a self-study and planned for evaluators to meet with faculty, students, and other constituents. All meetings and observations were virtual, however. Platforms such as Zoom, Microsoft Teams, Google Meet, and GoToMeeting were available for meetings between evaluators and students, faculty, and other constituents. Visitors received supporting documentation via an electronic format, such as a USB drive, or through the institution's learning management system (LMS). Using the LMS was advantageous because of password security and date restriction for access. This alleviates concerns about loss, damage, or unauthorized access to documents (especially student documents) on a USB drive (Cobourne & Shellenbargar, 2021).

Within 24 months of the virtual visit, each program will have an on-site follow-up visit, which the USDE mandates as necessary to meet statutory and regulatory requirements (CCNE, 2020). As of this writing, scheduling these visits has yet to be determined and depends on COVID-19 status and recommendations from national health bodies. The ACEN has decided to conduct onsite visits in fall 2021 (www.acenursing.net/resources/Overview_of_Fall_2021_Site_Visits.pdf); at this writing, there is no information about CCNE site visits for the fall of 2021.

Approval by Regulatory Bodies

While accreditation is a voluntary process for nursing education programs, approval by regulatory bodies such as state boards of nursing (BON) is not; it is mandatory. Only students who graduate from BON-approved programs can take the National Council Licensure Examination (NCLEX). The primary mission of a state BON is to protect the public, and nursing program approval ensures the program provides the knowledge and skills graduates need to pass the NCLEX and practice competently and safely (Spector et al., 2018). Although each state has individual requirements for program approval in its Nurse Practice Act (NPA), there are standard key components that BON regulators evaluate:

- The governing entity (institutional support, regional accreditation of the institution, nursing specialty accreditation)
- Program leadership (qualifications of the chief nurse administrator and their ability to make autonomous decisions about the program)
- Faculty qualifications and governance, curriculum (elements and teaching–learning strategies)
- Adequacy of clinical learning experiences, physical and fiscal resources
- A plan for CQI (Spector et al., 2018)

Most BONs require submission of an executive summary or self-study document that illustrates the strengths and challenges of the program, current enrollment data, curricular materials such as syllabi, and the preparation and specialty areas of current faculty. Site evaluators visit new nursing programs to ensure they meet state regulations. Depending on the state, periodic reports (usually annually), or site visits may be required for established nursing programs to ensure continuous compliance with the state's NPA (Spector et al., 2018).

Approval by the state BON is necessary for a school to admit students. New programs must provide evidence of need, assurance that resources, including clinical sites; are available (many BONs require clinical site contracts to be in place before the program admits students); and evidence of an adequate student pool (Spector et al., 2018). This approval and measurements such as high completion rates and strong

NCLEX and specialty certification scores reflect the quality of a nursing program. It can create, however, a limited perspective on how well a program is meeting its mission, goals, and expected outcomes (Halstead, 2017). Accreditation of a nursing program goes beyond this perspective and provides public recognition of a nursing program's quality determined by a peer-review, standards-based process (Halstead, 2017).

Benefits to Accreditation

There are multiple benefits to accreditation. The nursing education program receives public acknowledgment of its quality. It is eligible to receive federal or state funding, which can be used for program initiatives (such as expanding graduate APRN specialty tracks to meet the needs of a program's community of interest). Accreditation also ensures that students are eligible for financial aid (Halstead, 2017). An increased number of nursing programs assess differential fees, an additional amount added to the institution's base tuition rate. These fees can place an extra burden on students; hence, financial aid may be integral to student success. Accreditation also facilitates academic progression for students; graduation from an accredited baccalaureate or master's program may be an admission criterion for further education. Graduates may be more marketable as some employers prefer to hire nurses who have graduated from an accredited program (Halstead, 2017).

CQI is a hallmark of the accreditation process. This process requires faculty to commit to the ongoing and systematic evaluation of the nursing program. This includes goal setting and reviewing how the nursing program has met expected outcomes related to governance, resources, faculty, students, and a community of interest, teaching–learning, and evaluation, all elements addressed in the standards of accrediting bodies (Halstead, 2017). CQI also allows faculty to highlight the nursing program, which can enhance student and faculty recruitment and attract donors and potential funding partners that invest in programs that demonstrate success in meeting their mission, goals, and outcomes.

Finally, accreditation supports innovation and program change. The written standards for both the ACEN and the CCNE are to support innovation through program self-assessment and implementation of evidence-based, reflective changes of the community of interests' needs. The standards support developing a curriculum that integrates societal and healthcare trends and incorporating multiple teaching, learning, and evaluation strategies (Halstead, 2020). Accrediting bodies and nursing programs have a common goal of ensuring quality nursing education that will benefit the profession by strengthening the quality of the nursing workforce (Halstead, 2020).

ACCREDITATION CASE STUDY

Chapter 14, "Program Evaluation and Accreditation," addressed program evaluation and the purpose of accreditation. This chapter has addressed the accreditation process, which is similar between the two nursing accrediting bodies, the ACEN and the CCNE. The following case study reviews the process for preparation for accreditation, including the development of a timeline, preparation of the self-study document, and hosting the site/evaluation visit. It incorporates changes in the process that resulted from the COVID-19 pandemic. The information applies to full program accreditation, specialty accreditation, or state board visits.

Getting Started

The accreditation process provides the opportunity for nursing faculty to illustrate the strengths of the educational program and validate current CQI processes.

Approximately 12 to 18 months before the site visit, the accrediting body notifies the chief nursing administrator regarding making arrangements for reaccreditation. At that time, the program confirms the dates for submission of the self-study and the site visit. It is essential, however, that the nursing program be aware of accreditation and accreditation expiration dates. It is ideal to begin preparing for accreditation approximately 3 years before the accreditation expiration date. Waiting until notification from the accrediting body may not leave the program adequate time to gather data needed for program analysis, write the self-study document, and prepare a resource room sufficient for the evaluators' needs.

◆ *Baccalaureate and master's degree nursing programs in a midsize school received accreditation in the spring of 2011; the dean and faculty are aware that the spring of 2021 is the program's next scheduled visit for reaccreditation in spring 2021. The baccalaureate program has approximately 260 prelicensure students and 110 master's students. At the first faculty/staff meeting in the fall semester of 2018, the dean informs the faculty that preparations for accreditation will begin that semester.*

The first step in the accreditation process is to determine the needed structures and processes for gathering program data, writing the self-study, and preparing for the evaluation visit. An effective committee structure and a robust systematic evaluation plan contribute to accreditation preparation (Haverkamp et al., 2017). A program evaluation committee (PEC), for example, can review outcomes in each program for congruency with accreditation standards. Undergraduate and graduate curriculum committees review and develop curricula that reflect accreditation and other professional standards and guidelines.

A robust systematic evaluation plan is part of CQI and delineates evidence needed to ensure the program meets its mission, goals, and outcomes; who is responsible for that evidence; and the location of that evidence. A PEC is integral to this process; it can determine what data are currently collected and additional needed information and supporting documents for the self-study and the site visit. The systematic evaluation plan is based on accrediting body standards; it also reflects the program's mission, goals, and outcomes. Accrediting bodies will want data that address those outcomes, such as NCLEX and national certification pass rates, employment rates, and student satisfaction ratings.

The chief nursing administrator typically appoints faculty to work on an accreditation committee that will prepare the self-study, set timelines, and prepare for the evaluation visit. The chair of the committee should be a senior faculty member who has previous experience with accreditation. One or more faculty members should attend training sessions offered by the accrediting body. Historically, these have been face-to-face sessions, but because of the COVID-19 pandemic, accrediting bodies provided a series of webinars that addressed the preparation of the self-study and hosting a virtual evaluation visit.

◆ *In the fall semester of 2018, the dean of the nursing program met with standing committees within the school to determine their role in preparation for accreditation. The dean appointed a senior faculty member who sat on the PEC to act as chair of the accreditation committee (an ad hoc committee), whose responsibility would be to prepare for accreditation. The dean appointed three other faculty to the committee: a curriculum committee member, a faculty member who taught primarily in the undergraduate program, and a faculty member who taught mainly in the graduate program. As a group, they decided to review each accreditation standard of the accrediting body and take a close look at how the program meets each standard. The committee decides to divide the workload and have committee meetings regularly.*

Timeline

A timeline for preparing the self-study and the evaluation visits depends on the expected date of reaccreditation. About 3 years before the evaluation visit, the nursing program should conduct a thorough assessment of the mission, goals, outcomes, curriculum, and evaluation plan. The accrediting body may require a progress report at the midpoint of the accreditation cycle, which is also a good time for this assessment (Haverkamp et al., 2017). The timeline is essential to keep the momentum and timeliness of a project such as accreditation moving forward. It is helpful to develop a "backward calendar" by looking at the date that the self-study report is to be submitted to the accrediting body.

◆ *The accreditation committee members meet to develop a master calendar/timeline. They work backward from the date of the accreditation visit, which will be in the spring semester of 2021. They set deadlines for gathering data, writing the self-study, and preparing the resource room. All faculty through a faculty retreat and assessment days built into faculty schedules undertakes a thorough assessment of the mission, goals, and outcomes; the curriculum; and the evaluation plan.*

The Accreditation Committee

The accreditation committee determines how program information will be gathered, shared, and stored for the evaluators and the site visit. While individual faculty members may be involved in preparing the self-study and resource room, the accreditation committee assumes major responsibility for these. It is critical that the self-study reads as one programmatic voice. The self-study focuses on topics specific to the accreditation standards. These specifics include the mission and vision of the organization, admission standards, enrollment data, student retention, employment of graduates, curriculum plan, pedagogical approaches, faculty preparation, faculty and preceptor preparation and competence, institutional functions that impact the school of nursing, program resources, administrative support, faculty resources, strategic planning processes, stakeholder needs, and an analysis of all program learning outcomes.

The committee will identify nonfaculty staff members who assist in accreditation through preparing the agenda and coordinating meetings between evaluators and students, faculty, and other stakeholders. They will also identify key members within the institution who will meet with evaluators such as the president, provost, relevant senate and committee members, librarian, informatics and data-processing administrators, and distance learning staff.

◆ ***2018–2020 (1–3 years prior to the site visit):*** *The accreditation committee reviews accreditation procedures to become familiar with the process. Changes in curricula generated from the assessment go through program and institution approval processes and are implemented with ongoing evaluation by the curriculum committee and PEC.*

◆ ***Spring 2020:*** *The accrediting body informs all nursing programs that, beginning in the fall of 2020, all evaluation site visits will be virtual because of the COVID-19 pandemic. The accreditation c works with the dean to evaluate how that change will affect the evaluation visit for the spring semester of 2021. All meetings with the evaluators will use Zoom, and the resource room will be virtual rather than on-site. The committee discusses the development of a virtual resource room to ensure ease of navigation for the evaluators and demonstrate the strengths of the nursing program. The committee plans for the structure of the resource room according to the accreditation standards, and documentation referenced in the self-study.*

The accreditation committee writes the first draft of the self-study. Faculty from standing committees within the program contribute to the draft. For example, the undergraduate and graduate curriculum committees take responsibility for reflecting on the key elements of the standard that addresses curricula (Standard III for CCNE, Standard 4 for ACEN) and highlighting the programs' successes. Faculty also audit materials integral to the programs, such as course catalogs, websites, syllabi, and grading criteria, to ensure accuracy. While the accreditation committee takes a major role in preparation for accreditation, all faculty are involved to ensure they understand the process and become knowledgeable about the standards and guidelines of the accrediting body.

◆ **Summer 2020:** *The accreditation committee views a series of webinars developed by the accrediting body that addresses the accreditation process, how the self-study will address accreditation standards, and what to expect in a virtual evaluation site visit.*

◆ **Fall 2020:** *The accreditation committee chair serves to be the consistent voice for writing subsequent drafts and the final version of the self-study, ensuring all faculty have the opportunity for feedback. The dean begins communication with the accreditation evaluators, creating an agenda that includes meetings with administrators, faculty, clinical partners, preceptors, and students. The dean's administrative assistant serves as the nonfaculty staff member who will work with the dean on the agenda and, during the site visit, initiates Zoom meetings between the evaluators and various constituents.*

Role of Faculty, Students, Administrators, and Stakeholders

Prepare all constituents who will participate in the site visit well in advance. Ensure that faculty know the evaluators will interview them about the program, courses, clinical settings, and students. All faculty members, full-time and part-time, should be familiar with the standards of the accrediting body, the curriculum, and their role in the delivery and evaluation of the program. Students should be aware of the accreditation process and familiar with their program and its goals and that they will have an opportunity to meet with the visitors. The chief nursing administrator of the program should ensure that all faculty members, including part-time clinical instructors and off-campus faculty, are available during the site visit.

The visitors may ask to speak to stakeholders and other institution members outside of the nursing department. In advance of the visit, the chief nursing administrator should work with the evaluators to determine with whom the evaluators wish to meet (president, provost, faculty, students, clinical partner representatives, and institutional support staff such as librarians, information technology, and student resources). Well before the site visit, the team develops a tentative agenda.

◆ **Spring and Fall Semesters 2020:** *For all faculty-meeting agendas, schedule the accreditation committee to provide updates on the accreditation process, the development of the self-study, and preparation for the site visit. The chair of the accreditation committee, provided two faculty development sessions in the fall semester of 2020 to help prepare faculty for the upcoming visit; discussion focused on the review of accreditation standards, how the program meets those standards, the review of the self-study, and the role of faculty in the accreditation evaluation visit. The chair also provided two sessions for undergraduate and graduate students to help prepare them for the site visit. The purpose and benefits of accreditation are discussed and students are provided possible questions (with answers) that evaluators might ask during the site visit.*

◆ **Spring Semester 2021:** *The dean, the dean's administrative assistant, and the chair of the accreditation committee prepare the agenda for the virtual site visit. People identified by the evaluators are scheduled. Because the site visit is virtual, consideration regarding the time zones of the evaluators when scheduling meetings were included on the agenda.*

◆ *The institution's LMS provided the location for a virtual resource room. Organizing the virtual resource room in accordance with the accrediting body's standards and key elements provided for ease of navigation by the evaluators. The resource room opened 1 week prior to the site visit, and the accreditation committee chair provided orientation for the evaluators. An information technology (IT) staff member served as a contact person for the evaluators should they have difficulties navigating the room. Materials that would have been placed in the on0site resource room (those referenced in the self-study, the program's systematic evaluation plan, course syllabi, faculty vitae and achievements, student work samples) were uploaded into the virtual room. Pictures of clinical sites were included. In addition, the evaluators viewed an uploaded, captioned pictorial of the campus physical facilities and student resources, and the school of nursing classrooms, labs, and faculty offices. Because evaluators were not onsite, creative approaches to the observation of students were developed. Videos of students in lab and simulation settings were developed and uploaded to the resource room. These videos included Skills Lab, medication administration, IV placement, and respiratory assessment. Actual simulation experiences (birthing, Code Blue) were videotaped and uploaded into the resource room including pre- and postbriefings with faculty and students. During the site visit, Zoom served as the platform for meetings between the evaluators and all constituents who met with them. The dean's administrative assistant began each meeting and then assigned host responsibilities to the designated evaluator once the meeting began. The last day of the evaluation, the accreditation team met with all faculty via Zoom to provide feedback on their findings.*

SUMMARY

The accreditation process ensures the public that a nursing program provides graduates with an education that prepares them not only to pass the licensing exam but also to practice safely and competently. Accreditation provides an endorsement that the program meets rigorous academic and professional standards developed by accrediting bodies recognized by the USDE. The accreditation process, from preparing the self-study to the site visit provides a nursing program opportunity to celebrate their successes and examine areas for improvement. The COVID-19 pandemic mandated changes in the process, moving parts, such as the site visit and the resource room, from a face-to-face to a virtual one.

END-OF-CHAPTER RESOURCES

DISCUSSION QUESTIONS

1. The COVID-19 pandemic dramatically changed the accreditation process. Historically, the site visit, including meeting with constituents, was face-to-face, and the resource room was on-site and available to evaluators during the visit. With the COVID-19 pandemic, the site visit, including meetings, took place via a platform such as Zoom, and the resource room became virtual, often through the institution's LMS. What are some of the advantages and disadvantages of each type of site visit and resource room? Think about the future of education, accreditation, and technology. Do you think that virtual visits should become the standard for accreditation? Why or why not?

2. Many educational systems in other nations in the world are under the direct supervision and regulations of the government. In the United States, accreditation is voluntary, although there are factors that curtail its activities if it is not accredited. Debate the pros and cons of voluntary versus regulated accreditation to ensure quality education. Do you believe the U.S. system of accreditation for higher education works? Explain the rationale for your answer.

LEARNING ACTIVITIES

Student-Learning Activities

1. Go to the websites of the ACEN, the CCNE, and the NLN CNEA and compare the standards for accreditation for each body according to the levels of education they accredit. What are the differences, if any, among the bodies?

2. Interview several faculty members for their perspectives on accreditation and its role in ensuring quality nursing education. Based on the interviews, do you think it is essential for all faculty members to be aware of accreditation processes? Why or why not?

Faculty Development Activities

1. Review the last self-study accreditation report for your nursing program. Identify changes in the program that took place after the visit. Were the changes a result of the accreditation process, or were there other factors that brought about the changes? Based on your review, what recommendations do you have for the next accreditation visit?

2. Identify the accreditation body for your nursing program. Review its standards/criteria for accreditation. What are strategies in your program in place to gather data that relate to the standards? Are current data in place and ready for analysis, evaluation, and follow-up on findings to ensure that the program meets the standards? What role in these strategies do you believe faculty has?

 SPRINGER PUBLISHING CONNECT™   A robust set of instructor resources designed to supplement this text is located at **http://connect.springerpub.com/content/book/978-0-8261-8686-7.** Qualifying instructors may request access by emailing **textbook@springerpub.com.**

REFERENCES

Accreditation Commission for Education in Nursing. (2020). *ACEN 2017 accreditation manual.* https://www.acenursing.org/Resources-for-Nursing-Programs/ACEN-Accreditation-Manual-General-Information.pdf

Beasley, S. F., Farmer, S., Ard, N., & Nunn-Ellison, K. (2019). A voice in the accreditation process: The role of peer evaluator. *Teaching and Learning in Nursing, 14,* A3–A5. https://doi.org/10.1016/j.teln.2019.06.001

Cobourne, K., & Shellenbarger, T. (2021). Virtual site visits: A new approach to nursing accreditation. *Teaching and Learning in Nursing Education, 16,* 162–165. https://doi.org/10.1016/j.teln.2020.11.001

Commission on Collegiate Nursing Education. (2018). *Standards for accreditation of baccalaureate and graduate nursing programs.* https://www.aacnnursing.org/Portals/42/CCNE/PDF/Standards-Final-2018.pdf

Commission on Collegiate Nursing Education. (2019). *Procedures for accreditation of baccalaureate and graduate nursing programs.* https://www.aacnnursing.org/Portals/42/CCNE/PDF/Procedures.pdf

Commission on Collegiate Nursing Education. (2020). *Frequently asked questions: Virtual evaluations nursing education programs.* https://www.aacnnursing.org/Portals/42/CCNE/News/Virtual-Evaluation-FAQs-for-Education-CCNE.pdf

Halstead, J. A. (2017). The value of nursing program accreditation. *Teaching and Learning in Nursing, 12,* 181–182. https://doi.org/10.1016/j.teln.2017.03.005

Halstead, J. A. (2020). Fostering innovation in nursing education: The role of accreditation. *Teaching and Learning in Nursing, 15,* A4–A5. https://doi.org/10.1016/j.teln.2019.10.003

Haverkamp, J., Ribar, A. K., Ball, K., Ballard, K., Butz, S., Chovan, J. D., Fried, E. M., Garrett, B., Hughes, K., Keane. P., Prusinski, R., & Shoemaker, J. R. (2017). A map for successful CCNE accreditation. *Journal of Professional Nursing,* 1–7. https://doi.org/10.1016/j.profnurs.2017.09.003

Spector, N., Hooper, J. I., Silvestre, J., & Hong, Q. (2018). Board of Nursing approval of registered nurse education programs. *Journal of Nursing Regulation, 8,* 22–31. https://doi.org/10.1016/S2155-8256(17)30178-3

U.S. Department of Education. (2020). *About ED.* https://www2.ed.gov/about/landing.jhtml

U.S. Department of Education. (2021, June). *Statement from the U.S. Department of Education on the status of recognition of nine accrediting agencies and withdrawal of recognition of the accrediting Council for Independent Colleges and Schools.* https://www.ed.gov/news/press-releases/statement-us-department-education-status-recognition-nine-accrediting-agencies-and-withdrawal-recognition-accrediting-council-independent-colleges-and-schools

SECTION V

RESEARCH, ISSUES, AND TRENDS IN NURSING EDUCATION

Stephanie Stimac DeBoor

OVERVIEW

This section provides a review of the current literature, existing issues, and trends in nursing education for their effect on curricula and the priorities derived from them that influence curriculum development and evaluation activities now and in the future. Chapter 16, "Research and Evidence-Based Practice in Nursing Education," reviews faculty's role in scholarship and the current state of research in nursing education, as it applies to curriculum development and evaluation. Identified are gaps in the literature and the need for further research on these topics, which provide the basis for evidence-based educational practice. A summary of the scholarly/research-based articles found in nursing and educational literature and presented throughout this text provides ideas for future research questions.

Chapter 17, "Issues and Challenges for Nursing Educators," summarizes the text chapters and reexamines some of the issues raised to offer possible solutions that could affect the future of nursing education. An examination of nursing education in hindsight leads to future forecasting of scenarios affecting the profession. If the pandemic showed us nothing else, it provided a way to dispense of stale educational teaching methods and embrace innovative, online delivery while maintaining mandates to produce knowledgeable, competent, and caring professionals. Ultimately, through creativity, nursing programs continue to educate nurses ready for the challenges of the current healthcare system. Nursing must continue to embrace higher education for practice entry or find itself out of step with other professionals and the healthcare system. This section begins the discussion for nursing educators and their role in meaningful research, scholarship, translational science, and evidence-based practice in nursing education to meet the challenges and plan for the future.

CHAPTER 16

Research and Evidence-Based Practice in Nursing Education

Teresa Serratt

CHAPTER OBJECTIVES

Upon completion of Chapter 16, the reader will be able to:

- Reflect on the faculty role in scholarship including research in nursing education and its influence on curriculum development and evaluation.

- Explore the utilization of research and translational science that can result in the development of evidence-based curriculum development and evaluation.

- Analyze current curriculum development and evaluation research in nursing education.

- Identify gaps in the body of literature pertaining to curriculum development and evaluation requiring further exploration through scholarly activity.

OVERVIEW

The role of nursing faculty typically encompasses three key activities: teaching, scholarship/research, and service. Although often described as separate activities, these activities often overlap. For example, faculty integrate their research findings into the courses they teach, identify areas for inquiry requiring the generation of new knowledge or the search for current evidence, and provide service within their departments to ensure the curriculum is updated and program outcomes are met. Although the emphasis on these areas may differ by faculty position/title, college, and/or university, the need for scholarship in curriculum development and evaluation is unquestionable. In this chapter, the faculty role as scholar is examined through the lens of curriculum development and curriculum evaluation. A more comprehensive definition of scholarly activity that embodies these overlapping areas of teaching, scholarship/research, and service is explored and key terms defined. Additionally, an overview of the current state of research related to curriculum development and curriculum evaluation is presented along with a reflection on the gaps in the literature, recommendations, and suggested topics for further examination.

Definitions of Scholarship, Research, and Evidence-Based Practice

Before we start our exploration of faculty roles and responsibilities related to scholarship, it is important to define commonly utilized terms. The American Association for Colleges of Nursing (AACN) defines *scholarship* as those activities that systematically advance the teaching, research, and practice of nursing through rigorous inquiry that (a) is significant to the profession, (b) is creative, (c) can be documented, (d) can be replicated or elaborated, and (e) can be peer-reviewed through various methods (AACN, 1999). This definition was influenced by the seminal publication *Scholarship Reconsidered: Priorities of the Professoriate* by Ernest Boyer (1990), who sought to examine what it meant to be an academic scholar. At the time, and still today in many universities, a scholar is considered to be someone who conducts research and is evaluated, in large part, by how many publications they have produced.

According to Boyer (1990), there are four components that promote faculty's integration of teaching activities, research, and scholarship: the scholarship of "discovery," "integration," "application," and "teaching." He describes the scholarship of "discovery" as those activities that result in the generation of new knowledge. For faculty educators, ideas can germinate from interactions between colleagues and students, during the facilitation of teaching and learning strategies, or from the experiences of developing and evaluating programs and/or curriculum. The scholarship of "integration" is bringing together knowledge, both within and outside of the discipline to foster understanding, communication, and collaboration that broadens the knowledge base. This interdisciplinary focus is particularly salient as nurse faculty prepare future nurses to successfully participate in interdisciplinary teams. The scholarship of "application" refers to the application of new knowledge to solve problems and can encompass a breadth of activities and issues. It is evidence-based practice and should be tested and evaluated as it evolves from theory to practice. This is the essence of translational science. The final component is "teaching" as scholarship. Teaching is a means of creatively sharing knowledge with the learner in ways that optimize learning and of exploring new knowledge and ways of applying models and strategies to the science of nursing education. Boyer's model provides a framework for faculty educators as they carry out their activities in teaching, scholarship/research, and service as these activities contribute to the discipline of nursing. Nursing education research findings should be disseminated so that faculty can develop and facilitate evidence-based practice into curriculum development and evaluation.

Now that *scholarship* has been defined, we turn to two other terms that need clarification. We often use the words *research* and *evidence-based* to imply a generalized meaning during informal conversations that may or not represent the true systematic processes involved. For the purpose of this discussion, *research* is defined as "the systematic inquiry designed to develop trustworthy evidence about issues of importance to the nursing profession, including nursing practice, education, administration, and informatics" (Polit & Beck, 2017, p. 2). Evidence-based practice is "a problem-solving approach to the delivery of healthcare that integrates best evidence from studies and patient care data with clinician expertise and patient preferences and values" (Melnyk et al., 2010, p. 51). While most definitions of *evidence-based practice* tend to utilize a clinical focus, studies exploring concepts and issues related to curriculum development and evaluation can inform evidence-based educational practice. Best practices are developed from a process of critical appraisal that incorporates relevant current research, expert opinion, clinical judgment, and patient values. Faculty utilize best practices that stem from evidence-based appraisals of teaching strategies, curriculum development, and evaluation and incorporate evidence-based content into their curricula.

Nursing Faculty Roles and Responsibilities Related to Scholarship

Scholarly activities are important components of the faculty role. Professional nursing organizations and nursing academia have embraced a broad definition of *scholarly activity* that is inclusive of nurse faculty with diverse educational preparation and institutional expectations. According to their education and expertise, nurse educators can participate in scholarly activities anywhere along the continuum from posing a research question to conducting a study to disseminating results or implementing evidence-based practices. Scholarly activities are particularly important for the development of relevant nursing programs and curriculum that center on learner competencies and program outcomes and meets the needs of the profession, healthcare system, and society. The National League for Nursing (NLN, 2021a) identifies scholarship as an essential part of the faculty role and established engaging in scholarship as one of the core competencies for nurse educators. Similar to AACN's (1999) position expressed in *Defining Scholarship for the Profession of Nursing*, the NLN includes teaching in its definition of *scholarly activity*.

A scholar seeks out the current state of knowledge and applies that knowledge to practice. They identify topics and issues needing additional investigation and share observations with others through discussion, debate, and presenting findings and/or writing scholarly publications based on evidence surrounding the topic. These activities lead to the generation of knowledge that builds and enhances the sciences of the profession and education and ultimately addresses nursing's social mandate to protect, promote, and optimize the health of people, populations, and communities (American Nurses Association [ANA], 2010).

In the absence of current knowledge, scholars raise questions and explore contextual factors that merit further investigation. Research questions are generated to guide inquiries and/or hypotheses that result in proposals for investigation. Studies are designed after a search of the literature that is designed to identify concepts and theories that relate to the topic and help provide a foundation for the proposed research. Study designs can vary from a pilot study to in-depth studies and include qualitative, quantitative, and mixed-methods approaches depending on the availability of resources and the type of research question being asked. Tenure-track nursing faculty are usually expected to engage in research as a component of their academic scholarship. Non-tenure-track faculty or those in multipurpose institutions typically do not have expectations of research but are expected to contribute to the profession through scholarship related to pedagogy and practice. It is imperative that nursing faculty understand the measures that will be used to evaluate their performance particularly as it relates to tenure and promotion.

A newly emerging area of scholarship is translational science, which utilizes research findings to develop evidence-based practice recommendations. It spans all disciplines and provides opportunities for multidisciplinary collaboration and interprofessional education of students in preparation for the collaborative relationships necessary to succeed in a multidisciplinary health system. Translational science has been described as "scientific findings or discoveries from basic laboratory, clinical, or population studies into new clinical tools, processes, or applications," thus, improving patient care and promoting public health. The intent is to build the bridge from "bench to bedside" (Grady, 2010, p. 164). As the call for stronger academic–clinical partnerships to advance healthcare transformation increases, translational science helps provide a natural connection between academia and healthcare entities. The DNP, as the nursing practice doctorate, has the knowledge and skills to translate evidence into practice. Partnering with academic health centers, academic nurse faculty (PhD or DNP) can help improve health outcomes by developing and disseminating their scholarship or by implementing evidence-based innovations in the clinical setting (Trautman et al., 2018).

CURRENT RESEARCH ON CURRICULA DEVELOPMENT AND CURRICULA EVALUATION

An exploration of available research on nursing curriculum development and evaluation in the United States and published over the last 10 years was performed to ascertain the current body of knowledge available to inform faculty practice. While many seminal studies remain relevant resources for faculty today, the proliferation of educational and clinical technologies, increasing diversity of students, and rapid changes in the U.S. healthcare system present new challenges for nursing faculty. Today's nurse educators are charged with meeting the needs of diverse students by developing curricula that meet the goals for diversity (the presence of difference), inclusion (people with different identities feeling/being welcomed and valued into a particular setting), and equity (everyone has access to the same opportunities to grow, develop and contribute). They also must assist their students in acquiring the knowledge, skills, and attitudes to foster these competencies in their nursing practice (AACN, 2017). Newer studies that address or consider these changes are necessary to help inform and guide innovative education solutions.

Curriculum Development and Revision

In this updated edition of this textbook, the literature was reviewed for current research and studies in curriculum development in nursing. Most of these were surveys or descriptive studies focused on models/frameworks for curriculum development/design or integrating concepts such as leadership, compassion, and end-of-life and culturally competent care into the curriculum. Notably, there was a paucity of studies that focused on interdisciplinary or graduate-level curriculum. Nonetheless, these surveys and studies can provide a foundation for further research that can be generalized across types and levels of programs. Reproducing and replicating studies help validate the findings and applicability beyond the original study (Polit & Beck, 2017). Table 16.1 lists some of the references reviewed in this text that relate to curriculum development. This review highlights the need for additional research-based studies that can inform faculty as they consider revising existing curricula or developing new programs. Particularly critical is the need for higher level studies that can provide stronger evidence supporting curriculum revision and development acknowledging that part of the challenge in conducting studies that are more robust are the constraints and design compromises inherent in conducting studies within an active curriculum.

Curriculum and Program Evaluation

Table 16.2 presents a summary of studies that were reviewed related to curriculum and program evaluation and includes recommendations for further study. A search of the current body of literature indicates a paucity of studies focused on nursing education programs and curriculum evaluation. All the studies in this review were either surveys or descriptive studies indicating the need for higher levels of evidence that can be used to inform formative and summative program and curriculum evaluation. Future research should focus on evaluative methods and *model* testing to validate their usefulness in measuring program outcomes and student learning. In the absence of nursing education research that informs evaluative models and methods, nursing faculty will need to explore studies generated by other disciplines to find and adapt those appropriate and applicable to nursing education.

TABLE 16.1: Curriculum Development Studies

Topic	Author(s)/Date	Type of Program	Type of Study	Recommendations
All Types				
National survey of accredited nursing programs in the United States to describe evidence-based teaching practices	Kalb et al. (2015)	All accredited nursing programs	National online survey of faculty in all accredited nursing programs in the United States	Revise by incorporating methods to achieve a more representative sample, especially within different programs. Provide information about types of evidence used. Consider incorporating indicators of student success (NCLEX® pass rates; advanced practice certification rates).
A model and recommendation to guide the integration of climate change into nursing education using Ecological Planetary Health Model	Leffers et al. (2017)	All accredited nursing programs	Recommendation for integrating concepts related to climate change into the curriculum	Utilize the model and analyze its effectiveness in curricular revision for similar programs. Compare to other models and programs.
Prelicensure				
National surveys of undergraduate programs to determine what physical examination skills are taught	Giddens et al. (2012)	Prelicensure	National survey of prelicensure programs	Replicate for changes in curricula, program outcomes, effect on patient care. Replicate through concept analyses of other specific concepts, e.g., patient safety, cultural competence.
A model to integrate leadership concepts and skills into the curriculum to develop leadership capacity and skills upon entry to practice	Miles and Scott (2019)	Prelicensure	Directed content analysis	Utilize the model and analyze its effectiveness in curricular revision for similar programs. Compare to other models and programs.
Survey of faculty in 98 nursing schools in New York, with a follow-up focus group to describe the integration of QSEN competencies within prelicensure programs	Pollard et al. (2014)	Prelicensure	Online survey of faculty and administrators in 98 member schools of the New York State Deans of Baccalaureate and Higher Degree programs and the Council for Associate Degree Nursing	Replicate incorporating methods to improve response rate and ability to evaluate generalizability. Expand sample to enable comparison of program types.

(continued)

TABLE 16.1: Curriculum Development Studies (*continued*)

Topic	Author(s)/Date	Type of Program	Type of Study	Recommendations
Undergraduate ADN, BSN, Second-Degree BSN, RN to BSN				
A curriculum development model using learning as central for all stakeholders; response to the NLN's call for curricular transformation	Davis (2011)	AND	Description of the curricular change process using a curriculum-development model	Utilize the model and analyze its effectiveness in curricular revision for similar programs. Compare to other models and programs.
Shared decision-making model for curriculum revision	D'Antonio et al. (2013)	BSN	Description of the curricular change process using the model	Utilize the model and analyze the effectiveness in curricular revision for similar programs. Compare to other models and programs.
Process for mapping an undergraduate program to the AACN Essentials	Dearman et al. (2011)	BSN	Process and how the model tied into NCLEX success rates	Review the literature for similar models, apply the model to several programs and compare results according to student demographics, type of program, student-learning outcomes, curricular differences, etc.
Incorporating workshops on bullying to reduce its impact on minority BSN students	Egues and Leinung (2014)	BSN	Quasi-experimental pre-posttest design using a survey of students attending workshops on bullying at a designated Hispanic- and minority-serving college	Incorporate an experimental design allowing comparison with a control group. Incorporate controls on intervention fidelity necessary for replication and comparative effectiveness of different evidence-based teaching methods.
Model for incorporating academic–clinical partnerships with the Veterans Administration (VA Nursing Academy)	Needleman et al. (2014)	BSN	Survey of faculty at partnership sites	Replicate in other academic–clinical partnership systems (e.g., schools of nursing within academic health centers).
Description of a Model Residency Program and its outcomes that resulted in increased confidence, competence, leadership, etc.	Goode et al. (2013)	BSN Residency	Evaluation of student-learning outcomes	Replicate for validity, reliability, and generalizability.

			Description of the curricular change process using the scaffolding model	Utilize the model and analyze the effectiveness in curricular revision in similar programs. Compare to other models and programs.
Cognitive Scaffolding Model for curricular revision (Task, metacognitive, and sociocommunicative)	Hagler et al. (2011)	BSN	Description of the curricular change process using the scaffolding model	Utilize the model and analyze the effectiveness in curricular revision in similar programs. Compare to other models and programs.
Incorporating technology into the curriculum from low- to high-fidelity technology	Skiba (2012)	Predominantly BSN	Recommendation for integrating technology into the curriculum when undergoing change	Conduct studies to demonstrate student-learning outcomes using various technologies. Survey schools for levels of integration of technology in the curricula and effects on student-learning outcomes and patient care.
Managers' perceptions of second-degree graduates' clinical skills; comparison of managers' and graduates' perceptions of performance	Rafferty and Lindell (2011), Ziehm et al. (2011)	Second-degree BSN	Survey of nurse managers of graduates	Replicate for reliability and validity and investigate for factors influencing perceptions, and generalizability.
Managers' perceptions of second-degree graduates' performance and retention rates	Weathers and Raleigh (2013)	Second-degree BSN	Survey of nurse managers of graduates	Replicate for reliability and validity and investigate for factors influencing perceptions, and generalizability.
A policy framework to integrate compassion into the curriculum	Younas and Maddigan (2018)	All undergraduate programs	Recommendation for integrating compassion into the curriculum	Integrate policy recommendations for integrating compassion into the curriculum and analyze its effectiveness in curricular revision and student outcomes for similar programs. Compare to other frameworks and programs.
Interdisciplinary				
An interdisciplinary curriculum for palliative care in oncology	Head et al. (2014)	Undergraduate and graduate interdisciplinary	Description of the program and methods used for formative feedback during development	Compare relevant student outcomes between students who have and have not participated in the curriculum.

(continued)

TABLE 16.1: Curriculum Development Studies (*continued*)

Topic	Author(s)/Date	Type of Program	Type of Study	Recommendations
Measure students' interprofessional attitudes across medicine, nursing, and pharmacy	Sheu et al. (2012)	Interdisciplinary	Mixed qualitative and qualitative on student interprofessional attitudes	Replicate for reliability and validity and investigate for factors influencing attitudes, and generalizability.
Entry-Level Master's				
Entry-level MSN students' lived experiences	McNiesh (2011)	Entry-level MSN	Qualitative survey of students	Investigate factors that apply to larger sample size and varying geographical areas.
Master's				
A master's-level curriculum that prepares nurse leaders to deliver culturally diverse and linguistic services in the healthcare system	Comer et al. (2013)	MSN	Description of the curriculum and report on outcomes	Integrate the model into comparable program curricula and measure outcomes and compare across programs, student demographics, and geographical locations.
Doctoral Programs				
A description of the intention of the practice doctorate for postmaster's and BSN to DNP programs	Grey (2013)	DNP	Description and need for studies that compare BSN to DNP and postmaster's DNPs to compare to the original intent(s) of the DNP	Conduct comparative studies of curricula, program outcomes, and graduates' practice across geographical locations, types of programs, and types of students.

AACN, American Association of Colleges of Nursing; NCLEX, National Council Licensure Examination; NLN, National League for Nursing; QSEN, Quality and Safety Education for Nurses.

TABLE 16.2: Program and Curriculum Evaluation Studies

Topic	Author(s)/Date	Type of Program	Type of Study	Recommendations
All Types				
Model for evaluating clinical simulation	Cummings (2015)	All types of schools of nursing	Descriptive	Test model and compare; multisite and multiple program types
Measure for evaluation of classroom teaching practices	Herinckx et al. (2014)	All types of schools of nursing	Descriptive/instrument development	Validate and test measure using independent samples
Summative evaluation of technology outcomes	Newhouse (2011)	All types of educational programs	Comparison of digital measures to written assessment tools applied to technology	Test model and compare
Survey of student attitudes and opinions about program during curriculum redesign	Ostrogorsky and Raber (2014)	All types of educational programs	Descriptive	Apply in other settings undergoing curriculum revision to guide improvement efforts; evaluate associations between ratings and student and program outcomes
Associate Degree/Community Colleges				
Models of program evaluation	Bers (2011)	Associate degree	Descriptive	Review for models to test, report of model, compare utilization of models across geographical areas and types and levels of educational programs
Prelicensure Programs				
Description of the use of Stufflebeam's CIPPS Model to evaluate nursing program	Lippe and Carter (2018)	Prelicensure nursing programs	Descriptive	Test model and compare between programs and sites

(continued)

TABLE 16.2: Program and Curriculum Evaluation Studies (*continued*)

Topic	Author(s)/Date	Type of Program	Type of Study	Recommendations
Description of the use of the OSCE for assessing clinical competency	Obizoba (2018)	Prelicensure nursing programs	Descriptive phenomenological study	Test framework and compare between programs and sites
Graduate Programs				
Description of models of evaluation to measure outcomes in schools of nursing	Horne and Sandmann (2012)	Graduate nursing programs	Integrative review of the literature	Review for models to test, report of model, compare utilization of models across geographical areas and types and levels of educational programs
Benchmarks and trends for DNP Programs	Udlis and Manusco (2012)	DNP programs	National survey of DNP programs	Replicate; investigate identified characteristics and benchmarks

CIPP, Context, Input, Process, Product; OSCE, Objective Structured Clinical Exam.

Potential Curriculum and Evaluation Topics for Further Inquiry

After reviewing the body of literature related to curriculum development and evaluation, the following is proposed list of topics for scholarly consideration:

◆ What is known about the use and effectiveness of cohort model program designs in graduate-level programs?
◆ How does the financing of programs impact program and curriculum development and evaluation?
◆ How do we garner support for and design an interprofessional curriculum that meets the needs of the disciplines involved?
◆ What evidence-based education practices can be leveraged to inform the design of BS-DNP and graduate programs?
◆ How can the formation of academic–clinical partnerships improve faculty, student, and patient outcomes?

These suggested topics are meant to be the starting point for generating ideas for scholarly reflection, discussion, and further inquiry. Additional ideas for research, translation of research, and scholarship in nursing education should be explored.

Next Steps for Curricula Development and Evaluation: Priorities and Challenges

Both the NLN and the AACN have identified and defined scholarship/research priorities. The aim of the NLN (NLN, 2021b) current research priorities is to support the utilization of nursing education and learning sciences as evidence to guide best practices for educators in the preparation of the next generation of nurses who will be tasked with supporting the health of those in their care. The NLN's research priorities for 2020–2023 follow:

◆ Build the science of nursing education through the generation and translation of innovative teaching and learning strategies.
◆ Build faculty-teaching practice.
◆ Create partnerships, including inter/intra-professional education (IPE) and global initiatives that advance learning, enhance health and client care.
◆ Build a nurse faculty workforce to meet the needs of nursing education, staff, administration, and healthcare.

"Research needs to focus on the generation and translation of evidence in the areas of innovative teaching and learning strategies, faculty teaching practice, educational partnerships, and nurse faculty workforce capacity" (NLN, 2021b, p. 1).

Similar to the NLN's aim and priorities for nursing education scholarship/research, the AACN (2018) advocates for the advancement of the scholarship of teaching within academic nursing through the conduct of evaluation research, application of theoretical concepts, and innovation. Selected examples within each of these three categories include

◆ evaluating the impact of teaching processes, methodologies, and curriculum on efficiencies and impact on student and program outcomes.
◆ utilizing theoretical concepts to guide teaching practices, curriculum development, and student success.
◆ innovating teaching strategies, development, and evaluation to improve education that meets the needs of students, the healthcare community, and the profession.

"Along with the need to determine what constitutes high quality education, the time is right to reconsider the role of the faculty in an increasingly complex learning environment where research, teaching, practice, and service are all of crucial importance. In today's academic setting, scholarship should be inclusive and applicable to scientists, as well as practice, education, and policy scholars" (AACN, 2018, p. 1).

Challenges in addressing these priorities begin with the availability of faculty scholars with the time and expertise to design, conduct, and disseminate findings from studies producing needed empirical evidence, and the skills and knowledge to then translate those findings into real-world nursing pedagogy. In the report *The Future of Nursing: Leading Change, Advancing Health,* the Institute of Medicine (IOM, 2011) called for the evaluation of teaching effectiveness and efficiency, advancement of evidence-based teaching and the development of IPE models that improve patient outcomes, regardless of setting, was made more than a decade ago and remains relevant today.

The second challenge is the lack of adequate funding for nursing education research. In the same IOM (2011) report , the need for additional funding was highlighted and echoed by the Carnegie Foundation for the Advancement of Teaching's *Educating Nurses: A Call for Radical Transformation* (Benner et al., 2010). The report called on entities such as schools, federal and state governments, and philanthropies to increase support for faculty to engage in the scholarship of teaching and learning. Ongoing advocacy by faculty, nursing academic and professional organizations, and other stakeholders for building the cadre of academic nurse scholars, funding nursing education research, supporting interdisciplinary research partnerships, conducting multisite studies, and leveraging academic–clinical partnerships that promote the dissemination and implementation of evidence-based care that improves health outcomes is necessary to meet the complex needs of our society.

SUMMARY

This chapter discussed the role of faculty in engaging in and with scholarly activities. Within the context of education, the terms *research, evidence-based,* and *translational science* were defined. The state of the science in curriculum development and evaluation was discussed along with an exploration of studies published over the last 10 years. Gaps in the literature and suggested areas for further inquiry were presented. Priorities and challenges for the next steps of nursing education research were discussed, along with a call for continued advocacy to support the efforts and meet the challenges as we continue to innovate through nursing education scholarly activities. As Diekelmann and Ironside (2002) said so eloquently, "without a science of nursing education, important knowledge of best practices in teaching, learning, and schooling, the efficacy of various approaches, and the meaning of these approaches to students and teachers remains unexplicated and anecdotal at best" (p. 379).

END-OF-CHAPTER RESOURCES

DISCUSSION QUESTIONS

1. In your opinion or experience, what are some of the challenges that negatively affect the faculty's role in scholarship and research? What strategies do you suggest to resolve some of these challenges?

2. Differentiate between scholarship, research, evidence-based practice, and translational sciences they apply to the faculty role. Provide examples for each.

LEARNING ACTIVITIES

Student-Learning Activities

1. Divide your class into groups and have each group choose one of the priorities identified by the NLN or the AACN for nursing education scholarship.

    a. Describe the existing factors that support meeting that priority.

    b. Identify existing barriers that impede meeting that priority and present potential solutions that may help resolve those barriers.

Faculty Development Activities

1. Identify a problem in your practice as a nursing educator. Discuss it among your colleagues and identify the necessary steps to begin investigating potential solutions. If potential evidence-based solutions do not currently exist, what should you do?

 SPRINGER PUBLISHING CONNECT™

A robust set of instructor resources designed to supplement this text is located at **http://connect.springerpub.com/content/book/978-0-8261-8686-7.** Qualifying instructors may request access by emailing **textbook@springerpub.com.**

REFERENCES

American Association of Colleges of Nursing. (1999). Defining scholarship for the discipline of nursing [Position statement]. https://www.aacnnursing.org/News-Information/Position-Statements-White-Papers/Defining-Scholarship

American Association of Colleges of Nursing. (2017). AACN diversity, inclusion & equity [Position statement]. https://www.aacnnursing.org/News-Information/Position-Statements-White-Papers/Diversity

American Association of Colleges of Nursing. (2018). *Defining scholarship for academic nursing task force consensus position statement*. https://www.aacnnursing.org/Portals/42/News/Position-Statements/Defining-Scholarship.pdf

American Nurses Association. (2010). *Nursing's social policy statement: The essence of the profession*. Nursesbooks.org.

Benner, P., Sutphen, M., Leonard, V., & Day, L. (2010). *Educating nurses: A call for radical transformation*. Jossey-Bass.

Bers, T. (2011). Program review and institutional effectiveness. *New Directions for Community Colleges, 152,* 63–73.

Boyer, E. (1990). *Scholarship reconsidered: Priorities for the professoriate*. The Carnegie Foundation for the Advancement of Teaching. https://www.umces.edu/sites/default/files/al/pdfs/BoyerScholarshipReconsidered.pdf

Comer, L., Whichcello, R., & Neubrander, J. (2013). An innovative Master of Science program for the development of culturally competent nursing leaders. *Journal of Cultural Diversity, 20*(2), 89–93. https://unr.idm.oclc.org/login?url=https://www.proquest.com/scholarly-journals/innovative-master-science-program-development/docview/1371387668/se-2?accountid=452

Cummings, C. (2015). Evaluating clinical simulation. *Nursing Forum, 50*(2), 109–115. https://doi.org/10.1111/nuf.12075

D'Antonio, P. O., Brennan, A. M. W., & Curley, M. A. Q. (2013). Judgment, inquiry, engagement, voice: Reenvisioning an undergraduate nursing curriculum using a shared decision-making model. *Journal of Professional Nursing, 29*(6), 407–413. https://doi.org/10.1016/j.profnurs.2012.10.003

Davis, B. W. (2011). A conceptual model to support curriculum review, revision, and design in an associate degree nursing program. *Nursing Education Perspectives, 32*(6), 389–394. https://doi.org/10.5480/1536-5026-32.6.389

Dearman, V., Lawson, R., & Hall, H. R. (2011). Concept mapping a baccalaureate nursing program: A method for success. *Journal of Nursing Education, 50*(11), 656–659. https://doi.org/10.3928/01484834-20110817-01

Diekelmann, N., & Ironside, P. M. (2002). Developing a science of nursing education: Innovation with research. *Journal of Nursing Education, 41*(9), 379–380. https://doi.org/10.3928/0148-4834-20020901-03

Egues, A., & Leinung, E. (2014). Antibullying workshops: Shaping minority nursing leaders through curriculum innovation. *Nursing Forum, 49*(4), 240–246. https://doi.org/10.1111/nuf.12083

Goode, C. J., Lynn, M. R., & McElroy, D. (2013). Lessons learned from 10 years of research on a post-baccalaureate nurse residency program. *Journal of Nursing Administration, 43*(2), 73–79. https://doi.org/10.1097/NNA.0b013e31827f205c

Giddens, J. F., Wright, M., & Gray, I. (2012). Selecting concepts for a concept-based curriculum: Application of a benchmark approach. *Journal of Nursing Education, 51*(9), 511–515. https://doi.org/10.3928/01484834-20120730-02

Grady, P. A. (2010). News from NINR: Translational research and nursing science. *Nursing Outlook, 58*, 164–166. https://doi.org/10.1016/j.outlook.2010.01.001

Grey, M. (2013). The doctor of nursing practice: Defining the next steps. *Journal of Nursing Education, 52*(8), 462–465. https://doi.org/10.3928/01484834-20130719-02

Hagler, D., Morris, B., & White, B. (2011). Cognitive tools as a scaffold for faculty during curriculum redesign. *Journal of Nursing Education, 50*(7), 417–422. https://doi.org/10.3928/01484834-20110214-03

Head, B. A., Schapmire, T., Hermann, C., Earnshaw, L., Faul, A., Jones, C., Kayser, K., Martin, A., Shaw, M. A., Woggon, F. & Pfeifer, M. (2014). The interdisciplinary curriculum for oncology palliative care education (iCOPE): Meeting the challenge of interprofessional education. *Journal of Palliative Medicine, 17*(10), 1107–1115.

Herinckx, H., Munkvold, J., Winter, E., & Tanner, C. (2014). A measure to evaluate classroom teaching practices in nursing. *Nursing Education Perspectives, 35*(1), 30–36. https://doi.org/10.5480/11-535.1

Horne, E. M., & Sandmann, L. R. (2012). Current trends in systematic program evaluation of online graduate nursing education: An integrative literature review. *Journal of Nursing Education, 51*(10), 570–576. https://doi.org/10.1089/jpm.2014.0070

Institute of Medicine. (2011). *The future of nursing: Leading change, advancing health.* National Academies Press. https://doi.org/10.17226/12956

Kalb, K., O'Conner-Von, S., Brockway, C., Rierson, C., & Sendelbach, S. (2015). Evidence-based teaching practice in nursing education: Faculty perspectives and practices. *Nursing Education Perspectives, 36*(4), 212–219. https://doi.org/10.5480/14-1472

Leffers, J., Levy, R. M., Nicholas, P. K., & Sweeney, C. F. (2017). Mandate for the nursing profession to address climate change through nursing education. *Journal of Nursing Scholarship, 49*(6), 679–687. https://doi.org/10.1111/jnu.12331

Lippe, M., & Carter, P. (2018). Using the CIPP model to assess nursing education program quality and merit. *Teaching and Learning in Nursing, 13*, 9–13.

Miles, J. M., & Scott, E. S. (2019). A new leadership development model for nursing education. *Journal of Professional Nursing, 35*, 5–11. https://doi.org/10.1016/j.profnurs.2018.09.009

National League for Nursing. (2021a). *Nurse educator core competency.* http://www.nln.org/professional-development-programs/competencies-for-nursing-education/nurse-educator-core-competency

National League for Nursing. (2021b). *Research priorities in nursing education.* http://www.nln.org/professional-development-programs/research/research-priorities-in-nursing-education

Needleman, J., Bowman, C., Wyte-Lake, T., & Dobalian, A. (2014). Faculty recruitment and engagement in academic-practice partnerships. *Nursing Education Perspectives, 35*(6), 372–379. https://doi.org/10.5480/13-1234

Newhouse, C. P. (2011). Using IT to assess IT: Towards greater authenticity in summative performance assessment. *Computers & Education*, *56*, 388–402. https://doi.org/10.1016/j.compedu.2010.08.023

Obizoba, C. (2018). Mitigating the challenges of objective structured clinical examination (OSCE) in nursing education: A phenomenological research study. *Nurse Education Today*, *68*, 71–74. https://doi.org/10.1016/j.nedt.2018.06.002

Ostrogorsky, T., & Raber, A. (2014). Experiences of first-year nursing students during an education redesign: Findings from the Oregon Consortium for Nursing Education. *Nursing Education Perspectives*, *35*(2), 115–121. https://doi.org/10.5480/12-854.1

Polit, D. F., & Beck, C. T. (2010). *Essentials of nursing research: Appraising evidence for nursing practice*. Lippincott, Williams & Wilkins.

Pollard, M., Stapleton, M., Kennelly, L., Bagdan, L., Cannistraci, P., Millenbach, L., & Odondi, M. (2014). Assessment of quality and safety education in nursing: A New York state perspective. *Nursing Education Perspectives*, *35*(4), 224–229. https://doi.org/10.5480/13-1104.1

McNiesh, S. G. (2011). The lived experience of students in an accelerated nursing program: Intersecting factors that influence experiential learning. *Journal of Nursing Education*, *50*(4), 197–203. https://doi.org/10.3928/01484834-20101029-03

Melnyk, B. M., Fineout-Overholt, E., Stillwell, S. B., & Williamson, K. M. (2010). Evidence-based practice: Step by step. The seven steps of evidence-based practice: Following this progressive, sequential approach will lead to improved health care and patient outcomes. *American Journal of Nursing*, *110*(1), 51–53. https://doi.org/10.1097/01.NAJ.0000390523.99066.b5

Rafferty, M., & Lindell, D. (2011). How nurse managers rate the clinical competencies of accelerated (second-degree) nursing graduates. *Journal of Nursing Education*, *50*(6), 355–357. https://doi.org/10.3928/01484834-20110228-07

Sheu, L., Lai, C. J., Coelho, A. D., Lin, L. D., Zheng, P., Hom, P., Diaz, V. & O'Sullivan, P. S. (2012). Impact of student-run clinics on preclinical sociocultural and interprofessional attitudes: A prospective cohort analysis. *Journal of Health Care for the Poor and Underserved*, *23*(3), 1058–1072. https://doi.org/10.1353/hpu.2012.0101

Skiba, D. (2012). Technology and gerontology: Is this in your nursing curriculum? *Nursing Education Perspectives*, *33*(3), 207–209. https://doi.org/10.5480/1536-5026-33.3.207

Trautman, D. E., Idzik, S., Hammersla, M., & Rosseter, R. (2018). Advancing scholarship through translational research: The role of PhD and DNP prepared nurses. *OJIN: The Online Journal of Issues in Nursing*, *23*(2), Manuscript 2. https://doi.org/10.3912/OJIN.Vol23No02Man02

Udlis, K. A., & Manusco, J. M. (2012). Doctor of nursing practice programs across the United States: A benchmark of information. Part I: Program characteristics. *Journal of Professional Nursing*, *28*(5), 265–273. https://doi.org/10.1016/j.profnurs.2012.01.002

Weathers, S. M., & Raleigh, E. D. (2013). 1-year retention rates and performance ratings: Comparing associate degree, baccalaureate, and accelerated baccalaureate degree nurses. *Journal of Nursing Administration*, *43*(9), 468–474. https://doi.org/10.1097/NNA.0b013e3182a23d9f

Younas, A., & Maddigan, J. (2018). Proposing a policy framework for nursing education for fostering compassion in nursing students: A critical review. *Journal of Advanced Nursing*, *75*(18), 1621–1636. https://doi.org/10.1111/jan.13946

Ziehm, S. R., Uibel, I. C., Fontaine, D. K., & Scherzer, T. (2011). Success indicators for accelerated master's entry nursing program: Staff RN performance. *Journal of Nursing Education*, *50*(7), 395–403. https://doi.org/10.3928/01484834-20110429-02

CHAPTER 17

Issues and Challenges for Nursing Educators

Stephanie Stimac DeBoor

CHAPTER OBJECTIVES

Upon completion of Chapter 17, the reader will be able to:

- Analyze the trends, issues, and challenges raised throughout the text that apply to curriculum development and evaluation.
- Consider some strategies for resolution of the issues raised and ways to meet the challenges with an eye to the future.

OVERVIEW

This chapter summarizes the text to provide the reader with an overview of the processes related to curriculum development and evaluation in nursing education. It begins with the major milestones in the history of nursing education in the United States to gain perspectives on its move into higher education in order to meet the needs of the current and future healthcare systems. The chapters provide guidelines from expert, experienced nursing educators and the latest literature and research on theories, concepts, and models that apply to curriculum building, evaluation, accreditation, and the roles of faculty in the processes. Major issues and challenges raised throughout the text are reviewed with some ideas for strategies to bring them to resolution. Some of the major challenges facing nursing education for the future are discussed in the following sections.

CHAPTER 1: HISTORY OF NURSING EDUCATION IN THE UNITED STATES

Chapter 1 raises many of the issues related to nursing's role in academe from the time of Nightingale, to hospital-based, apprentice-type programs, and ultimately, to higher education institutions including the associate degree, baccalaureate, master's, and doctorate levels. Provided is a review of the influence of major wars and resulting federal support of nursing education. It is interesting to see the influence of wars and the major changes in the healthcare system and society had on nursing education. What will the future hold in relation to global conflicts? The 21st century continues to see a growth in all levels of nursing education, bolstered by *The Future of Nursing 2020–2030* initiative by the National Academy of Medicine (NAM, 2019). DNP programs continue to outpace PhD enrollment and entry into practice continues to evolve based on curriculum revisions and new program development. Major factors influencing the future of nursing education include the need for more students into the PhD as the discipline's research and theory-building degree, healthcare legislation, technology, recruitment, and educating a diverse nursing workforce.

CHAPTER 2: CURRICULUM DEVELOPMENT AND APPROVAL PROCESSES IN CHANGING EDUCATIONAL ENVIRONMENTS

Chapter 2 reviews the importance of faculty in relation to processes that schools of nursing undergo to bring about curriculum revision or to develop new programs. It includes some of the issues encountered with these processes and the importance of incorporating research into the development and evaluation of curriculum, specifically, the issues that occurred during the COVID-19 pandemic and changes to online formats and use of technology. The pandemic led us to explore innovations for implementing a curriculum, such as innovative conceptual learning approaches, technology, high-fidelity simulations, and virtual patients and community.

The chapter discusses the roles and responsibilities of faculty for ensuring curriculum integrity and its currency with existing and future practice in both nursing and education. Presented are consideration for the various levels of approval for curricular revision or proposals for new programs and the need for the resources to support the processes. Stakeholders such as students, healthcare partners, and other disciplines serve as consultants for curriculum design helping secure the ultimate success. Ideas for faculty development are presented especially as they relate to new and part-time faculty members who may have minimal preparation for the role of educator in academe. Changes within healthcare systems and evidence-based practice lead to the issue of content saturation. The temptation to overcrowd the curriculum beyond the point of reason will overwhelm students' learning capacity.

CHAPTER 3: NEEDS ASSESSMENT: THE EXTERNAL AND INTERNAL FRAME FACTORS

Chapter 3 introduces the frame factors model, a conceptual model that describes the major external and internal factors that influence, facilitate, or impinge upon the curriculum. It reviews the major components of a needs assessment that include analyses of these factors. A needs assessment guides faculty in the curriculum plan, implementation, evaluation, and the final program outcomes. Faculty members sophisticated in the assessment of frame factors are at an advantage to view the curriculum and its place in the scheme of financial security, position within the healthcare system and the profession, the role in meeting the healthcare needs of the community and industry, and its significance to the parent institution. The author recommends that nursing educators use the frame factors model when evaluating and revising a current curriculum or initiating new programs. While nursing administrators may take a leadership role in conducting needs assessments, faculty should participate in the decision-making for what type and how much data to collect and what decisions affect the curriculum based on the assessment. An updated version of the case study found in the Appendix illustrates the application of the frame factors model. It proposes a collaborative, international program between two schools of nursing, one in the United States and one in Africa. With the expanding use of distance education through the internet, it provides some ideas about the challenges and the eagerness related to developing these types of curricula.

CHAPTER 4: FINANCIAL SUPPORT AND BUDGET MANAGEMENT FOR CURRICULUM DEVELOPMENT OR REVISION

Chapter 4 reviews the resources and costs related to the financial support and budget planning for curriculum development, evaluation, and accreditation activities. Specific costs include faculty release time, administrative and staff support, office equipment, technology support, and supplies. These are costs over and above the usual budget demands and must be planned for in advance. The challenge is to earmark funds for these activities to avoid unexpected shortfalls and an impact on other program expenditures, such as start-up costs for a new program. Knowledge of possible resources external to the program is useful for generating funds that help initiate and support new programs. Provided are potential funding sources. The COVID-19 pandemic caused significant changes to academic budgets, thus affecting development and revision planning as well as the hiring of faculty to support these curricular changes. In addition, the roles and responsibilities of administrators and faculty and the importance of faculty participation and contributions to budgetary planning are noted.

CHAPTER 5: THE CLASSIC COMPONENTS OF THE CURRICULUM: DEVELOPING A CURRICULUM PLAN

Chapter 5 discusses the various types of educational institutions and levels of nursing education. It includes how formal and informal curriculum promotes or impedes relations ships between the faculty and students. In addition, when planning curriculum faculty must examine the campus environment (in person or virtual) and how that fosters student belonging. This chapter organizes the components of the curriculum in detail concerning the mission/vision, philosophy, goal, organizational framework, student-learning outcomes (objectives), and implementation plan. These components provide a logical order and an organizing framework for initiating or revising a nursing educational program. It is important to examine the curriculum by its major components when considering planning and evaluation. Examination of major concepts related to the underlying philosophy and the beliefs faculty hold about nursing and education considering their contribution to the philosophy and their role in the curriculum contribute to potential issues. It is best to review the curriculum from a holistic approach to avoid a "domino" effect. Always question how a change may lead to consequences within the program as a whole.

CHAPTER 6: IMPLEMENTATION OF THE CURRICULUM

Chapter 6 continues the discussion of curriculum planning by reviewing the processes necessary to implement the curriculum once the mission, vision, philosophy, goals, and student-learning outcomes are in place. It provides synopses of common learning theories and taxonomies that specifically apply to nursing education. Crucial to the process is the faculty's knowledge and beliefs concerning learning theories and the foundational basis of a curriculum.

Moving from learning theories, the chapter discusses their application to student-focused instructional strategies. The strategies include problem-based learning, team-based learning, the flipped classroom, and simulation. The chapter concludes with the process of student evaluation, measuring student learning outcomes, and benchmarking program goals.

CHAPTER 7: USING EDUCATIONAL TAXONOMIES TO PROMOTE CRITICAL THINKING

Chapter 7 provides an overview of educational taxonomies and learning domains in relation to a nursing curriculum and evaluating student learning. Included are current revisions of the presented educational taxonomies and examples of their use in student-learning outcomes. Provided is a table for educators' use that shows the alignment taxonomy and educational outcomes, which assists in identifying and preventing any curricular gaps. This chapter examines critical thinking, clinical reasoning, and clinical judgment skills through the lens of taxonomy. The ability of nursing educators to foster critical thinking in nursing students promotes evidence-based responses to healthcare issues.

CHAPTERS 8 THROUGH 10: CURRICULUM PLANNING FOR UNDERGRADAUTE AND GRADUATE PROGRAMS

Chapter 8: Undergraduate Programs

Chapter 8 discusses the current trends in prelicensure nursing education, that is, the ADN and the baccalaureate/BSN. Diploma programs continue to exist but are decreasing in numbers. There are articulation agreements with community colleges offering bachelor's degrees (depending on state regulations) and those that are looking beyond. Due to the number of community colleges, universities may serve as partners to multiple community colleges, allowing for the sharing of resources such as faculty and space. Thus, there remains a continued need for collaboration of curricula that provide seamless entry from ADN to BSN programs and BSN to doctorates.

This chapter describes new *Essentials: Core Competencies for Professional Nursing Education* of the American Association of Colleges of Nursing (AACN, 2021) in curriculum development and provides an example of utilization of the domains, competencies, and subcompetencies in a traditional BSN course. Offered are examples of student-learning outcomes and measures (rubric) for grading competencies. Continued advances in educational technologies and virtual learning platforms are altering the delivery of entry level to practice education. With these changes come issues in curriculum development, evaluation, and faculty preparedness. Ongoing competition for clinical sites provides a challenge for educators to ensure clinical experiences that prepare nursing students for "real-life" practice. With simulation approved as an alternative for learning experiences, colleges and universities need to assess budgetary and faculty resources when considering this option. At the national level, there is a call to recruit a nursing student body that resembles the demographics of populations in the United States. Also discussed is recruitment. This chapter concludes with an examination of generic and accelerated BSN entry to practice programs and RN-to-BSN completion programs.

Chapter 9: Curriculum Planning for Specialty Master's Nursing Degrees and Entry-Level Graduate Degrees

Chapter 9 provides a brief history of master's-level graduate education. The various current master's programs are described including the RN to MSN, entry-level MSN (for nonnursing college graduates, the clinical nurse leader, advanced practice programs, and functional roles such as case management, nursing administrators, and nurse educators).

Like the previous chapter, an example of AACN's (2021) new *Essentials: Core Competencies for Professional Nursing Education* provides the reader with information on the utilization of the domains, competencies, and subcompetencies in curriculum development for an MSN course. Issues related to master's programs are raised such as the remaining question about entry into practice, at what level advanced practice belongs, and the standardization and regulations for advanced practice through licensing, accreditation, certification, and education.

Chapter 10: Planning for Doctoral Education

This chapter presents an overview of the historical beginnings of the PhD and DNP degrees in nursing. A comparison of the degrees shows differences in curriculum development and evaluation of educational programs. The DNP continues to outpace the PhD degree in enrollments, thus creating a deficit in nursing scientists. As the graduates of DNP programs increase and the political atmosphere continues calling for legislative changes affecting healthcare delivery systems, the role of nursing becomes even more crucial.

It is the first option for exploring how faculty roles are defined to provide high-quality instruction that prepares professionals who meet current and future healthcare needs and remain current in practice, provide service, and maintain research and scholarship. Graduate programs are particularly hard hit by the continued shortage of doctorally prepared teachers as faculty members and mentors for PhD students. Additionally, the DNP degree is replacing the master's in response to the AACN (2004) and the National Organization of Nurse Practitioner Faculties' (NONPF; 2018) recommendation that the DNP be the terminal practice degree by 2025. A challenge to this recommendation is whether to "grandparent in" those already in practice with a master's degree.

An issue related to doctorally prepared faculty is the debate that continues about the DNP versus the research-focused degrees (DNS/PhD) and their places in nursing education. Those with a research-focused doctorate, who can generate funding from their research agenda, continue to hold most tenure-track positions (Auerbach et al., 2015). Yet in looking to the future, a collaboration of these doctorates will lend to changes in healthcare policy and provide evidence-based practice built on research and translational science. Finally, as with the previous chapters, an example of AACN's (2021) new *Essentials: Core Competencies for Professional Nursing Education* provides the reader with information on the utilization of the domains, competencies, and subcompetencies in curriculum development for a DNP advanced practice course.

CHAPTER 11: A PROPOSED UNIFIED NURSING CURRICULUM

Entry into practice as an RN remains multilayered with graduates of diploma, ADN, BSN, and entry-level master's degrees eligible for licensure. These multiple pathways continue to confuse the public and those seeking education to become RNs. Chapter 11 provides an update of Keating's (2018a) Unified Nursing Curriculum. With a continued debate and issues related to the numerous points of entry into nursing practice, this serves as an example of an educational continuum. Students have an option of entering and "stepping out" for licensure and then returning later for upper division and graduate levels of nursing education. A unified nursing curriculum offers a nonstop program from the baccalaureate level or one that accommodates a student's personal and professional goals. The advantages of the unified curriculum are numerous. It facilitates high school graduates' entry into a nursing program with graduation 8 years away, thus producing expert clinicians, researchers, and educators who are relatively young in age.

The chapter ends with a list of characteristics for nursing education that promotes the preparation of nursing leaders, policy initiators, faculty, researchers, and advanced practice clinicians and practitioners. As the healthcare system continues to rapidly change, it is important for nursing educators to prepare students on health policy, public and global health, leadership, and interprofessional collaboration to provide safe, high-quality, and evidence-based care.

CHAPTER 12: FROM STAFF DEVELOPMENT TO THE SPECIALTY OF NURSING PROFESSIONAL DEVELOPMENT

Chapter 12 applies the principles of curriculum development and evaluation to the role of staff development, or more currently known as, nursing professional development (NPD) in the healthcare setting. This chapter provides readers with the historical beginnings of NPD, qualifications, roles, and responsibilities of the position. Provided are theories of adult learning for consideration in creating learning activities and educational programs. Included are the components for planning and evaluating a curriculum, along with examples of formal and informal approval processes. The NPD specialist provides educational opportunities for the staff in the maintenance of competency with changing standards, policies, and equipment.

Accreditation and regulatory standards influence educational requirements in healthcare settings. Another issue of concern is the rapidly changing technology used in electronic medical records and healthcare equipment. Institutional budgetary cuts often affect the NPD department, thus leading to constant justification of the financial worth. Due to the nature of a small unit, often there is a lack of ability to mentor new specialists as they come into the position, which leaves the new NPD specialist guessing the priorities and full responsibilities of the position.

CHAPTER 13: DISTANCE EDUCATION, ONLINE LEARNING, INFORMATICS, AND TECHNOLOGY

Chapter 13 offers an overview of the factors to consider along with budgetary considerations in relation to technology. Current formats for delivering the curriculum through onsite campuses and web-based online learning are described and their advantages and disadvantages are discussed. The pandemic required colleges and universities across the country to rapidly transition to online learning and institute new options for clinical experiences. This abrupt change in educational delivery identified shortfalls in faculty competencies at providing online learning and using the technologies required. Assessment of budgetary constraints levied by the pandemic requires consideration for those institutions who wish to continue an online format. It will be important to continue monitoring NCLEX® and national certification results for an assessment of the potential impact of these changes. With future expansions of technology and its application to nursing and education, it becomes the responsibility of nursing educators to become or stay savvy in the use of informatics, clinical simulations, and other technological applications.

This chapter provides a review of research findings related to the efficacy of distance education programs as well as a discussion of the identified trends and issues. Some current issues raised include the challenges for providing cost-effective programs, the increasing market of learning management systems, and the maintenance of quality through evaluation processes including meeting professional and accreditation standards.

CHAPTER 14: PROGRAM EVALUATION AND ACCREDITATION

Chapter 14 provides an analysis of common definitions, concepts, and theories related to evaluation and quality assurance of accreditation. Nursing education evaluation is evolving from the past use of models of evaluation to the adaptation of business and healthcare benchmarks to measure productivity, outcomes, cost-effectiveness, and quality. This chapter discusses accreditation agencies, their purpose, and their role in total quality management. While accreditation is voluntary, it carries certain advantages for the institution and its students and graduates. For an accredited institution, it signifies to the community that the programs meet quality standards set by education and the nursing profession. For students and graduates, an accredited program identifies eligibility for certain financial aid programs and meets requirements, in most cases, when pursuing higher levels of education at other institutions.

Two issues for consideration in regards to accreditation, first keeping the program standards up-to-date. Owing to many accreditation standards, educational programs usually have a strategic or master plan of evaluation in place to facilitate the process of collecting and analyzing data. While the burden of this activity falls mainly to the program administrator, faculty are responsible for participating in program approval and review processes in academe by being a member of curriculum and program evaluation committees for the nursing program and or institution. These kinds of activities contribute to faculty's professional development and the ability to keep abreast of changes occurring in education and the profession that call for modifications of program outcomes, accreditation, and regulatory standards and criteria. Second is the timely notification of new programs and revisions. Both national accreditation and state regulatory agencies require notification of substantive program revision and the development of new programs. Agencies have specific timelines for meeting these notifications and any delay or lack of notification can result in a program's suspension or loss of accreditation.

CHAPTER 15: PLANNING FOR ACCREDITATION

Chapter 15 provides an overview of accreditation processes for nursing education programs and a case study is presented that describes the processes a nursing faculty undergoes for preparing for an accreditation visit, including preparation of the self-study. Due to the pandemic, accreditation visits were held virtually and the case study identifies the differences of a virtual visit from that of a face-to-face site visit. In the United States, there are three accreditation bodies for nursing programs; the Accreditation Commission for Nursing Education (ACEN), the Commission on Collegiate Nursing Education (CCNE) and, recently, as of this writing, the National League for Nursing (NLN) Commission for Nursing Education Accreditation (CNEA). In addition, there are two accrediting agencies for nurse midwives and nurse anesthetists. PhD programs are not accredited by a nursing accreditation program but are usually housed in institutions of higher education that have regional accreditation.

CHAPTER 16: RESEARCH AND EVIDENCE-BASED PRACTICE IN NURSING EDUCATION

With the reduction in enrollment in PhD programs, there are fewer nursing scientists. This consequently impacts the research of curriculum development and evaluation. Chapter 16 discusses the role of faculty scholarship in nursing education for evidence-based practice. It reviews how the three key roles of faculty, teaching, scholarship, and service overlap to fill gaps in current nursing curricula. The appeal for faculty is to rely on past strategies for developing curricula and instructional strategies. However, with the rapid changes in the healthcare delivery system and the impact of technology, as seen during the COVID-19 pandemic, educators must provide preparation for the nursing workforce through curricula that respond to these changes. This chapter provides the most up-to-date research for curriculum development and education through a literature review. It concludes with next steps and challenges of the future, faculty scholars, and funding.

SUMMARY

Each chapter of this text reviews the classic and recent literature related to curriculum development and evaluation in nursing. This chapter summarized each of the previous chapters in the text and raised issues from each topic. Although this text focuses on curriculum development and evaluation in nursing in the United States, we contemplate the future regardless of challenges. There is a need to envision a broader, global perspective about nursing and the education required for its professionals. The global pandemic gave us the opportunity to share knowledge and expertise with students and colleagues. Literature published during this time shows our international colleagues share the same concerns of U.S. nursing educators for preparing quality health professionals to meet the needs of the world's populations. While predicting the future due to rapid changes in healthcare is a difficult task, there remain challenges that impact the development and evaluation of nursing curricula. Preparation of educators for these changes shape policy and care of the future. Keating (2018b) identified that nursing educators have a responsibility to prepare curricula with their colleagues that "prepares nurses for the future, who are competent and caring, excellent clinicians and practitioners, leaders and change agents, and scholars and researchers" (p. 262).

END-OF-CHAPTER RESOURCES

DISCUSSION QUESTIONS

- What challenges do you envision over the next 5 to 10 years based on nursing and faculty shortages and the rapid changes in the healthcare and educational systems?

- Are there past strategies in nursing education that can be applied to the current needed changes in nursing education today? What are the lessons from the past that prohibited nursing from moving its educational agenda forward? How can today's nurse educators use these lessons to bring about change?

LEARNING ACTIVITIES

Student-Learning Activities

1. Synthesize the information in this text into a "Dream School of Nursing." Develop a curriculum that prepares nurses for practice 10 years hence, keeping in mind that practice and the setting in which it is delivered will be different. Be imaginative and think way outside the box!

Faculty Development Activities

1. Hold a faculty meeting focused on brainstorming and let creative thoughts flow freely. List the characteristics of the ideal nurse you would like to care for you in the future. Examine these characteristics and decide how a curriculum can be developed that provides the kind of education necessary to prepare this kind of nurse. Focus on creativity and newer theories of learning. Compare these ideas to your existing curriculum. How can it be transformed into the one you envision and still meet accreditation and professional standards and criteria?

A robust set of instructor resources designed to supplement this text is located at **http://connect.springerpub.com/content/book/978-0-8261-8686-7.** Qualifying instructors may request access by emailing **textbook@springerpub.com.**

REFERENCES

American Association of Colleges of Nursing. (2004). *AACN position statement on the practice doctorate in nursing.* http://www.aacnnursing.org/Portals/42/News/Position-Statements/DNP.pdf

American Association of Colleges of Nursing. (2021). *The essentials: Core competencies for professional nursing education.* https://www.aacnnursing.org/Portals/42/AcademicNursing/pdf/Essentials-2021.pdf

Auerbach, D. I., Martsolf, G., Pearson, M. L., Taylor, E. A., Zaydman, M., Muchow, A. N., Spetz, J., & Dower, C. (2015). *The DNP by 2015: A study of the institutional, political, and professional issues that facilitate or impede establishing a post-baccalaureate doctor of nursing practice program.* https://www.rand.org/content/dam/rand/pubs/research_reports/RR700/RR730/RAND_RR730.pdf

Keating, S. B. (2018a). A proposed unified nursing curriculum. In S. B. Keating & S. S. DeBoor (Eds.), *Curriculum development and evaluation in nursing education* (4th ed., pp. 171–184). Springer.

Keating, S. B. (2018b). Issues and challenges for nursing educators. In S. B. Keating & S. S. DeBoor (Eds.), *Curriculum development and evaluation in nursing education* (4th ed., p. 262). Springer.

National Academy of Medicine. (2019). *The future of nursing 2020–2030: Charting a path to achieve health equity.* https://nam.edu/publications/the-future-of-nursing-2020-2030/

National Organization of Nurse Practitioner Faculties. (2018, May). *The doctor of nursing practice degree: Entry to nurse practitioner practice by 2025.* https://cdn.ymaws.com/www.nonpf.org/resource/resmgr/dnp/v3_05.2018_NONPF_DNP_stateme.pdf

APPENDIX

Case Study

Sarah B. Keating

Updated by Stephanie Stimac DeBoor

The case study presented in this Appendix is fictitious and is used to illustrate a needs assessment and the development of a proposed curriculum based on the assessment. It includes the collection of data related to external and internal frame factors, their analyses, a curriculum decision based on the findings, and a proposed program of study.

CHAPTER OBJECTIVES

Upon completion of the Case Study, the reader will be able to:

- Analyze a needs assessment of two fictitious schools of nursing considering expansion of their degree programs through a collaborative arrangement.

- Identify gaps in the data collected for the needs assessment and other possibilities for development from the data analysis.

- Practice curriculum development based on the case study's needs assessment by refining the proposed program or developing a new one.

EXTERNAL FRAME FACTORS

Description of the Community

An existing baccalaureate and higher degree nursing program whose home campus is located in a suburban town of 22,000 adjacent to a large U.S. state capital with a population of more than 1,500,000 is about to undertake a needs assessment to determine if the program should expand. The U.S. home institution is a private, sectarian, multipurpose higher education institution. It has a long history of liberal arts education and recently developed a partnership with a higher education university in Kenya, Africa, supported by the same religiously based organization. Presently, the Kenyan university offers a bachelor of arts (BA) in general studies and is the home institution to a bachelor of science in nursing (BScN) program with master's degrees in business and education that are available online. The purpose of the partnership between the two universities is to increase and diversify the student population, develop exchange programs, and promote international higher education. The U.S. institution's home campus has several professional schools, including business, education, engineering, nursing, and the performing arts with baccalaureates and master's degrees in those majors, and there are three doctorate programs, in education (PhD), business administration (DBA), and nursing practice

(DNP). The undergraduate population numbers 8,000, and there are 3,000 graduate students. Faculty include 850 on-campus faculty members, with 350 of them in part-time positions. In the past 5 years, the institution and, specifically, its professional schools increased the number of online course offerings, and with the onset of the global pandemic, all programs were adapted to distance and online learning.

Nursing faculty and administrators are aware of the continuing and projected nursing workforce shortage in the nation and in the region, the changes in the healthcare system and their effect on the nursing workforce, and the trend for increasing the basic entry level of nursing education to the baccalaureate and entry level for practitioners to the DNP. Anecdotal information indicates employers of nurses prefer baccalaureate or higher degree nurses. Owing to the complexity of the acute care setting, the shortages of nurses prepared to practice in primary care and community settings, and the recommendation of the Institute of Medicine (IOM, 2010, now known as the National Academy of Medicine) in *The Future of Nursing*, a need for a baccalaureate as the entry for professional nursing.

Responding to this need, 3 years ago, the nursing program developed a track in the baccalaureate program for RNs to complete their BSN degrees totally online in addition to its on-campus undergraduate bachelor's program (BSN). At the same time, it expanded its master's family nurse practitioner (FNP) and adult/geriatric acute care nurse practitioner (AGACNP) advanced practice options into a DNP program. The majority of the master's and DNP theory courses are offered online and the DNP is open to master's-prepared advanced practice nurses as a DNP completion track. The master's program offers postbaccalaureate community health nursing (CHN), and administration (ADM) tracks, as well as an entry-level clinical nurse leader (CNL) program for non-nursing college graduates. The ADM and CHN master's and the completion DNP are totally online. The graduate program recently experienced an increase in applications from nurses in practice in the United States and from the graduates of the BScN program of the parent institution's partner in Kenya.

The nursing program is clinically affiliated with a religious-based healthcare organization of the same denomination as its parent organization. The healthcare organization is a managed care system and has nationwide and regional facilities and some international services in East Africa and Kenya. It is supportive of the nursing program and offers clinical sites for student practice. It has scholarship or loan forgiveness programs for its staff and for students who come to its facilities after graduation. Recently, there has been interest in the graduate program from other nations' healthcare systems and nursing programs affiliated with the supportive religious organization. With this information in hand, the dean of nursing asks the faculty to conduct a needs assessment for expanding the nursing program by increasing enrollments for entry-level nurses and/or expanding the graduate program to provide additional advanced practice nurses both nationally and internationally. The dean appoints the two associate deans of undergraduate and graduate nursing programs to serve as leaders of a needs assessment task force.

Using the guidelines for assessing external and internal frame factors (see Chapter 3, Tables 3.1 and 3.2); the task force initiates a needs assessment. The U.S. campus includes the town, nearby city, six major suburban areas, and an adjacent three-county rural area. The major industries and employers near the home campus include the state government, two alternative-energy manufacturers, several food-processing plants, a large inland port, a railroad center, a rocket engineering and manufacturing plant, the primary and secondary educational systems, and several large healthcare systems that serve the city, suburbs, and rural neighbors. In addition to the home campus nursing program, a state-supported baccalaureate and higher degree program with a nursing program are located in the city. There are three state-supported community college nursing programs and there is one large university-based medical center with a PhD nursing program. Other than the home campus DNP program, there are no other DNP programs in the nearby region.

Results from statewide achievement tests reveal that the city's kindergarten through 12th-grade system ranked in the 60th percentile. Most of its students prefer to remain in the local area and the majority of those who continue schooling after high school (40%) go to the local community colleges. Of the suburban students, 55% continued their education in either community colleges or higher educational institutions; however, only 15% of students in rural areas continued their education after high school.

The public transportation system within the region includes buses and a light rail system. Three major highways intersect with the city, providing easy access for automobile travel. There is a middle-sized airport with commuter planes and major airlines and AMTRAK services are available. Greyhound Bus has a terminal in the city, with buses providing interstate transportation. There is one major daily paper, several suburban papers, at least 25 radio stations, five major television stations, TV cable service, and telecommunication services for computer access. There are four major healthcare systems. There are public health clinic services for those who do not have health coverage and who are eligible for state-supported healthcare programs. The city has an elected city council with a mayor, while the smaller incorporated cities are managed through part-time mayors and city councils with full-time city managers. The counties have elected boards of supervisors and each has a sheriff department supplemented by state highway patrol services.

The campus in Kenya is located outside of the largest major metropolis and capital of the nation in a rural countryside. The campus is somewhat isolated by its location and the surrounding countryside by its boundary of fences and walls with security systems in place. The campus is located about 10 miles outside of the capital city and there is a weekly, daily bus service that leaves at 7 a.m. in the city and departs campus at 5 p.m. Students needing transportation on other days and times must provide their own transportation. The adjacent cosmopolitan city has an international airport, public transportation consisting of minibuses, buses, and trains. It is a media hub for Kenya, East Africa, and international broadcasting groups.

The Kenyan government operates the constitution of 2010 with the president as chief executive, a deputy president, an attorney general, and 21 cabinet secretaries. Kenya has a legislature, senate, and judiciary arm. There are 47 decentralized counties within the country, led by the county governor. The official language in Kenya is English (from its time as a British colony) and the national unifying language is Kiswahili (Swahili). The population of Kenya is about 54.9 million, 59% of the population under 24 years and 33.7% in the 25–54 years of age group, with a median age of 20.1 years. The life expectancy is 69.3 years. Approximately 85% of the population is Christian, 11% Muslim, 1.8% other, and the remainder is other or unknown (The World Factbook, 2021).

Agriculture is Kenya's main economic resource and it is an economic and transportation hub for East Africa. Tourism is another attraction; however, terrorism incidents over the past few years led to a decrease in tourism. The lack of infrastructure within the country due to a weak government hampers its economic growth (The World Factbook, 2021). Kenya's educational system consists of an 8-year public, government-supported, primary school system for children starting at 6 years of age followed by a secondary system that runs for 4 years. Its purpose is twofold: to provide education for children who will terminate their education at age 18 and to provide for those who intend to continue into higher education. The country has eight public universities with an emphasis on technology and science. There are other private universities with a variety of degree offerings supervised by the commission on higher education (Embassy of the Republic of

Kenya, 2021). Three of the universities in the city, including the institution's partner, offer nursing programs that award the BScN, and one offers a master's degree in nursing. (The majority of nurses in Kenya have a diploma in nursing.)

Kenya's healthcare system consists of faith-based, private, governmental, and non governmental organizations. The major components of the healthcare system include the Ministry of Health at the national level, divided into the Ministry of Medical Services and the Ministry of Public Health and Sanitation. Health facilities are distributed publicly and through private and faith-based organizations regionally, with the most sophisticated services available in the major cities and at the national level. The tertiary National, Referral, and Teaching Hospitals (NRTH), such as Kenyatta National Hospital in Nairobi, have premier levels of services. The next level of care is found in the secondary county hospitals, followed by primary hospitals. Beneath the primary level there are health centers, dispensaries, maternity centers, and nursing homes, and at the base, community health services at the village, household, and family levels. As is common in most countries, private care provides the highest quality of care, while public services are crowded and difficult to access, especially in rural areas (Oyugi, 2019; World Health Organization, 2017).

Preliminary Conclusions

The infrastructure of the home campus region and the population base for potential student and healthcare services support the existing campus program and could accommodate additional nursing students and graduates. The Kenyan campus infrastructure supports the nursing program, and there is potential for growth.

Demographics of the Populations

The total population of the city adjacent to the U.S. home campus is a little over 1.2 million. The racial breakdown for the urban region is as follows: White: 45.3%, Native American: 1.3%, African American/Black: 8.6%, Asian: 10.9%, Hispanic: 12.6%, two or more races: 6.3%, and other race: 15.0%. The age distribution is as follows: 19 years and younger: 30.2%, 20 to 34: 23.0%, 35 to 44: 15.0%, 45 to 59: 15.9%, 60 to 74: 10%, and 75 and older: 5.9%. Of the population, 77.3% hold a high school diploma, and 23.7% have a baccalaureate or higher. The unemployment rate is 5.6%. The median household income is $41,200. In contrast, the populations of the three surrounding counties are quite different. The racial breakdown averages over 70% White, 7% African American, 2% Native American, 9% Asian, 12% Hispanic, and 1% other. The average median income is $51,000, and less than 5of % households are below the poverty level. The average age distribution in the counties reveals a somewhat older population than the city. About 23% of the counties' residents hold a high school diploma, 17% hold baccalaureates, and 31% had some college education but no degree.

The population of Kenya is 54.9 million and reflects an overall increase as births exceed deaths; if external migration continues, there will be a decrease of 12,555 per year (Country Meters, 2021). There are about 11 African ethnic groups in Kenya, with their specific languages spoken in rural areas and in places where they live. In addition to the African tribes, there are Asian, Arab, and European groups. The population of the multicultural, cosmopolitan city near the campus is over 3.5 million. Half of its population lives in slums; however, the other half live in high-income estates or good housing with new apartment buildings rising in response to the economic growth and resultant expanding middle-income group.

Unemployment rates in Kenya are high (40%), particularly among the young, and are leading to high rates of emigration to seek better employment opportunities. Major employment sectors in Kenya include agriculture with Kenya exporting tea, coffee, fruits, and vegetables; the service industry to support tourism; telecommunications; and mining for soda ash, salt, gold, and some precious stones. Poverty in both rural and urban areas remains high, for example, two thirds of Nairobi's population live in the slums. As mentioned previously, children must enroll in the publicly supported school system from age 6 until the end of the secondary school system, about age 18. However, parents must pay for books, supplies, uniforms, and transportation putting a burden on the poor, and thus the dropout rates from primary to secondary schools are high. Owing to the mandated primary education, the literacy rate is 87%, and there has been an improvement in the rates of education for females.

Preliminary Conclusions

Overall, the population surrounding the home campus in the United States is growing and is economically stable. Its diverse ethnic population meets the program's goal to increase cultural diversity in its student population. There is a large percentage educated beyond high school and who are potential students, faculty, and staff for the program. The situation in Kenya is vastly different. Emigration rates for the young are high, and completion rates for secondary education that provides potential students are low. Higher education opportunities are very limited owing to the lack of available programs and financial support.

Political Climates and Bodies Politic

The town in which the U.S. home campus is located has a mayor and a town council, while the capital city has a mayor and city council. The democrats are the political party in control for both the town and city. The adjacent counties have mayors and council governments for the smaller cities and boards of supervisors for the county government that are predominantly Republican. A review of the political climate reveals that while there are no major health issues currently, key members of the governing bodies and political action groups are aware of the nursing program and its role in the preparation of health professionals for the region. The director of extended education felt that most of the cities' and counties' populations were aware of the parent institution from the college's media campaign. Extended education runs spot announcements on the radio and advertisements in the local newspaper, usually a month before the semesters start. The director described his role on the committee on higher education for the city council, which gives him the opportunity to meet other key educators in the community. It was his overall impression that the reputation of the institution and its quality were gaining in the community.

Although the parent institution's board of regents has only one representative in the public government, the president of the college meets periodically with ad hoc committees of the city councils and boards of supervisors to discuss higher education issues that affect their populaces. He told the survey team that the institution enjoys a high regard in the town and city (students provide income for local businesses) and as a private, high-quality educational institution faculty from the university are often called in as consultants on issues in the region.

The dean of nursing in Kenya shared that he and the dean of pharmacology hold positions in the faculty governance (the senate) and that they serve on the advisory board for the academic vice president. Nationally, nursing is well respected and is beginning to increase its educational preparation at the BScN and master's levels, although the predominant nursing workforce is diploma prepared. Kenyan law allows independent practice for RNs, who must be reviewed and licensed by the National Council. The president of the college is well aware of the need for nurses and in his role as a member of the advisory board to the Commission on Higher Education is educating the commission about the need to raise expectations for the level of preparation for nurses. He serves on the Advisory Board of the Kenyan National Commission for Higher Education that accredits all private higher education institutions in the country (accreditation by the commission is not required for public institutions). Through his membership, he is aware of changes and issues in the government and the political milieu that could affect the institution. At the same time, he is able to have some influence in decisions that affect higher education.

Preliminary Conclusions

The faculty team concluded that key members of the body politic and the public surrounding the U.S. home campus recognize the quality of the institution and are familiar with its programs. The presidents of both institutions and the director of extended education in the United States have key roles in promoting the universities in the community. In Kenya, the nursing program is respected on the university campus, and the dean holds influential positions on campus. Nursing as a profession is respected nationally in Kenya; for example, nurses can practice independently.

The Healthcare Systems and Health Needs of the Populaces

There are four major healthcare systems serving the U.S. home city and surrounding home campus region. Data collection from the websites of the American Hospital Association, the National Association for Home Care, *Morbidity and Mortality Weekly Report* (www.cdc.gov/mmwr/index.html), the state health department's health statistics, and GIS Inventory maps (www.gisinventory.net/index.php?page_id=624) provide the region's health indicators to national and statewide data. One of the systems is a large nonprofit healthcare organization that has a nationwide network. There are two nonprofit regional healthcare systems providing enrollees with a wide array of services. One is sponsored by the same religious-based organization as that of the nursing program's parent institution. The other is a federation of former independent nonprofit community hospitals that merged to share resources for cost savings. There is one public hospital in addition to the state-supported university medical center.

The Veterans Administration (VA) has a large medical center with acute care for all specialties (except maternity and pediatrics, which it subcontracts to other regional hospitals), outpatient services, a nursing home unit, and a rehabilitation center. It prefers RNs with baccalaureates for staffing and employs master's- and DNP-prepared CNLs, clinical nurse specialists, acute care and primary care nurse practitioners, managers, and administrators. It provides clinical practice sites for both undergraduate and graduate students in the region and encourages its staff to continue its education with released time and educational stipends as incentives. It is especially supportive of the master's CNL program and uses many of the school's graduates including administrators and DNP graduates in advanced practice roles. There are three for-profit agencies, and there is one nonprofit visiting nurse association for home healthcare and hospice care. Most school districts have one school nurse, there is a nurse practitioner with four RNs assigned to the city jail, and three of the major industries have occupational health nurses.

The major healthcare problems of the populace match those of the morbidity and mortality statistics of the state and the nation. The population is aging and thus, the need for health services for seniors and chronic diseases is expected to rise. The systems appear to meet the acute care needs of the populace. Additional nurse practitioners are needed in the near future to staff primary care services owing to the increased numbers of insured clients.

The majority of staff nurses are associate degree graduates. All the large healthcare systems employ clinical nurse specialists or acute care nurse practitioners and those with primary care services employ nurse practitioners. The university-based medical center has an all RN staff and employs more clinical nurse specialists and acute care nurse practitioners than the other systems. The public health clinics use public health nurses prepared at the baccalaureate and master's levels for follow-up visits and for health promotion and disease prevention programs. Nurse practitioners staff the few primary care clinics. The visiting nurse organization uses both public health nurses and RNs for home visiting and hospice services. The administrators reported that they welcome nursing students and have existing clinical placement agreements with the regional nursing schools. The affiliating system was especially open to having additional students in their agencies and indicated that the program's students would receive priority placements.

Kenya's healthcare system is organized from the top down, and healthcare services are distributed regionally. The city adjacent to the university has a large teaching hospital where private and public healthcare at the tertiary care level is provided and which provides clinical experiences for the nursing students. Counties provide the next level of care; however, the quality of care drops significantly. In smaller regional health centers, complex health problems are referred to the larger institution with the health centers focusing on primary care, counseling, and maternity, and child health services. Only 20% of Kenyans have health insurance, and over half of the population lives in poverty. Major health problems include malaria, communicable diseases, HIV (although rates have slowed somewhat), malnutrition, high maternal and infant mortality rates, poor sanitation, and a lack of affordable medications. Kenya has a shortage of health professionals, with providers poorly distributed throughout the country (Child Fund International, 2021).

Preliminary Conclusions

There is a wide variety of healthcare agencies with a plethora of potential clinical experiences available for students enrolled in the U.S. home campus nursing program. Nursing administrators welcomed the idea of expanded programs to increase the numbers of baccalaureate and higher degree nurses in the region. The healthcare problems and needs of the populace are not unique and match the existing content of the curriculum. Kenya has major health and socioeconomic problems to address, and except for large metropolitan areas, tertiary healthcare services are limited and of lesser quality. With so many Kenyans living in poverty, minimal health insurance coverage of the population, major health problems requiring primary care, maternal and child health, and community/public health services, and the concomitant shortage of nurses, there is a critical need to expand nursing education opportunities.

Characteristics of the Academic Settings

A survey of the U.S. schools' websites provides the types of nursing programs and tracks offered, enrollments, graduation rates, licensure examination (National Council Licensure Examination [NCLEX]) pass rates, and where the majority of graduates works. In the area, three community colleges offer associate degrees in nursing (ADNs), and the state-supported school offers an entry-level BScN program as well as an RN-to-BSN program. It has two master's specialty tracks: one in education and an FNP program. The three community colleges are about equal in size and their total enrollments are approximately 150, with 50 graduates each year. Their qualified applicant pool numbers 350 each, although they believe they may be drawing from the same applicant pool. The vast majority of their graduates remain in the local area to practice in acute care, nursing homes, or home health agencies. The state-supported school has a total enrollment of

300 students in the basic BSN program, 60 RNs in the RN-to-BSN program, and 90 in the graduate programs. The master of science in nursing (MSN) nurse practitioner program is the most popular, with the educational tracks enrolling approximately 10 to 12 students each year. The basic BSN program graduates approximately 65 each year. About 80% of its graduates remain in the area to practice. The qualified applicant pool for the basic BSN program is 350, and again, the administrator believes some of the applicants may be in the same pool as the ADN programs.

The U.S. university academic health sciences center currently has medical, dental, pharmacy, and nursing programs. It is a research extensive institution and therefore offers a research-focused degree (PhD) in nursing. Graduates of the nursing program hold positions as researchers in medical centers and as faculty in schools of nursing. It has about 36 students enrolled in the program in various stages of doctoral study, graduates about 10 students each year and admits approximately 8 to 10 students per year.

In the city near the Kenyan campus, there are seven private universities and one state-supported university that has a BScN and MSN program. Two of the private universities have BScN programs that are in competition for applicants to the partner university. The campus is about 10 miles outside one of the major cities in Kenya. It has a traditional campus with academic, ADM, library, sports and recreational complexes, and student housing. It holds accreditation by the Kenyan Commission on Higher Education and regional accreditation from one of the accreditation commissions in the United States. It is an international campus, and students from other countries enroll in its programs with many coming from those nations affiliated with the sponsoring religious organization. Recently, the Kenyan government fostered a partnership with private universities to support Kenyan students' tuition at private institutions. There are four major areas of study in the institution including the Colleges of Social Studies and Humanities, Science and Technology, Health Sciences, and Engineering and Agriculture. Within the College of Health Sciences are the Schools of Pharmacology and Nursing. Nursing awards a BScN in basic nursing practice and is accredited by the National Council of Kenya (NCK; for nursing). There are 100 students in the undergraduate program, with 25 graduating each year. It experiences about 100 applications each year.

Preliminary Conclusions

In the United States, the region has six nursing programs, three ADN, two baccalaureate and master's degree programs (includes the home campus), one DNP program offered on the home campus, and one PhD in nursing program. There appears to be an adequate qualified applicant pool for the regional programs. In Kenya, there are three higher degree programs in nursing programs that are in competition with the partner school; however, there is an adequate applicant pool each year.

The Need for the Program

In the region of the U.S. home campus, the nursing workforce has 1,450 RNs of whom 1,250 are employed. The four major healthcare systems report a vacancy rate of 10% and the schools, public health clinics, and home care agency report a total of 50 vacant positions. The number of vacancies does not account for the numbers of nurses in the workforce who plan to retire within the next 5 years. In addition to entry-level positions, 100% of the administrators of the nursing services programs told the team that they anticipated increasing their staff owing to the growing demand and complexity of healthcare. The administrators indicated a preference for baccalaureate-prepared nurses and when informed about the entry-level master's, RN-to-BSN online program, and the DNP program, their interest increased, especially if the programs are accelerated.

In Kenya in 2016, there were 19,994 nurses employed in 4,287 healthcare facilities. Notable is a decrease in the number of students enrolling in nursing by the end of 2015 (Ministry of Health, 2015). The ratio of nurses in Kenya in 2018 was about 1.1 per 1,000 population (The World Bank, 2021), compared to approximately 12.6/1,000 in the United States (NurseJournal, 2021).

Preliminary Conclusions

There is a documented need for entry-level nurses in the United States and an increased need for baccalaureate-prepared graduates and advanced practice nurses. There is a shortage of nurses at all levels to meet the healthcare needs of the population in Kenya. The needs thus far match the types of options of the home campus nursing program and there is a need for all levels of nurses in Kenya. Since the university in Kenya has only the entry-level BScN, there are possibilities for expanding their program for RNs to BSN and possibly a master's program through collaboration with the home campus online.

The Nursing Profession

In the United States, nursing is responding to the National Academy of Medicine, 2021 (previously known as the Institute of Medicine) recommendations calling for advanced nursing education and to the effects of the Affordable Healthcare Act (U.S. Department of Health and Human Services, 2021) that resulted in more of the population having health insurance. According to the American Association of Colleges of Nursing (AACN, 2019), the numbers of students enrolled in BSN, particularly in degree completion programs, master's, and the doctorate in nursing practice continue to increase.

In the United States, about 60% of the employed nurses work in acute care, the remainder are in community-based agencies. About 60% of the working nurses have an ADN or diploma, 31% have a BSN, 8% have a master's, and fewer than 1% have a doctorate. It was difficult to match the educational preparation of the nurses to the type of position they held although anecdotal information demonstrated that the majority of master's-prepared nurses were top administrators (vice presidents), clinical nurse specialists, CNLs, or nurse practitioners. The BSN nurses were employed in public health, schools, home care, or as case managers or administrators.

The latest information on the nursing workforce in Kenya came from the Kenya Nursing Workforce Report (Ministry of Health, 2015). At that time, hospitals employed 67.9% of the nursing workforce, dispensaries 17.7%, and 3.1% were in government management offices. Of the nursing workforce, 13% had postbasic specialty training and 79.5% received basic midwifery training. Out-migration continues to be a problem with nurses applying to migrate out of the country. As previously stated, enrollments in schools of nursing have decreased. In 2015, there were 3,077 seeking licensure following graduation, with 271 in certificate programs, 2,552 in diploma programs, and 254 in BScN programs.

Preliminary Conclusions

In the United States, there is a shortage of nurses in the region, state, and nation. The majority of the workforce practices in acute care and is prepared at the ADN level, although enrollments in baccalaureate and higher degree programs are increasing. The current workforce in the United States does not meet the preferred need for baccalaureate and advanced practice–prepared nurses. The existing regional schools of nursing cannot meet the current demand for nurses, and employers of nurses forecast an increasing need in the future. In Kenya, there is a critical shortage of nurses and particularly those prepared at the baccalaureate and higher degree levels. Seventy percent of the workforce is employed in acute care, with only 17.7% employed in dispensaries in spite of the need for nurses in primary care, maternal and child health, and public health nursing roles to match the health needs of the populace.

Regulations and Accreditation Requirements

The U.S. program is due for a Commission on Collegiate Nursing Education (CCNE) reaccreditation visit in 2 years. CCNE requires that educational programs planning new programs must submit a substantive change report to the commission no earlier than 90 days prior to implementation or no later than 90 days after its implementation. The U.S. nursing program has the approval of the state board of nursing. The board must approve any expansions of the program that affect any of the licensure or state certification requirements and must be presented to the board at least 6 months in advance. Board guidelines include a list of qualified faculty, adequate student services including library facilities, approved clinical facilities, and adequate classroom and learning laboratories.

The nursing program on the Kenyan campus is accredited by the NCK. Schools in Kenya must submit an application form and a copy of the curriculum. Faculty teaching in degree programs must have at least a master's degree and 2 years of clinical training, while those teaching in diploma programs must have at least a baccalaureate, 2 years of clinical practice, and preparation in education and curriculum development. Schools are inspected to ensure that standards are maintained such as tutor capacity, physical facilities, transportation, bed capacity, and bed occupancy.

Both parent institutions in the United States and Kenya have regional accreditation. New degree programs must be preapproved by the agency at least 6 months prior to the enrollment of the first class. The criteria for approval are much the same as the state board of nursing. In addition to the requirements of the board, the regional agency looks for evidence of infrastructure feasibility and educational effectiveness. The usual turn-around time for a response to a proposal is 2 months.

Preliminary Conclusions

Both the parent institutions and the nursing programs are accredited regionally and nationally. The home campus nursing program is accredited by the state b of nursing. If the faculty and administrators of the home campus revise or develop new tracks in the program or develop a partnership with Kenya, the proposal for the changes must be completed and submitted to the state board of nursing and the regional accrediting agency at least 6 months prior to start-up of the program. A description of the program should be submitted to CCNE and the NCK in Kenya 90 days prior to its initiation.

Financial Support

The assessment team prepares a report and business case on the financial resources of the parent institution and the nursing program. The parent institution has an endowment fund of over $120 million. It has an active alumni association and raises at least $2 million each year for scholarships. Its capital operating costs match that of the tuition and fees income each year. It has several million-dollar grants from private and federal sources for research in science and for program development in education. The nursing program has one federal grant ($600,000) for the DNP program, $10,000 from the federal advanced education nursing traineeships, one healthcare system grant for $10,000 for preparing RNs to BSNs, and several scholarship funds totaling $5 million in endowments. The financial-aid programs include a statewide tuition assistance program for needy students, the federally sponsored work-study programs and traineeships, PELL grants, nursing loan programs, and a forgivable loan program from a healthcare agency for students who agree to work for that agency for 2 years upon graduation. In addition, there are numerous private scholarships that are available to nursing students from external sources. The university in Kenya has an endowment fund through the religious-based organization of $10 million (U.S. equivalent dollars). Industry in Kenya in the metropolitan areas provides tuition support for students majoring in agriculture, engineering, and business. The healthcare organization through which students have clinical experiences offers three full scholarships for students in nursing on a rotating basis.

The U.S. comptroller ensures the team that the institution will provide a business plan for the nursing program to calculate start-up costs and the economic feasibility of an expanded program and that he will share it with his counterpart in Kenya. If the program appears to be economically sound, the institutions will provide the start-up costs. The four major healthcare systems indicate to the assessment team that they will continue to provide clinical sites, and scholarships or loans for nursing students are possible. The affiliate system has some labs that students could use for clinical skills practice, and they are quite interested in scholarship programs or forgivable loans for students who commit to a 2-year contract upon graduation.

The dean of nursing in Kenya indicates that he will investigate additional resources for nursing students such as the Ministry of Health and the sectarian healthcare system that provides clinical experiences for students. He reminds the team that the Kenyan government recently put a tuition assistance program in place for students in private institutions of higher education.

Preliminary Conclusions

The parent institutions in the United States and Kenya and the nursing programs are financially stable. There is the promise of start-up funds and professional consultation from the home campus for a business plan if the decision to expand the program is realized. In addition to the traditional economic resources, there are potential sources of income and support from the healthcare systems in both places, and the government in Kenya recently put a tuition assistance program in place for students enrolled in a private institution.

INTERNAL FRAME FACTORS

Description and Organizational Structure of the Parent Academic Institutions

The most recent accreditation reports for the CCNE and the board of nursing, the regional accreditation report, and the report for the NCK provide a description including the organizational structure for both universities and schools. The home school of nursing shares offices, classrooms, and several laboratories with the science department. In addition, it has one clinical skills lab, one low- and one high-fidelity simulation lab under its control. Nursing represents about 4.5% (350 BSN, 100 master's, and 60 DNP) of the student body and was the first professional school in the university. The institution averages an enrollment of 8,000 undergraduate students each year, with the graduate school enrollment at 3,000. It has six schools: Arts and Sciences (40% of the enrollment), Business Administration and Economics (20%), Computer Science (10%), Education (10%), Extended Education (4%), and Nursing. All but the Arts and Sciences school have graduate programs and Education is a graduate-only school. The highest degree that the institution awards is the doctoral degree (PhD, DBA, and DNP), and it awards the BA, bachelor of science, master of arts, and master of science degrees.

Although the original purpose of the university had strong liberal arts and religious foci, the institution became multipurpose with the addition of the professional schools. The School of Extended Education offers distance education programs in business administration, computer sciences, and education from the home campus and works collaboratively with nursing on the RN-to-BSN program. Each school has a dean and the school of nursing dean has been in his position for 12 years and therefore has a strong voice in the council of deans. There is an academic provost to whom the deans report. The president is its chief executive officer. There is a comptroller, a dean of student affairs and enrollment services, directors of human resources, the library, and information services and instructional support.

The academic senate is composed of two representatives from each school's faculty, three members-at-large, undergraduate and graduate student representatives, a presidential appointee, and the academic provost. There are three major committees of the senate: curriculum, graduate, and faculty affairs. There is one nursing faculty member on the graduate committee, one nurse is chair of the faculty affairs committee, with another, a member-at-large of the senate. The school of nursing faculty and the senate curriculum committee must approve new academic programs and curriculum revisions. If the proposals emanate from graduate programs, the graduate committee recommends approval after review and sends them to the senate with recommendations.

The school of nursing faculty numbers 40 full-time tenured/tenure-track faculty and 15 part-time clinical faculty, not including the dean, and five administrative support staff (approximately 1–11 faculty–student ratio). There are two administrators for instructional support and information systems. A part-time clinical instructor serves as the clinical placement coordinator. There are two associate deans, one each for the graduate program and the undergraduate program. The three track coordinators for the BSN, master's, and DNP programs have 20% released time for these functions. The part-time faculty's teaching role occurs primarily in supervising students during their clinical experiences. The faculty members teach in both undergraduate and graduate programs, although some are predominantly assigned to one or the other depending on their clinical expertise and academic preparation. Seventy-five percent of the full-time tenure track faculty members have doctorates and there are currently three enrolled in doctoral programs. The school of nursing faculty meets once a month during the academic year and there are four major committees: curriculum, graduate, peer evaluation, and student affairs. All program and curriculum revisions must be approved through the appropriate nursing committee structure, approved by the faculty as a whole, with final administrative review and approval by the dean. Approved proposals are forwarded to the appropriate senate committee that makes recommendations to the senate that votes for approval or disapproval. Upon approval of the senate, the provost completes a final review and makes recommendations to the president.

The dean of nursing in Kenya provided an organizational chart for his university and the school of nursing. Like the home campus, the university, as a private, sectarian institution, has a strong reputation in the region and with its accreditation by the Commission on Higher Education in Kenya, as well as the U.S. regional accreditation, carries high regard in academic circles. The university numbers a total of 6,000 students (5,500 undergraduate and 500 graduate) with nursing accounting for 2% (100 students) of the total and pharmacology 3% for a total of 5% for the College of Health and Human Services, social studies and humanities, 25%; science and technology, 20%; and agriculture and engineering, 50%. There are 260 full-time faculty members and 40 part-time. In nursing, there are 10 full-time and 5 part-time faculty members, with an approximate 1-to-8 faculty-to-student ratio. The part-time faculty members supervise students in clinical settings. There are 1.5 administrative assistants and one clinical faculty coordinator who staffs the learning lab. All the full-time faculty members have master's degrees, and the part-time faculty members have BScNs that meet the requirements of the National Council. The faculty meets as a whole once a month and task forces are assigned ad hoc according to program needs. For curricular changes, an ad hoc committee reviews proposals, refines them, and then presents them to the faculty for approval. If approved, a proposal moves to the curriculum committee of the university senate that, upon approval, moves it forward for full senate approval. The vice president for academic affairs makes a recommendation to the president who must approve or disapprove the program. A nursing faculty member serves on the senate, and the dean of nursing is a member of the president's advisory council.

Preliminary Conclusions

Both universities have strong reputations for high-quality liberal arts and professional educational programs and the nursing programs and their faculty members have significant roles within the institutions. There are clear hierarchal lines of communication for administrative decisions and for gaining curriculum and program approval. While the nursing schools account for only a small proportion of the total academic offerings, they are highly regarded by others. The schools have representatives on the governing senates and the deans of nursing have influential roles in the administrative systems.

Mission and Purpose, Philosophy, and Goals of the Parent Institution

Owing to the institution's religious base, both nursing programs' missions are congruent with those of their parent institutions' missions and goals that focus on the preparation of compassionate and responsible citizens for society and professionals who provide services to the community.

Preliminary Conclusions

The nursing programs' missions and purposes, philosophies, and goals are in congruence with those of the parent institutions.

Internal Economic Situation and Its Influence on the Curriculum

When conducting the assessment of the external frame factors, faculty found that both schools of nursing are financially stable. The U.S. comptroller will develop a business case for a proposed program, and there are potential external funding resources for new programs should they start. The sponsoring religious organization and its healthcare system both in the United States and in Kenya indicated an interest in donating some start-up funds and possible scholarships. However, this requires released time for faculty to write the grants. It is calculated that two faculty members from the U.S. campus and one from Kenya each need 10% released time for the next semester to write these grants. The comptroller refers both deans to their respective provosts/vice presidents, who agree to provide a total of $10,000 in the United States and $5,000 equivalent dollars in Kenya for faculty to write grant proposals.

A concern of the deans and faculty is the need to provide released time for curriculum development when and if expansion is approved. This would involve at least three faculty members and would take about 5% of their workload in assigned time activities to develop or revise the existing curriculum. The comptroller suggests that the deans place this on their agendas when the next year's budgets are proposed.

Preliminary Conclusions

The schools of nursing are economically stable. Their administrations indicate support for developing a business case for an expanded and/or revised program. The provost and the vice president will provide funds for the next semester for faculty to write grants for program development. The deans will include the cost for faculty-released time for curriculum development into next year's budget.

Resources Within the Institution and Nursing Programs

Since proposed changes or new programs must match the resources of the existing programs and yet meet the needs of students who may be at a distance from the schools, the assessment team surveys resources needed for possible distance outreach. The home campus classrooms, learning and computer laboratories, and classrooms, although not under the U.S. school's control, are adequate in size and number for the current on-campus student enrollment. There is a need to upgrade the clinical practice laboratory and add at least one additional simulation lab with high-fidelity mannequins. The library has one of the largest holdings in the region for nursing journals and texts as well as for other disciplines. The director of the library and the administrators for information systems and instructional support services meet with the team and indicate that nursing will continue to have access to these technologies.

The Kenyan school of nursing shares general classrooms with the total university and has no problems with scheduling lecture classes. There is one science lab that is shared with the school of pharmacy and nursing has its own skills lab with four hospital beds, mannequins, and equipment; a low-fidelity lab to practice additional skills; and a computer lab with 10 computers donated from the healthcare system. The university library is well stocked with texts and journals from the arts and sciences and recently, through a grant from industry, increased its online access to more than 100 databases, including PubMed, Cumulative Index to Nursing and Allied Health Literature (CINAHL), and EBSCO Information Services. For the present undergraduate students, the campus offers adequate learning labs, classrooms, and library facilities although a new high-fidelity simulation lab would help meet clinical skills demands as healthcare becomes more complex. As mentioned before, the schools of business and education have online programs for students, thus the infrastructure for web-based learning has been initiated. The Kenyan faculty representative indicated an interest in web-based learning and is currently enrolled in a U.S. online doctoral program. She is interested in exploring possibilities for nursing to collaborate with the schools of business and education in distance education. The dean and the faculty member met with the deans of business and education and information systems and instructional support administrators to share information about the possibility of expanding their program in collaboration with the U.S. campus. The deans are interested in the proposal and agree to meet again when plans are in place to initiate a program.

In the United States, the team meets with the director of enrollment services and discusses recruitment, student records, counseling services, financial aid programs, and work-study options for nursing students. The proposed program calls for at least one additional staff member in enrollment services for all of the services mentioned previously. The faculty member in Kenya discusses the possible expansion of the nursing program with student services. Since it is more than likely that the expansion will be web-based, additional recruitment, financial aid, and online access to databases are indicated.

Home Campus	*Kenya Campus*
Upgrade clinical skills lab	*High-fidelity simulation lab*
High-fidelity simulation lab	*Additional staff for student services*
Additional staff for web-based learning, and other student services	*Faculty development for web-based program*
Additional faculty depending on enrollments	*Additional faculty depending on enrollments*
	Expansion of web-based systems

Preliminary Conclusions

Current facilities and services for the schools of nursing are adequate for the on-campus programs in the United States and in Kenya, including the current online programs in the United States. However, the following is a list of needs if the program expands or an outreach web-based program is decided on.

Potential Faculty and Student Characteristics

The team agrees that a full-time coordinator for a new program or additional faculty for expanded program(s) is necessary during the planning stages as well as for managing the program when it commences. If tracks are expanded, and depending on enrollments, additional faculty members will be added with increased released time for the coordinators of the expanded programs. Educational levels, clinical expertise, scholarship and research, and teaching experience qualifications of new faculty must be matched to the needs of new programs, university expectations, and accreditation standards. If the Kenyan program adds graduate tracks, it will need master's and preferably doctorate-prepared faculty. At the present time, the dean in Kenya has his doctorate and one faculty member is earning her doctorate in nursing practice online from an American university. The size of the faculty will be determined by the choice of program, specialty, prelicensure program or not, and the delivery mode of the program. Currently, the faculty-to-student ratio of 1 to 11 on the home campus and 1 to 8 in Kenya is acceptable.

Like the faculty, the characteristics and size of the student body depend on the decision to expand or to offer new programs and the types of programs. A calculation is necessary for the critical mass of students needed to meet the cost of mounting the program. With these factors in mind, the team looks at enrollment patterns over the past 5 years. The undergraduate program enrollments have been stable; however, the applicant pool decreased on the home campus by 5%. The entry-level MSN program applicant pool increased by 15%. The DNP program is very popular, and the admission rate was about 20% (30 admissions to 150 applicants) with a waiting list for up to 1 year. Graduates of the home campus BSN program have priority for admission to the DNP program with up to 15 admitted each year. In Kenya, the applicant pool for the BScN increased slightly over the past 2 years. There have been increased inquiries about a graduate program. Establishing a partnership with the Kenya School of Nursing would require additional staff on both campuses to coordinate recruitment and admission activities.

Preliminary Conclusions

While the current overall nursing faculty-to-student ratio is good for both schools, any new or expanded programs will require additional faculty and staff depending on enrollments and the nature of the programs. Support staff for the programs, admissions, and enrollment services will be necessary. Applications to the existing programs on both campuses remain steady and in fact, are increasing for the graduate-level programs on the home campus. The applicant pool remains steady in Kenya, and there have been increased inquiries for a graduate program.

See Appendix Table 1 for a summary of the findings for external and internal frame factors of the needs assessment.

SUMMARY OF THE NEEDS ASSESSMENT

A needs assessment of external and internal frame factors revealed a positive environment for an expanded program when compared to the desired outcomes of the guidelines for assessing external and internal frame factors found in Chapter 3, Tables 3.1 and 3.2. Both physical environments of the universities in the United States and Kenya are supportive of the schools of nursing and the surrounding communities have resources available to the academic communities. The universities hold U.S. regional accreditation, and the Kenyan university is accredited by the Commission on Higher Education in Kenya. Both schools of nursing are accredited nationally: in the United States, by the CCNE and, in Kenya, by the NCK. The schools of nursing are highly regarded on the home campuses, their missions and goals match those of the institutions, and the administrators and faculty of the programs hold influential positions on campus and in the community. Because of the efforts on the part of the institutions' leaders and faculty in the community, the broader body politic supports the universities and the schools of nursing.

Competition from neighboring schools of nursing seems negligible owing to the large applicant pool, and the need for nurses and the PhD program in the United States have the potential for providing faculty from its graduates. Potential applicants to all U.S. programs reflect a diverse population, and the applicant pool in Kenya is steady, but the population base for entry-level baccalaureate programs is small. The healthcare systems indicate a need for nurses prepared at the baccalaureate and higher degree levels and continue to support both schools of nursing. Healthcare needs are very high in Kenya, and there is a shortage of nurses. In addition, with the great majority of nurses prepared at the diploma level, there is a need for degree programs for the existing workforce. The potential for a collaborative online program exists as Kenya has experience with master's education in business and education and the United States. RN-to-BSN, master's, and doctorate programs are all online.

The financial health of both institutions is good and there are possible additional resources available for program expansion. There are multiple grants and scholarships available to nursing programs and students in the United States and there is tuition support from the national government in Kenya as well as possible scholarships from the healthcare systems. Both schools of nursing currently have adequate classrooms, clinical labs, and technology support; however, if the Kenyan program were to offer web-based courses, it would need to link to the existing web system for business and education. Library and instructional support systems are adequate at this time, although additional staff and faculty may be needed if enrollments increase and there is an increased need for technical support.

The organizational structures of the two universities are such that faculty members develop the curriculum and the governing bodies of the universities (the senates) review and approve the proposals prior to administrative approval by either the provost (U.S.) or academic vice president (Kenya) and, finally, the presidents with assent from the respective boards of trustees. The parent institution indicated support by offering to develop a business case and start-up funds should the faculty recommend an expanded program, and it will work with the Kenyan campus. The provost and the academic vice president promised funds for faculty to write grants for program development.

TABLE A.1: Analysis of the Case Study's Needs Assessment: External and Internal Frame Factors and Decision-Making

External Frame Factors	Findings			Conclusions
	Positive	**Negative**	**Neutral**	
Community description	Size, location, and infrastructure of the home region support potential expansion. In Kenya, the infrastructure of the BScN program is supportive and there is potential for growth.			*Positive* In the United States, the community location and support systems, including the online program, can accommodate an expansion of the program. The Kenyan program has infrastructure support.
Demographics	There is an adequate diverse regional applicant pool in the United States and the economy is stable. There is a pool of potential faculty and staff in the United States. The applicant pool for the Kenyan BScN is good.	In Kenya, graduation rates from secondary schools are low, and there is a high emigration rate of the educated youth.		*Positive* Applicant pools for the home campus and Kenya are good. In the United States, there is a diverse population in the region. In the United States, there is a pool of potential faculty. *Negative* The potential applicant pool for an expanded BScN program in Kenya is uncertain.
Political climate and the body politic	The parent institution and Kenyan campus are recognized in their respective communities. Representatives in leadership positions from both campuses have influential contacts in the community.			*Positive* Both nursing programs and their parent institutions are respected in their communities. Relationships with leaders in both locales are influential and good.

(continued)

TABLE A.1: Analysis of the Case Study's Needs Assessment: External and Internal Frame Factors and Decision-Making (*continued*)

External Frame Factors	Findings			Conclusions
	Positive	**Negative**	**Neutral**	
Healthcare system and health needs of the population	There is a wide variety of healthcare agencies for learning experiences. Nursing administrators favor and support BSN or higher degree programs. Healthcare needs match curriculum content. There is a critical need to expand nursing education in Kenya.	Multiple health and social problems face the population of Kenya.		*Positive* The healthcare system is supportive and offers many learning opportunities for students. Healthcare needs match the existing curriculum. There is a critical need for nurses to meet the healthcare needs of the Kenyan population. *Negative* There is a critical need to address the healthcare and social needs of the population of Kenya.
Academic settings	Adequate, diverse applicant pool for all six U.S. area schools. The Kenyan campus offers only BScN and has an adequate applicant pool.			*Positive* In the United States, there is an adequate, diverse applicant pool. In Kenya, there is an adequate applicant pool to the BScN.
Need for the program	In the United States, there is a need for additional entry-level nurses in light of current and future shortages. There is a demand for BSN+-prepared nurses. Existing program offerings match the demand. In Kenya, there is a need for all levels of nursing, specifically, degree prepared.			*Positive* An expanded program could meet the regional and Kenyan demand for additional nurses at the professional entry- and advanced practice levels.

Nursing profession	There is a shortage of nurses prepared at the baccalaureate and higher degree levels in the United States. There is a critical shortage of nurses in Kenya. The majority of nurses in Kenya are prepared at the diploma level.	*Neutral* As stated in the need for the program, nursing workforce shortages at higher degree levels continue in the United States. There is a critical shortage of nurses in Kenya. The majority of nurses are prepared at the diploma level in Kenya.
Regulations and accreditation	Both parent institutions and the nursing programs are accredited. A proposal for a new degree program must be submitted to the regional accrediting body and the state board of nursing.	*Positive* Both parent institutions and the nursing programs are accredited. *Neutral* Proposals must be submitted to the accrediting and regulating bodies in advance of initiation if the assessment of external and internal frame factors is favorable toward an expanded program.

(continued)

TABLE A.1: Analysis of the Case Study's Needs Assessment: External and Internal Frame Factors and Decision-Making (*continued*)

External Frame Factors	Findings			Conclusions
	Positive	**Negative**	**Neutral**	
Financial support	Financial reports indicate economic health and stability in both places. The parent institution will provide start-up funds. At least two healthcare systems offered financial assistance.		There are other potential financial resources to be investigated.	*Positive* The financial picture is good. *Neutral* There are future potential resources that need to be explored further.

Internal Frame Factors	Findings			Conclusions
	Positive	**Negative**	**Neutral**	
Description and organizational structure of the parent institution	Both schools are held in high regard by their parent institutions. Organizational and hierarchal communication lines are clear for curriculum approval. There are nursing representatives on the senates. The deans have influence in the universities.			*Positive* The organizational structures and administrators are supportive. The deans have influence in the universities. Nursing representatives are on the senates.
Mission and purpose, philosophy, and goals of the parent institution	Both nursing programs' missions, purposes, philosophies, and goals match those of their home institutions.			*Positive* The nursing programs' missions, purposes, philosophies, and goals match those of their home institutions.

Internal economic situation and its influence on the curriculum	Both schools are economically stable. There is administrative support and funds for grant proposals. A business plan will be developed.		*Positive* A business plan will be developed. The schools are financially stable. There are funds for grant writing.
Resources within the institution and nursing program	Current facilities are adequate on both campuses. Library resources are adequate. A web-based system exists in the United States.	There is potential for a web-based system in Kenya.	*Positive* Current facilities are adequate on both campuses. Library resources are adequate. A web-based system exists in the United States.
	On-campus facilities may need updating if entry-level programs are added. Additional staff and faculty may be required.		*Negative* On-campus facilities may need updating if entry-level programs are added. Additional staff and faculty may be required. *Neutral* There is potential for a web-based system in Kenya.

(continued)

TABLE A.1: Analysis of the Case Study's Needs Assessment: External and Internal Frame Factors and Decision-Making (*continued*)

External Frame Factors	Findings			Conclusions
	Positive	Negative	Neutral	
Potential faculty and student characteristics	Faculty to student ratios are good. Faculty are qualified. Applications to the programs are increasing except for the entry-level BSN on the home campus.		Additional faculty and staff will be necessary with program expansion.	*Positive* Faculty are qualified. Present faculty ratios are good. Overall, application rates are good. *Neutral* Additional faculty and staff will be necessary if the program expands.
Overall conclusions				28 Positive 4 Negative 7 Neutral

Final Decision Statement

Based on the needs assessment of the external and internal frame factors that surround the schools of nursing on the U.S. campus and in Kenya, the needs assessment team recommends the development of a partnership between the two schools to maintain the viable offerings in the U.S. curriculum and to increase the numbers of baccalaureate and higher degree level nurses in Kenya through web-based education.

The assessment team offered several recommendations to the deans for their consideration and action based on the analysis and summary. Possible strategies for developing specific plans to implement the recommendations were included:

1. Open the online RN-to-BSN program to diploma graduates in Kenya.
   a. The School of Nursing in Kenya should take the lead in recruitment and enrollment services for Kenyan nurses to enroll in the online U.S. program.
   b. The U.S. campus provides its expertise and experience in online education so that the campus in Kenya assumes responsibility for its own program at least 3 years following its implementation.
2. Expand the RN-to-BSN program into an accelerated RN-to-MSN online program for both schools.
   a. Review both schools' baccalaureate programs to ensure that core concepts and content meet accreditation and professional standards.
   b. Review the current master's program and its options for an accelerated master's for RNs.
3. Open the online DNP advanced practice tracks to Kenyan BScN graduates.
   a. If there is interest in the program from Kenya, add up to five slots in the program with at least three targeted for qualified BScN graduates.
   b. Explore the possibility of an additional advanced practice track in maternal/child health to meet the critical healthcare needs of Kenya and its potential in the United States.

CASE STUDY: CURRICULUM FOR ACCELERATED RN-TO-MSN PROGRAM

The following is a description of a curriculum that opens the U.S. RN-to-BSN program to diploma-prepared RNs from Kenya and revises the RN-to-BSN program to accelerate both U.S. and Kenyan students into the master's ADM or CHN tracks. The administrative track prepares leaders for management roles in the healthcare system that applies to both nations. The CHN track prepares professional nurses to provide high-level, coordinated community/public health nursing care. It includes public health sciences that are especially useful to nurses in Kenya, where rural areas, poverty factors, and inadequate infrastructures cause major health problems. It was decided that the RN-to-BSN and the accelerated RN-to-MSN programs have priority and will serve as a pathway, at a later time, to the DNP program. Opening the RN-to-BSN track to Kenyan nurses will require consultation, planning, and coordination with the dean and faculty in Kenya and the financial officers on both campuses. For this case study's purposes, the following is a sample curriculum plan for the RN to MSN, online, CHN track.

After a review of the existing missions, visions, and overall goals of the two parent universities and the schools of nursing, both faculties find them similar and broad enough to encompass the existing end-of-program objectives for the RN-to-BSN and master's CHN programs. The overall master's end-of-program outcome serves as the guide for the student-learning outcomes (SLOs) throughout the RN-to-MSN program and states, "the master's prepared nurse provides advanced practice nursing and interprofessional leadership within the evolving and complex healthcare system to prevent disease, promote health, and elevate care for groups, communities, and populations in various settings."

In order to move into graduate-level courses, RNs complete the equivalent of upper-division–level BSN courses having completed lower division courses in their entry-level nursing programs (ADN or diploma). Individual assessment of the RNs' associate degrees or diplomas must take place to ensure that the lower division courses or their equivalents have been completed. The U.S. home campus has articulation agreements with the regional associate degree programs so that ADN graduates directly transfer in credits. For the remaining RNs, if prerequisite discrepancies are found, individual academic plans are made to either enroll in equivalent courses or receive credit for them through challenge or portfolio through their home campus in the United States or Kenya. It should not take any longer than one or two semesters for them to complete the prerequisites.

It is planned that the accelerated RN-to-MSN program will take 3 years full-time to complete (a part-time option will be available). The first year (Level 1) is 1 calendar year (three semesters) and students complete the equivalent of upper division nursing courses in the BSN program. Therefore, the level objectives for Level 1 of the program are the same as the SLOs for the basic BSN. The outcomes are those that already exist on the U.S. campus and were compared to the Kenyan BScN nursing program and found to be similar enough to be approved by the Kenyan nursing faculty, the academic senates, and the administrations of the parent institutions. They are consistent with the new AACN (2021), *The Essentials for Professional Nursing Practice*:

The RN-to-MSN Level 1 student will:

1. Apply a liberal education and the sciences to the practice of professional nursing.
2. Demonstrate leadership in providing high-quality care and patient safety in the healthcare system.
3. Provide professional nursing care that is based on the translation of evidence.
4. Manage information and technology in the provision of quality patient care.
5. Participate in health promotion and disease prevention practice to improve population health.
6. Influence healthcare policy, financing, and regulations as they affect professional nursing practice.
7. Improve healthcare outcomes through interprofessional communication and collaboration.
8. Demonstrate professional values that include altruism, autonomy, human dignity, integrity, and social justice.
9. Respect the variations of professional practice that apply to the care of individuals, families, groups, communities, and populations across the life span.

To meet the SLOs, the RNs take many of the same courses that junior and senior students in the BSN program take; however, like the RN-to-BSN students, the courses are offered online. The courses are pathophysiology, genetics, health assessment, interprofessional healthcare practice: communication and collaboration, introduction to nursing research, nursing leadership, CHN theory and practice, and analysis of the healthcare system. The practicum takes place in the nurses' home communities under the supervision of the faculty and mentorship of an approved, qualified CHN mentor in the community. A professional nursing course is the first course that RNs take to bridge concepts from lower-division to upper division courses. Three advanced science courses are included in preparation for the master's tracks, which for the community/public health nursing track, are Public Health Sciences, Biostatistics, and Epidemiology.

After completing Level 1 courses, the RNs spend two semesters in the first level of the MSN program (Level 2, of the RN-to-MSN program). They select the advanced practice option in which they wish to major, that is, ADM or CHN. Upon completion of Level 2, the student moves to Level 3.

Note the adaptation of the objectives in italics for the CHN track. Similar adaptation occurs for the ADM track.

The RN-to-MSN Level 2 student will:

1. Integrate knowledge from the sciences and humanities into advanced nursing practice in the care of groups, communities, and populations.
   - *Integrate knowledge from the sciences, humanities, and public health sciences into advanced nursing practice in the care of groups, communities, and populations.*
2. Provide nursing leadership in healthcare organizations and systems.
   - *Same*
3. Participate in patient safety and quality improvement strategies in the care of groups, communities, and populations.
   - *Same*
4. Translate scholarship and research into advanced practice nursing.
   - *Translate scholarship and research into advanced practice nursing in the community setting.*
5. Apply informatics and healthcare technologies to advanced practice nursing.
   - *Same*
6. Advocate for change in healthcare systems and policy that benefits the health of groups, communities, and populations.
   - *Same*
7. Participate in interprofessional collaboration to improve group, community, and population health outcomes.
   - *Same*
8. Provide advanced practice nursing strategies for clinical prevention and health promotion for groups, communities, and populations.
   - *Same*

The RN-to-MSN Level 3[a] student will:

1. Apply knowledge from the sciences and humanities to advanced nursing practice in the care of groups, communities, and populations.
   - *Integrate knowledge from the sciences, humanities, and public health sciences into advanced nursing practice in the care of groups, communities, and populations.*
2. Provide leadership in healthcare organizations and systems.
   - *Same*
3. Initiate patient safety and quality improvement strategies in the care of groups, communities, and populations.
   - *Same*
4. Integrate scholarship and research into advanced practice nursing.
   - *Integrate scholarship and research into advanced practice nursing in community settings.*

5. Apply informatics and healthcare technologies to advanced practice nursing.
   - *Same*
6. Institute change in healthcare systems and policy that benefits the health of groups, communities, and populations.
   - *Same*
7. Provide leadership for interprofessional collaboration to improve group, community, and population health outcomes.
   - *Same*
8. Improve the health of groups, communities, and populations through advanced practice nursing strategies for clinical prevention and health promotion.
   - *Same*

These outcomes are the same as the end-of-program outcomes/objectives of the MSN program.

MSN students have core courses in nursing theory, research, healthcare systems policy, and advanced pathophysiology, pharmacology, and health assessment. Their specialty courses consist of three core science courses and three didactic courses with clinical preceptorships for each. Students complete 600 hours of supervised clinical practice by the end of the program. In addition, students complete a project as a capstone experience. A sample program of study for the MSN, CHN track program follows the summary.

SUMMARY

The faculty agrees that the level objectives for the RN-to-MSN programs come from the SLOs (end-of-program objectives) and are learner-focused, contain the content of what is to be learned, and specify when they are to be completed and to what extent. The level objectives imply mastery of the content; they must be met by the end-of-course work for each level and are arranged in sequential order. All the objectives are measurable and serve as guides for developing course objectives and for collecting data for formative (course, faculty, and level reviews) and summative evaluation (program review and accreditation).

SAMPLE PROGRAM OF STUDY MSN, CHN TRACK

Level 1: Nursing Courses (equivalent to BSN program outcomes) and Core Public Health Courses

Semester 1	Semester 2	Semester 3
Pathophysiology (3)	Interprofessional Health Practice (3)	Nursing Leadership (3)
Professional Nursing (2)		Practicum (2)
Health Assessment (2)	Practicum (2)	Community Health Nursing (2)
Practicum (1)	Analysis of the Healthcare System (3)	Practicum (4)
Genetics (3)	Introduction to Nursing Research (3)	Epidemiology (3)
Public Health Sciences (3)	Biostatistics (3)	
Total credits 14	*14*	*14*

Level 2: MSN Advanced Community Health Nursing Courses

Semester 1

Nursing Theory (3)

Advanced Pathophysiology (3)

Advanced Health Assessment (1)

[a]Practicum (2)

Total credits 9

Semester 2

Translational Research (3)

Advanced Pharmacology (3)

Leadership and Political Action (2)

[a]Practicum (1)

9

Level 3: Advanced Community Health Nursing Courses

Semester 1

Community Health Nursing (3)

[a]Practicum (3)

Interprofessional Leadership in the Community (2)

[a]Practicum (1)

Total credits 9

Semester 2

Community Health Nursing (3)

[a]Practicum (3)

Capstone (3)

9

[a]*600 hours of supervised clinical practice @ 4 hours/credit.*

END-OF-CHAPTER RESOURCES

DISCUSSION QUESTIONS

1. As you read the case study, what gaps in the information did you identify, and what additional data would you like to have? Were there redundancies, or too much information in the data that you viewed as unnecessary to the needs assessment?

2. What, in your opinion, are the pros and cons of collaboration with another school of nursing in a region, nationally, and/or internationally?

SUGGESTED LEARNING ACTIVITIES

Student Project

Identify another possible collaborative program that the two schools of nursing in the case study could develop. Summarize the data that justify developing the program and identify any gaps in the data that you believe need further assessment. Develop a program of study for your selection.

Faculty Project

Analyze the needs assessment from the case study and determine how easy or difficult it would be for you to collect similar data for your nursing program. Do you believe nursing programs should routinely conduct needs assessments for evaluation purposes and to identify the need for changes in the future? Why or why not?

A robust set of instructor resources designed to supplement this text is located at **http://connect.springerpub.com/content/book/978-0-8261-8686-7.** Qualifying instructors may request access by emailing **textbook@springerpub.com.**

REFERENCES

American Association of Colleges of Nursing. (2019). *2019 Annual report*. https://www.aacnnursing.org/Portals/42/Publications/Annual-Reports/Annual-Report-2019.pdf

American Association of Colleges of Nursing. (2021). *The essentials: Core competencies for professional nursing education*. https://www.aacnnursing.org/Portals/42/AcademicNursing/pdf/Essentials-2021.pdf

Child Fund International. (2021). *Struggles facing the Kenyan health care system*. https://www.childfund.org/Content/NewsDetail/2147490088

Country Meters. (2021). *Kenya population*. http://countrymeters.info/en/Kenya

Embassy of the Republic of Kenya. (2021). *Education in Kenya*. https://kenyaembassy.com/aboutkenyaeducation.html

Ministry of Health. (2015). *Kenya health workforce report: The status of healthcare professionals in Kenya, 2015*. https://taskforce.org/wp-content/uploads/2019/09/KHWF_2017Report_Fullreport_042317-MR-comments.pdf

NurseJournal. (2021, May). *The U.S. nursing shortage: A state-by-state breakdown*. https://nursejournal.org/articles/the-us-nursing-shortage-state-by-state-breakdown/

Oyugi, C. (2019). *Kenya's health structure and the six levels of hospitals-an overview*. https://roggkenya.org/2019/07/22/kenyas-health-structure-and-the-six-levels-of-hospitals-an-overview/

U.S. Department of Health and Human Services. (2021). *About the affordable care act*. https://www.hhs.gov/healthcare/facts-and-features/key-features-of-aca-by-year/index.html#

The World Factbook. (2021). *Kenya*. https://www.cia.gov/the-world-factbook/countries/kenya/

World Health Organization. (2017). *Primary health care systems (PRIMSYS). Case study of Kenya, abridged version*. https://www.who.int/alliance-hpsr/projects/alliancehpsr_kenyaabridgedprimasys.pdf?ua=1

Glossary

Accelerated programs: Programs consisting of intensive full-time study with no breaks, giving students the opportunity to finish the program in a shorter time than traditional programs. They include accelerated RN to BSN, RN to MSN programs, and entry-level BSN and MSN programs for graduates with bachelor's (or higher) degrees not in nursing.

Accreditation: A process that education programs undergo to receive recognition for meeting basic standards or criteria set by national, regional, or state organizations. Although it is voluntary, most programs undergo accreditation to demonstrate their quality to the consumers (students, parents, alumni, employers) and to meet certain requirements for financial aid and academic requirements.

Adult learning theory, andragogy: A model of instruction geared toward adult learning that takes into account the adult's autonomy, life experiences, personal goals, and need for relevancy and respect.

Articulation agreements: Renewable agreements negotiated to ensure equivalency between college and university courses, support educational mobility, and facilitate the seamless transfer of academic credit between ADN and BSN programs (American Association of Colleges of Nursing [AACN], 2019).

Asynchronous: Learning activities that occur at various times.

Behaviorism, behaviorist learning theory: A group of learning theories, often referred to as stimulus–response, that view learning as the result of certain conditions that stimulate the responses (behaviors) that follow.

Benchmark: A reference point in similar organizations/institutions that is used to compare quality and to identify gaps that drive improvement measures.

Body politic: The people/power(s) behind the official government within a community. It is composed of the people and major political forces that exert influence within the community.

Brain-based learning: Learning that is enhanced by creating conditions where the brain learns best such as relaxed alertness, immersion in complex multiple experiences, and actively engaging in experiences that help develop meaning. Also known as neuroeducation and educational neuroscience.

Clinical nurse leader: Master's prepared generalist who evaluates, assesses, and coordinates care for clients or groups of clients across all settings within a microsystem (AACN, 2021a).

Cognitive learning theory: Focuses on learning as an internal process including thinking, understanding, information organizing, and consciousness (McSparron et al., 2019).

Concept analysis/mapping: A detailed analysis of a concept and its relationships within the curriculum depicted into a map with arrows signifying relationships.

Concept-based curriculum: A theoretical or organizational curriculum model that guides the teaching of core ideas (concepts); it unifies the curriculum and creates a coherent approach across courses and levels deepening critical thinking. Integrating concepts throughout the curriculum promotes greater understanding and application (Repsha et al., 2020).

Constructivism, constructivist learning theory: A learning perspective that argues that individuals construct much of what they learn and understand, which produces knowledge based on their beliefs and experiences.

Content mapping: Similar to concept mapping, it tracks specific content's placement throughout the curriculum.

Continuous quality improvement (CQI): A system designed to provide for ongoing evaluation, analysis of findings, and implementation of plans for improvement within an organization.

Critical thinking: "The skill of using logic and reasoning to identify the strengths and weaknesses of alternative healthcare solutions, conclusions, or approaches to clinical or practice problems" (AACN, 2021c, p. 65).

Curricular framework: An organizational or conceptual framework that guides the development and evaluation of the curriculum plan according to the program mission/vision, overall goal, philosophy, and student learning outcomes and responds to professional educational standards.

Curriculum: The formal plan of study that provides the philosophical underpinnings, goals, and guidelines for delivering a specific educational program.

Deep learning: Allows students to dig deeper into complex and challenging learning situations. It is intentional and creates new meaning for the learner (Candela, 2020).

Demographics: Data that describe the characteristics of a population, for example, age, gender, socioeconomic status, ethnicity, education levels, and so on.

Distance education: Any learning experience that takes place a distance away from the parent institution's home campus.

Doctor of nursing practice (DNP): A doctorate degree that "prepares nurse leaders at the highest level of nursing practice to improve patient outcomes and translate research into practice" (AACN, 2021b).

Educational taxonomies: Provide the terminology on which to focus for the main domains of learning: cognitive, psychomotor, behavioral, and affective.

End-of-program objectives (see also Student learning outcomes): Reflect the framework of the curriculum and define the specific expectations or competencies of graduates upon completion of the nursing program.

Entry-level master's/generic master's/accelerated master's for nonnurses/second-degree master's programs: Programs that prepare nonnursing college graduates for eligibility to take NCLEX. Programs vary from generalist degrees to specialty or functional roles.

Entry-level/generic programs: Programs that prepare students for eligibility to take the licensure examination (NCLEX) for RNs. The programs include diploma, associate degree, baccalaureate, master's, and doctoral levels. Students entering master's entry-level programs have a baccalaureate in another field as a minimum. Students in entry-level programs do not have previous education in nursing.

Evidence-based practice: Discipline-specific (nursing) practice that is research-based and reflects the entirety of nursing practice and research.

Flipped classroom: A reversed instruction model in which students complete preclass assignments and use in-class time for active learning activities (Youhasan et al., 2021).

Formal curriculum: The planned program of studies for an academic degree or discipline.

Formative evaluation: Evaluation "intended by the evaluator as a basis for improvement" (Scriven, 1996, p. 4). The assessment takes place during the implementation of the program or curriculum. It can also be viewed as a process evaluation. In education, this type of evaluation is often linked to course or level objectives.

Frame factors: The external and internal factors that influence, impinge upon, and/or enhance educational programs and curricula. As a conceptual model, they serve to collect, organize, and analyze information that is useful for the development and evaluation of curricula. There are two major categories of frame factors: external and internal factors.

> **External frame factors**—Factors outside of the home institution in which the nursing program is housed.

> **Internal frame factors**—Factors within the institution and in the nursing program that influence the curriculum.

Goal: Overall statement(s) about what the program prepares the graduates for. Statements are usually long term and stated in global terms.

Goal-based evaluation: Evaluation based on the stated goals of the entity undergoing evaluation. It is frequently used in education and tied to the stated goals, purpose, and end-of-program objectives (student learning outcomes) of the program or curriculum.

Goal-free evaluation: A method to assess and judge some thing or entity. The evaluator has no prior knowledge of the entity (program or curriculum) that they are evaluating. The person must be an expert in the field of evaluation and the type of entity that is evaluated. The value of this type of evaluation is that it is relatively bias free.

Graduate education: Education that takes place after completion of the baccalaureate, that is, master's and doctorate levels.

Humanism, humanistic learning theory: An approach to teaching and learning that assumes people are inherently good and possess unlimited potential for growth; therefore, it emphasizes personal freedom, choice, self-determination, and self-actualization.

Hybrid distance education: Utilizes a blend of synchronous and asynchronous formats for learning.

Immersion (as in web-based with immersion): The student comes to the home campus for one or more days during a semester or academic year to test and participate in hands-on practice, utilizing standardized patients, simulation manikins, and task trainers. Students are able to interact face to face with faculty and peers of their cohort during this time.

Informal curriculum: Sometimes termed as the hidden curriculum, co-curriculum, or extracurricular activities; planned and unplanned influences on students' learning.

Institutional accreditation: A comprehensive review of the functioning and effectiveness of the entire college, university, or technical institution. The state mandate or institutional mission provides the lens used to guide the review.

Learning: "change in behavior (knowledge, attitudes, and/or skills) that can be observed or measured and that occurs . . . as a result of exposure to environmental stimuli" (Bastable, 2021, p. 14).

Massive open online courses (MOOCs): Open enrollment for access to online higher education courses with some offering to academic credit if certain course requirements are met.

Mission statement: The institution's beliefs about its responsibility for the delivery of programs through teaching, service, and scholarship.

M1 and M2 master's programs: The size of master's programs according to the Carnegie classification of educational institutions.

Multiple intelligences: Presents seven constructs of intellects: bodily-kinesthetic, visual-spatial, verbal-linguistic, logical-mathematical, musical-rhythmic, interpersonal, and intrapersonal (Gardner, 1983).

Needs assessment: The process for collecting and analyzing information that can influence the decision to initiate a new program or revise an existing one.

Nonsectarian: Not associated with a religious organization.

Objectives: The steps necessary for reaching the overall goal of the program that include a description of the learner, a behavior that is measurable, a timeframe, at what level of competency, and the topic or behavior expected.

Course objectives: Have the same properties as end-of-program and midlevel objectives but apply to specific courses and relate to and lead toward midlevel and end-of-program objectives.

End-of-program objectives: Highest level of learner behaviors that demonstrate the characteristics, knowledge, and skills expected of the graduate and relate to the overall goal. They focus on the learner and must include a behavior that is measurable, a timeframe, at what level of competency, and the topic or behavior expected. These can also be defined as student learning outcomes.

Example: X School of Nursing prepares competent, compassionate nurse clinicians and leaders who serve the healthcare needs of the people of the state and the healthcare systems.

Level (intermediate) objectives: Have the same properties as end-of-program objectives but occur midway through an educational program and are usually higher than the first-level objectives.

Student (individual) learning outcomes: All of these objectives are student or individual learning outcomes and should be learner-centered and describe what behavior (outcome) is expected.

Example: At the end of the Health Assessment course, the student will present a complete health assessment of a client that includes an accurate health history, a write-up of all components of the physical examination, a list of problems and actual or potential nursing diagnoses, and a plan for follow-up of the problems and diagnoses.

Pedagogy: Teaching methods; although it originally applied to methods used to educate children, it can be used to apply to all age groups.

PhD program or, in the case of nursing, the PhD or DNS: Degrees that emphasize nursing theory and research and educate nurses prepared to conduct research and foster the development of new knowledge in healthcare and nursing.

Private educational institution: An institution supported through private funding.

Problem-based learning: A mechanism for teaching students that focuses on clinical problems and professional issues that the nurse may face in practice.

Program approval: A process whereby regulating bodies review programs to ensure consumer safety. Nursing education programs are subject to state regulations that are usually administered by the state board of nursing.

Programmatic or specialized accreditation: Focuses on the functioning and effectiveness of a particular program or unit within the larger institution (e.g., medicine, nursing).

Public institution: An institution whose main financial support comes through governmental funds.

Quality: Measured as "purposeful, transformative, exceptional, and accountable" (Schindler et al., 2015, p. 8).

Quality assurance: The process of collecting data on how well the institution or program meets its defined standards, criteria, goals, and mission.

Regional accreditation agency: One of seven private, voluntary accreditation agencies within six defined regions of the United States, formed for the purpose of peer evaluation and setting of standards for higher education.

Regulatory: A form of approval, recognition, or accreditation required by a federal, state, or provincial government agency.

R1, R2, and R3 doctoral programs: The level of research conducted in doctoral programs according to the Carnegie classification of educational institutions.

Satellite campuses: Programs that offer the curriculum as a whole or in part on off-campus sites from the parent institution. While they may incorporate technology and the internet, learning still takes place in classrooms with in-person participation of the instructor and students.

Scholarship of teaching: Application of teaching activities to scholarship that includes four components: discovery, integration, application, and teaching (Boyer, 1990).

Sectarian: Associated with or supported by a religious organization.

Simulation: Allows students to participate in activities that mimic real-life scenarios or situations.

Standardized patients: Individuals who have been trained to portray a patient with a specific medical condition; often hired to teach and evaluate students' performances in a simulated clinical setting.

State regulatory agencies: Agencies that recognize or approve colleges, universities, or programs for operation within the state as governed by state statutes.

Student learning outcomes (see also end-of-program objectives): Reflect the framework of the curriculum and define the specific expectations or competencies of graduates upon completion of the nursing program.

Summative evaluation: A holistic approach to the assessment of a program that uses results from formative evaluation (Scriven, 1996). Summative evaluation takes place at the end of the program and measures the final outcome.

Synchronous: Learning activities that take place simultaneously.

Team-based learning (TBL): A structured, active learning strategy involving a sequence of three key phases: preclass preparation; readiness assurance process; and application.

Total quality management: Continuous assessment of an educational program, correcting errors as they occur, thus improving the quality of the program.

Translational science: Research findings that are translated and applied into practice.

Undergraduate education: Postsecondary education from the associate degree (traditionally 2 years) to the baccalaureate (traditionally 4 years) levels.

Virtual learning environment (VLE): Educational programs offered online in cyberspace.

Vision statement: A statement that is outlook-oriented and reflects the institution's plans and dreams about its direction for the future.

Web-based learning: Education offered online and the student interacts with faculty and other students via computer.

REFERENCES

American Association of Colleges of Nursing. (2019). *Articulation agreements among nursing education programs.* https://www.aacnnursing.org/News-Information/Fact-Sheets/Articulation-Agreements

American Association of Colleges of Nursing. (2021a). *Clinical nurse leader toolkit.* https://www.aacnnursing.org/Education-Resources/Tool-Kits/Clinical-Nurse-Leader-Tool-Kit

American Association of Colleges of Nursing. (2021b). *Developing a DNP program tool kit.* http://www.aacnnursing.org/Education-Resources/Tool-Kits/DNP-Tool-Kit

American Association of Colleges of Nursing. (2021c). *The essentials: Core competencies for professional nursing education.* https://www.aacnnursing.org/Portals/42/AcademicNursing/pdf/Essentials-2021.pdf

Bastable, S. (2021). Overview of education in health care. In S. Bastable (Ed.), *Nurse educator: Principles of teaching and learning for nursing practice* (5th ed., pp. 3–29). Jones & Bartlett.

Boyer, E. L. (1990). *Scholarship reconsidered: Priorities of the professoriate.* The Carnegie Foundation for the Advancement of Learning. http://depts.washington.edu/gs630/Spring/Boyer.pdf

Candela, L. (2020). Theoretical foundations of teaching and learning. In D. Billings & J. Halstead (Eds.), *Teaching in nursing: A guide for faculty* (5th ed., pp. 247–269). Elsevier.

Gardner, H. (1983). *Frames of mind.* Basic Books.

McSparron, J. I., Vanka, A., & Smith, C. C. (2019). Cognitive learning theory for clinical teaching. *The Clinical Teacher, 19,* 96–100. https://onlinelibrary.wiley.com/doi/pdf/10.1111/tct.12781?casa_token=yP-4bcLCLboAAAAA:xZiOdw1DYt6v4dRYcOdB4BMum7rKOiwKvwVDK45RKJu3xsHMvnWUFNXp2zbR_Nh9O5ZBYCvzoCkfZTs

Repsha, C. L., Quinn, B. L., & Bostian Peters, A. (2020). Implementing a concept-based learning curriculum: A review of the literature. *Teaching and Learning in Nursing, 15*(1), 66–71. https://doi.org/10.1016/j.teln.2019.09.006

Schindler, L., Puls-Elvidge, S., Welzant, H., & Crawford, L. (2015). Definitions of quality in higher education: A synthesis of the literature. *Higher learning research communication, 5*(3), 3–13. https://doi.org/10.18870/hlrc.v5i3.244

Scriven, M. (1996). Types of evaluation and types of evaluators. *Evaluation Practice, 17*(2), 151–161. https://doi.org/10.1177/109821409601700207

Youhasan, P., Chen, Y., Lyndon, M., & Henning, M. A. (2021). Exploring the pedagogical design features of the flipped classroom in undergraduate nursing education: A systematic review. *BMC Nursing, 20,* 1–13. https://doi.org/10.1186/s12912-021-00555-w

Index